CW01072457

Current Topics in Pathology
89

Managing Editors

C.L. Berry   E. Grundmann

Editorial Board

W. Böcker, H. Cottier, P.J. Dawson, H. Denk
C.M. Fenoglio-Preiser, Ph.U. Heitz, O.H. Iversen
U. Löhrs, F. Nogales, U. Pfeifer, N. Sasano
G. Seifert, J.C.E. Underwood, Y. Watanabe

D. Harms D. Schmidt (Eds.)

Soft Tissue Tumors

Contributors

P.W. Allen · M. Brockmann · A.O. Cavazzana
E. Durieux · C.D.M. Fletcher · R. Frunzio · D. Harms
H. Hashimoto · D. Katenkamp · H. Kosmehl · V. Krieg
I. Leuschner · P. Meister · W. Mellin · A. Montaldi
M. Morgan · W.A. Newton · A. Niezabitowski · V. Ninfo
F. Pedeutour · J. Ritter · D. Schmidt · R. Tirabosco
J. Treuner · T.J. Triche · C. Turc-Carel · P. Wuisman

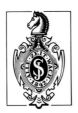

Springer-Verlag
Berlin Heidelberg New York
London Paris Tokyo
Hong Kong Barcelona
Budapest

D. Harms, Professor Dr.
Institut für Paidopathologie
Klinikum der Christian-Albrechts-Universität
Michaelisstr. 11, 24105 Kiel, Germany

D. Schmidt, Professor Dr.
Institut für Pathologie
A2,2, 68159 Mannheim, Germany

With 150 Figures, Some in Colour, and 37 Tables

ISBN 3-540-55150-6 Springer-Verlag Berlin Heidelberg New York
ISBN 0-387-55150-6 Springer-Verlag New York Berlin Heidelberg

Library of Congress Cataloging-in-Publication Data. Soft tissue tumors/D. Harms, D. Schmidt (eds.). p. cm.—(Current topics in pathology; v. 89) Includes bibliographical references and index. ISBN 3-540-55150-6 (alk. paper).—ISBN 0-387-55150-6 (alk. paper) 1. Soft tissue tumors. I. Harms, Dieter. II. Schmidt, D. (Dietmar), 1952– . III. Scries. [DNLM: 1. Soft Tissue Neoplasms. W1 CU821H v. 89 1994/WD 375 S68113 1994] RB1.E6 vol. 89 [RC280. S66] 616.07 s—dc20 [616.99'4] DNLM/DLC for Library of Congress. 94-29977

This work is subject to copyright. All rights are reserved, whether the whole or part of the material is concerned, specifically the rights of translation, reprinting, reuse of illustrations, recitation, broadcasting, reproduction on microfilm or in any other way, and storage in data banks. Duplication of this publication or parts thereof is permitted only under the provisions of the German Copyright Law of September 9, 1965, in its current version, and permission for use must always be obtained from Springer-Verlag. Violations are liable for prosecution under the German Copyright Law.

© Springer-Verlag Berlin Heidelberg 1995
Printed in Germany

The use of general descriptive names, registered names, trademarks, etc. in this publication does not imply, even in the absence of a specific statement, that such names are exempt from the relevant protective laws and regulations and therefore free for general use.

Product liability: The publishers cannot guarantee the accuracy of any information about dosage and application contained in this book. In every individual case the user must check such information by consulting the relevant literature.

Typesetting: Best-set Typesetter Ltd., Hong Kong

SPIN: 10058623   25/3130/SPS – 5 4 3 2 1 0 – Printed on acid-free paper

List of Contributors

ALLEN, P.W., Dr.   Histopathology Department
The Queen Elizabeth Hospital
Woodville Road
Woodville South, South Australia
5011

BROCKMANN, M., Dr.   Institute of Pathology
Krankenanstalten Bergmannsheil
University of Bochum
44789 Bochum, Germany

CAVAZZANA, A.O., Dr.   Department of Surgery
Institute of Anatomic Pathology
II. University of Rome
Tor Vergata
Via Carnevale
00173 Rome, Italy

DURIEUX, E., Dr.   Université de Nice
Faculté de Médecine
CNRS URA 1462
Avenue de Valombrose
06034 Nice Cédex, France

FLETCHER, C.D.M.,
Dr., MB, BS, MRCPath   Department of Histopathology
St. Thomas' Hospital
London SE1 7EH, England

FRUNZIO, R., Dr.   Universita di Padova
Cattedra di Anatomia e Istologia
Pathologica III
Via A. Gabelli 01
35121 Padova, Italy

HARMS, D., Prof. Dr.   Institut für Paidopathologie
                            Klinikum der Christian-Albrechts-
                            Universität
                            Michaelisstraße 11
                            24105 Kiel, Germany

HASHIMOTO, H., Prof. Dr.   Department of Pathology and
                            Oncology
                            School of Medicine
                            University of Occupational and
                            Environmental Health
                            1-1 iseigaoka, Yahatanishi-ku
                            Kitakyushu 807, Japan

KATENKAMP, D., Prof. Dr.   Institut für Pathologische Anatomie
                            Friedrich-Schiller-Universität
                            Ziegelmühlenweg 1
                            07743 Jena, Germany

KOSMEHL, H., Dr.   Institut für Pathologische Anatomie
                            Friedrich-Schiller-Universität
                            Ziegelmühlenweg 1
                            07743 Jena, Germany

KRIEG, V., Dr.   Clinical Cancer Registry
                            Münster, Germany

LEUSCHNER, I., Dr.   Abteilung Allgemeine Pathologie
                            und Pathologische Anatomie
                            Klinikum der Christian-Albrechts-
                            Universität
                            Michaelisstraße 11
                            24105 Kiel, Germany

MEISTER, P., Prof. Dr.   Institut für Pathologie
                            Städtisches Krankenhaus Harlaching
                            Sanatoriumsplatz 2
                            81545 München, Germany

MELLIN, W., Priv.-Doz.   Institut für Pathologie
Dr.   Otto-von-Guericke-Universität
                            Leipziger Straße 44
                            39120 Magdeburg, Germany

MONTALDI, A., Dr.   Universita di Padova
                                     Cattedra di Anatomia et Istologia
                                     Patologica III
                                     Via A. Gabelli 01
                                     35121 Padova, Italy

MORGAN, M., Dr.   Abteilung Hämatologie und
                                     Onkologie
                                     Olgahospital Kinderklinik
                                     Bismarckstraße 8
                                     70176 Stuttgart, Germany

NEWTON, JR., W.A., Dr.   Intergroup Rhabdomyosarcoma
                                     Study Pathology Center
                                     Children's Hospital
                                     700 Children's Drive
                                     Columbus, OH 43205, USA

NIEZABITOWSKI, A., Dr.   Department of Pathology
                                     Oncological Center
                                     University of Cracow
                                     Cracow, Poland

NINFO, V., Prof. Dr.   Universita di Padova
                                     Cattedra di Anatomia e Istologia
                                     Patologica III
                                     Via A. Gabelli 01
                                     35121 Padova, Italy

PEDUTOUR, F., Dr.   Université de Nice
                                     Faculté de Médecine
                                     CNRS URA 1462
                                     Avenue de Valombrose
                                     06034 Nice Cédex, France

RITTER, J., Dr.   Pediatric Clinic
                                     University of Münster
                                     Münster, Germany

SCHMIDT, D., Prof. Dr.   Institut für Pathologie
                                     A2,2
                                     68159 Mannheim, Germany

TIRABOSCO, R., Dr.   Universita di Padova
                                  Cattedra di Anatomia e Istologia
                                  Patologica III
                                  Via A. Gabelli 01
                                  35121 Padova, Italy

TREUNER, J., Prof. Dr.   Abteilung Hämatologie und
                                  Onkologie
                                  Olgahospital Kinderklinik
                                  Bismarckstraße 8
                                  70176 Stuttgart, Germany

TRICHE, T.J., MD, PhD   Department of Pathology and
                                  Laboratory Medicine
                                  Children's Hospital Los Angeles
                                  4650 Sunset Boulevard
                                  Los Angeles, CA 90027, USA

TURC-CAREL, C., Dr.   Université de Nice
                                  Faculté de Médecine
                                  CNRS URA 1462
                                  Avenue de Valombrose
                                  06034 Nice Cédex, France

WUISMAN, P., Dr.   Orthopedic Clinic
                                  University of Münster
                                  Münster, Germany

Preface

Soft tissue tumors are a very heterogeneous group of tumors in terms of histogenesis, morphology, cytogenetics, molecular biology, clinical manifestation, and prognosis. Their spectrum is fascinating for morphologists and basic scientists alike. Yet precisely this variability in the morphologic manifestation of soft tissue tumors, specifically their histologic and cytologic patterns, presents great difficulties to any effort to categorize them.

Although many soft tissue tumors are today defined not only by histology but also by immunohistochemical, cytogenetic, and molecular biological findings, the histogenesis of many soft tissue tumors, in particular malignant ones, continues to be unknown. This is associated with the fact that the actual precursor cells that lead to these tumors have frequently not yet been identified. For this reason, the customary classification of malignant soft tissue tumors is primarily not histogenetic, but actually according to the dominant phenotype, however characteristic it is. Of course, an exact morphologic examination of soft tissue tumors continues to be an essential prerequisite for making a diagnosis and determining a therapy. The use of a wide range of additional modern examination techniques, however, can make a substantial contribution toward more precisely defining the biological behavior of a tumor, which without doubt can have therapeutic implications.

This volume covers the entire spectrum of examination techniques that are currently available, including those in modern molecular biology. Nonetheless, in many chapters conventional light microscopy, together with immunohistochemistry and electron microscopy, are dominant, just as is the case in daily practice in the diagnosis of tumors. For this reason, modern molecular biology and cytogenetics are covered in special chapters; the same is true of questions on tumor grading and heterogeneity.

As a consequence, this volume contains first a thematically organized "general" pathology of soft tissue tumors, including clinical manifestations, and second a "special" pathology of important tumor groups. Naturally it has not been possible to systematically present all tumor entities; it was necessary for us to make a selection, both on the basis of topicality and of space.

We have left the authors, who come from different countries and schools, great liberty in the selection of their material and in the method of presentation; nevertheless, we, and with us the authors, are confident that the individual chapters combine to form an informative whole.

We would like to thank the authors for their collaboration, and Springer-Verlag for its assistance during the editorial and production phases of the preparation of this book.

Kiel and Mannheim   D. HARMS and D. SCHMIDT
September 1994

Contents

Incidence of Soft Tissue Sarcomas in Adults

H. Hashimoto

1 Introduction

Soft tissue sarcomas are relatively uncommon neoplasms. The annual incidence rate is about one or two per 100 000 population (CUTLER and YOUNG 1975; RANTAKOKKO and EKFORS 1979; AGNARSSON et al. 1991). The American Cancer Society placed the estimated number of new soft tissue cancers in the United States in 1991 at 5800 (0.5%) out of a total of 1 100 000 new cancers in all sites, and 3300 deaths (0.6%) per year were caused by these tumors out of a total of 514 000 cancer deaths (BORING et al. 1991). Other data from Brazil indicated that 3759 soft tissue cancers were diagnosed during the period 1976–1980, and accounted for 1.0% among a total of 369 767 cases of cancers in all sites (BRUMINI 1982). The Annual of the Pathological Autopsy Cases in Japan included 493 deaths caused by malignant soft tissue tumors (0.4%) out of a total of 128 002 cancer deaths in all sites during the period 1984–1988, compared with 19 538 deaths of lung cancer and 18 567 deaths of gastric cancer (JAPANESE SOCIETY OF PATHOLOGY 1984–1988) (Table 1).

The relative frequency of malignant to benign soft tissue tumors is difficult to estimate accurately because the emphasis in the literature has

Current Topics in Pathology
Volume 89, Eds. D. Harms/D. Schmidt
© Springer-Verlag Berlin Heidelberg 1995

Table 1. Autopsy cases of cancers in Japan by site for 5 years.
(Data from the Japanese Society of Pathology 1984–1988)

Site	Cases (n)
Lung	19 538
Stomach	18 567
Lymphoid and hematopoietic system	15 000
Breast	2 931
Central nervous system	2 684
Skin	731
Soft tissue	493
Bone and joint	409
	128 002

been laid disproportionately on the malignant ones. According to the data recorded in the Second Department of Pathology, Faculty of Medicine, Kyushu University, benign tumors outnumber malignant ones at an approximate ratio of 15:1 (18 000 benign and 1200 malignant).

In recent years, a more exact classification of soft tissue sarcomas has evolved, and the criteria of each entity have now been established. In addition, there have been many elaborate reports of a large series of each tumor, from a clinicopathologic point of view. Regrettably, however, most of the previous statistical data on overall soft tissue sarcomas have been on only a relatively small number of cases, generally including fewer than 300 (LIEBERMAN and ACKERMAN 1954; HARE and CERNY 1963; HORN 1963; CRAWFORD et al. 1970; FERRELL and FRABLE 1972; GAILLARD et al. 1974; SUIT et al. 1975; MYHRE-JENSEN et al. 1983; COSTA et al. 1984; TROJANI et al. 1984; EILBER 1984; TSUJIMOTO et al. 1988; FISHER 1989; AGNARSSON et al. 1991; MYHRE-JENSEN et al. 1991), with the exception of the following five cases. One was the STOUT (1953) series with 1349 malignant mesenchymal tumors of the soft tissues recorded in his laboratory at Columbia University up to 1951. Another large single series included 1215 cases of soft tissue sarcomas collected from 13 institutions by the Task Force on Soft Tissue Sarcoma of the American Joint Committee for Cancer Staging and End Results Reporting (RUSSELL et al. 1977). More recently, the Commission on Cancer of the American College of Surgeons carried out a nationwide survey of soft tissue sarcomas in adults, excluding patients under the age of 18 year, using data obtained from 504 hospitals in 1977–1978 (2355 patients) and 645 institutions in 1983–1984 (3457 patients) (LAWRENCE et al. 1987). Two other larger series recently reported were the data from the Memorial Sloan-Kettering Cancer Center, which analyzed 565 cases of soft tissue sarcomas (TOROSIAN et al. 1988), following the previous series from the same institution (HAJDU 1979), and from the University of Illinois, which tabulated the histologic classification of 681 cases of soft tissue sarcomas (DAS GUPTA 1983). Reviewing these data, however, it should be kept in mind that, since the formulation of the concept of malignant fibrous histiocytoma, some of the previously described lesions would no longer be considered as appropriately categorized.

The present observations involve a statistical review of 1002 cases of soft tissue sarcomas in Japanese adults by modern histologic concepts. These cases were selected from a total of 1116 cases of various soft tissue sarcomas collected at the Second Department of Pathology, Kyushu University over a 30-year period, excluding patients under the age of 15 years.

2 Histologic Distribution of Soft Tissue Sarcomas in Adults

Soft tissue sarcomas comprise a heterogeneous group of malignant tumors that are classified principally on a histogenetic basis according to the normal tissue they resemble. The criteria of malignant fibrous histiocytoma (MFH) have recently been extended to include assorted variants in addition to its classic form, since an epochal publication on this tumor by WEISS and ENZINGER (1978). A nationwide survey in the United States of soft tissue sarcomas in adults, which was carried out under the auspices of the Commission on Cancer of the American College of Surgeons during two separate 2-year periods, indicated that MFH increased in the frequency of histologic diagnosis over the two periods (LAWRENCE et al. 1987) (Table 2). As well as in the above survey, MFH (27.8%) and liposarcoma (13.0%) were the two most common soft tissue sarcomas, followed by leiomyosarcoma (10.2%), synovial sarcoma (6.7%), malignant schwannoma (6.3%), rhabdomyosarcoma (5.4%), and fibrosarcoma (4.1%) among the 1002 soft tissue sarcomas in adults in our series (Table 3). The apparent increase of MFH compared to earlier reports is due principally to the fact that many of these tumors were previously diagnosed as pleomorphic rhabdomyosarcoma, pleomorphic or myxoid liposarcoma, or fibrosarcoma (ENJOJI et al. 1980).

The majority of soft tissue sarcomas may be easily diagnosed by light microscopy. However, in 5%–15% of soft tissue sarcomas, their cellular origin is less clear and there is no evidence of differentiation either by light or electron microscopy or by immunohistochemistry (RUSSELL et al. 1977; MYHRE-JENSEN et al. 1983; COSTA et al. 1984; ENJOJI and HASHIMOTO 1984; LAWRENCE et al. 1987; TSUJIMOTO et al. 1988; KYRIAKOS 1990; FLETCHER 1990; AGNARSSON et al. 1991) (Table 2). Unclassified sarcomas accounted for 7.5% of the cases in our series (Table 3).

3 General View of Soft Tissue Sarcomas

There were 514 males and 488 females among the 1002 patients 15 years or older with a sex ratio approaching 1:1 (Table 3). The mean age of the

Table 2. Frequency distribution of soft tissue sarcomas in the literature

Histologic types	Hare and Cerny (1963) (n = 200) (n)	(%)	Russell et al. (1977) (n = 1215) (n)	(%)	Hajdu (1979) (n = 2489) (n)	(%)	Myhre-Jensen et al. (1983) (n = 261) (n)	(%)	Costa et al. (1984) (n = 163) (n)	(%)	Lawrence et al. (1987) (1977–78) (n = 2355) (n)	(%)	Lawrence et al. (1987) (1983–84) (n = 3457) (n)	(%)	Torosian et al. (1988) (n = 565) (n)	(%)	Fisher (1989) (n = 200) (n)	(%)
Malignant fibrous histiocytoma	23	11.5	128	10.5	392	15.7	73	28.0	34	20.9	348	14.8	897	25.9	114	20.2	57	28.5
Liposarcoma	13	6.5	221	18.2	416	16.7	24	9.2	38	23.3	547	23.2	611	17.7	121	21.4	38	19
Leiomyosarcoma	5	2.5	79	6.5			6	2.2	19	11.7	324	13.8	513	14.8	113	20.0	7	3.5
Synovial sarcoma			84	6.9	187	7.5	17	6.5	19	11.7	87	3.7	126	3.6	54	9.6	21	10.5
Malignant schwannoma			60	4.9	141	5.7	23	8.8	14	8.6	76	3.2	138	4.0	26	4.6	12	6
Rhabdomyosarcoma	10	5.0	234	19.3	546	21.9	11	4.2	3	1.8	167	7.1	124	3.6	42	7.4	26	13
Fibrosarcoma	86	43.0	231	19.0	358	14.4[a]	36	13.8	6	3.7	262	11.1	228	6.6	62	11.0	4	2
Dermatofibrosarcoma protuberans	6	3.0					19	7.3										
Extraskeletal chondrosarcoma																		
Angiosarcoma			33	2.7	212	8.5	18	6.9	2	1.2	29	1.2	42	1.2			3	1.5
Malignant hemangiopericytoma									2	1.2	48	2.0	103	2.9	11	1.9	4	2
Clear cell sarcoma							3	1.1	1	0.6							1	0.5
Epithelioid sarcoma																	2	1
Alveolar soft part sarcoma					51	2.0	2	0.8	1	0.6	10	0.4	20	0.6	5	0.9	7	3.5
Extraskeletal Ewing's sarcoma																	3	1.5
Extraskeletal osteosarcoma							8	3.1[b]			10	0.4	21	0.6			5	2.5
Malignant mesenchymoma							3	1.1			32	1.4	36	1.0			3	1.5
Kaposi's sarcoma							2	0.8										
Malignant granular cell tumor									1	0.6								
Other types			24	2.0	186	7.5					332	14.1	441	12.8	17	3.0		
Sarcoma, type undetermined	57	28.5	121	10.0			16	6.1	23	14.1	127	5.4	186	5.4			7	3.5

[a] Cases including desmoid tumors.
[b] Cases including extraskeletal chondrosarcomas.

Table 3. Frequency and sex distribution of 1002 soft tissue sarcomas in adults ($\geq$15 years of age)

Histologic types	Patients (n)	(%)	Male (n)	Female (n)
Malignant fibrous histiocytoma	279	27.8	165	114
Liposarcoma	130	13.0	78	52
Leiomyosarcoma	102	10.2	39	63
Synovial sarcoma	67	6.7	26	41
Malignant schwannoma	63	6.3	28	35
Rhabdomyosarcoma	54	5.4	34	20
Fibrosarcoma	41	4.1	20	21
Extraskeletal chondrosarcoma	35	3.5	16	19
Angiosarcoma	32	3.2	15	17
Malignant hemangiopericytoma	26	2.6	9	17
Malignant mesothelioma	22	2.2	10	12
Clear cell sarcoma	20	2.0	10	10
Malignant neuroepithelioma	14	1.4	4	10
Epithelioid sarcoma	11	1.1	6	5
Alveolar soft part sarcoma	9	0.9	2	7
Extraskeletal Ewing's sarcoma	8	0.8	6	2
Extraskeletal osteosarcoma	6	0.6	2	4
Malignant mesenchymoma	3	0.3	1	2
Malignant rhabdoid tumor of soft parts	3	0.3	3	0
Kaposi's sarcoma	2	0.2	1	1
Sarcoma, type undetermined	75	7.5	39	36
	1002	100	514	488

patients in our total series (1116 cases) was approximately 46 years (median 49 years), and the peak was composed of patients in their sixth decade of life, with the base of the patients after the age of 40 years constituting 63% of the total patients (Table 4). Of the 1116 cases, 114 (10%) were in the pediatric age group under 15 years and included 54 rhabdomyosarcomas, 17 fibrosarcomas, six synovial sarcomas, five malignant neuroepitheliomas, and five extraskeletal Ewing's sarcomas (Table 4).

The anatomic location most often involved was the lower extremities (39%) and the thigh was the most frequent primary site (24%) (Table 5). The next most frequent sites were the retroperitoneum and mesentery (18%) and the trunk (14%), followed by the upper extremities (13%). The anatomic distribution reflected a frequency similar to that of three large series done by the American Joint Committee for Cancer (1215 cases) (RUSSELL et al. 1977), by the Commission on Cancer of the American College of Surgeons (4550 cases) (LAWRENCE et al. 1987), and by TOROSIAN et al. (1988) who reported 565 cases of soft tissue sarcoma from the Memorial Sloan-Kettering Cancer Center.

Table 4. Age distribution of overall soft tissue sarcomas (1116 cases)

Histologic types	Age Mean	Age Median	0–14	15–19	20–29	30–39	40–49	50–59	60–69	70–79	80–89	90+	Total
Malignant fibrous histiocytoma	60	62	1	4	6	22	25	74	63	64	20	1	280
Liposarcoma	51	51	0	1	9	18	35	33	20	7	7	0	130
Leiomyosarcoma	57	59	0	0	3	10	15	25	32	12	5	0	102
Synovial sarcoma	37	37	6	9	9	16	15	12	4	1	1	0	73
Malignant schwannoma	42	43	3	5	10	14	9	16	2	5	2	0	66
Rhabdomyosarcoma	14	15	54	18	24	11	1	0	0	0	0	0	108
Fibrosarcoma	33	37	17	1	5	9	10	9	4	3	0	0	58
Extraskeletal chondrosarcoma	42	42	2	4	6	6	4	6	6	3	0	0	37
Angiosarcoma	58	65	1	2	3	2	0	5	9	6	4	1	33
Malignant hemangiopericytoma	45	42	0	2	1	8	5	6	0	3	1	0	26
Malignant mesothelioma	56	56	0	0	0	2	6	6	4	3	1	0	22
Clear cell sarcoma	43	39	0	0	4	6	2	5	3	0	0	0	20
Malignant neuroepithelioma	21	18	5	5	6	1	1	1	0	0	0	0	19
Epithelioid sarcoma	33	27	2	2	3	2	1	1	1	1	0	0	13
Alveolar soft part sarcoma	27	24	2	2	5	0	0	1	0	1	0	0	11
Extraskeletal Ewing's sarcoma	22	20	5	1	3	3	1	0	0	0	0	0	13
Extraskeletal osteosarcoma	62	66	0	0	0	1	1	0	2	3	0	0	6
Malignant mesenchymoma	34	40	1	0	0	1	1	1	0	0	0	0	4
Malignant rhabdoid tumor of soft parts	24	18	3	0	0	2	0	0	0	1	0	0	6
Kaposi's sarcoma	71	71	0	0	0	0	0	1	0	0	1	0	2
Sarcoma, type undetermined	46	49	12	4	4	10	14	13	16	13	1	0	87
	46	49	114	60	101	144	145	215	166	126	43	2	1116

Table 5. Anatomic distribution of soft tissue sarcomas in adults (≥15 years of age)

Histologic types	Head and neck	Shoulder	Upper arm and elbow	Forearm and hand	Chest wall	Abdominal wall	Back	Mediastinum	Buttocks	Thigh and knee	Lower leg and foot	Retroperitoneum and mesentery	Urogenital tract	Spermatic cord	Other sites	Total
MFH	27	12	29	11	13	9	18	1	23	72	24	37	1	2	0	279
Liposarcoma	3	4	2	1	2	3	6	2	10	49	3	38	0	6	1	130
Leiomyosarcoma	2	0	2	1	0	4	3	1	3	19	4	61	0	2	0	102
Synovial sarcoma	2	2	7	6	1	0	0	0	5	33	10	0	0	0	1	67
Malignant schwannoma	7	1	9	5	3	0	5	4	9	10	4	5	0	1	0	63
Rhabdomyosarcoma	13	0	1	6	3	1	2	0	5	3	4	2	12	0	2	54
Fibrosarcoma	7	6	2	1	2	8	8	0	1	5	0	1	0	0	0	41
Extraskeletal chondrosarcoma	4	1	1	1	0	3	2	0	5	11	4	2	0	1	0	35
Angiosarcoma	16	0	2	0	3	1	0	0	1	5	1	3	0	0	0	32
Malignant hemangiopericytoma	4	0	0	0	2	1	1	1	2	7	0	6	2	0	0	26
Malignant mesothelioma	0	0	0	0	8	0	0	0	0	0	0	12	1	0	1	22
Clear cell sarcoma	0	0	0	3	0	0	0	0	3	6	7	1	0	0	0	20
Malignant neuroepithelioma	1	0	0	1	2	0	2	0	2	3	2	0	1	0	0	14
Epithelioid sarcoma	1	0	0	5	0	1	0	0	0	0	3	0	1	0	0	11
Alveolar soft part sarcoma	0	0	1	2	1	0	0	0	1	3	1	0	0	0	0	9
Extraskeletal Ewing's sarcoma	0	1	0	0	1	1	1	0	0	4	0	0	0	0	0	8
Extraskeletal osteosarcoma	0	2	1	0	1	0	0	0	1	0	0	1	0	0	0	6
Malignant mesenchymoma	0	0	0	0	0	1	0	0	0	1	0	1	0	0	0	3
Malignant rhabdoid tumor of soft parts	1	0	0	0	0	1	0	0	0	0	0	1	0	0	0	3
Kaposi's sarcoma	1	0	0	0	0	0	0	0	0	0	1	0	0	0	0	2
Sarcoma, type undetermined	15	0	3	3	8	5	2	1	4	13	5	14	1	1	0	75
	104	29	60	46	50	39	50	10	75	244	73	185	19	13	5	1002

4 Specified Soft Tissue Sarcomas

4.1 Malignant Fibrous Histiocytoma

Malignant fibrous histiocytoma comprised 27.8% of 1002 adult soft tissue
sarcomas in our series (Table 3). The ages of the 279 patients (165 men and
114 women) ranged from 15 to 93 years, with a mean of 60 (median 62)
years (Table 4). A total of 201 tumors (72%) were present in patients who
were in their sixth, seventh, and eighth decades of life, and MFHs accounted
for 40% of patients 50 years or older with soft tissue sarcomas.

The thigh and buttocks were the sites of 95 (34%) of the tumors (Table
5); 119 tumors (43%) were located in the lower extremities, 52 (19%) in the
upper extremities, 40 (14%) on the trunk, 37 (13%) in the retroperitoneum
and mesentery, and 27 (10%) on the head and neck.

Referring to the criteria suggested by ENZINGER and WEISS (1988a), the
tumors in our series were subclassified into 188 ordinary or storiform-
pleomorphic type tumors (177 predominantly pleomorphic and 11 predominantly storiform tumors), 65 myxoid type, 14 inflammatory type, ten
giant cell type, and two angiomatoid type tumors. As has been noted by
others, however, there tended to be an overlap or mixture of these various
types.

4.2 Liposarcoma

Liposarcomas constituted the second largest group both in the files of the
Second Department of Pathology, Kyushu University (Table 3) and in the
survey of the Commission on Cancer of the American College of Surgeons
during the 2-year period 1983–1984 (LAWRENCE et al. 1987) (Table 2), and
accounted for 13.0% and 17.7%, respectively. There was a slight male
predominance with 78 men and 52 women (Table 3). The majority of
patients were in their fourth to seventh decades (106 cases, 82%), and our
soft tissue sarcoma file included no patients under 15 years of age (Table 4).
Indeed, liposarcomas in childhood are extremely rare (SHMOOKLER and
ENZINGER 1983).

The lower extremities were the most commonly involved sites in our
series, as was the case in the other series (Table 5) – 59 occurred in the thigh
or buttocks comprising 95% of the 62 lower extremity tumors and 45% of all
liposarcomas. The retroperitoneum was the next most frequently involved
site, comprising 28% (36 cases). Thus, the great majority of liposarcomas
occurred in two areas: the thigh and the retroperitoneum.

An attempt was made to classify the liposarcomas into five histologic
types (HASHIMOTO and ENJOJI 1982), and a review of the cases disclosed

that 57 (44%) were classified as myxoid, 40 (31%) as well differentiated, 16 (12%) as dedifferentiated, nine as pleomorphic, four as round cell, and the remaining four as mixed. It is of particular interest that the vast majority of myxoid liposarcomas occurred in the thigh while the majority of well-differentiated or dedifferentiated tumors was seen in the retroperitoneum.

4.3 Leiomyosarcoma

A total of 102 patients had leiomyosarcoma, the third most commonly encountered sarcoma in this series as well as in the largest recent series (LAWRENCE et al. 1987), comprising 10.2% in our series (Tables 2 and 3). The leiomyosarcomas were further classified into ordinary type in 79 cases, epithelioid in 17, and dedifferentiated in six. Female patients predominated over males in both internal and external soft tissue leiomyosarcomas in our series with a sex ratio of 1:1.6 (39 men and 63 women) (HASHIMOTO et al. 1986), although a few other reports have commented on the predilection of superficial leiomyosarcomas for men (DAHL and ANGERVALL 1974; FIELDS and HELWIG 1981; WILE et al. 1981) (Table 3). The incidence was highest for patients in their sixth and seventh decades (57 cases, 56%) with the mean age of 57 (median 59) years. This sarcoma has also been considered to be extremely rare in childhood (Table 4).

The tumor occurred most often in the retroperitoneum (35 cases, 34%), and other sites of occurrence were the mesentery in 26 (25%), and either the thigh or knee in 19 (19%) (Table 5). A review of our 198 cases with soft tissue sarcomas arising in the retroperitoneum and mesentery revealed that leiomyosarcoma was the most frequently encountered sarcoma (31%), followed by liposarcoma (19%), and MFH (19%) (HASHIMOTO et al. 1985).

4.4 Synovial Sarcoma

Synovial sarcoma comprised 6.7% of the cases in our series and ranked fourth in frequency (Table 3), and this rate of incidence was comparable to that of 10% (CADMAN et al. 1965), 6.9% (RUSSELL et al. 1977), 3.6% (LAWRENCE et al. 1987), and 9.6% (TOROSIAN et al. 1988) by others. The tumors were divided into biphasic and monophasic synovial sarcomas, consisting of 28 and 39 cases, respectively. Our data showed a slight female predominance with 26 men and 41 women (Table 3) (TSUNEYOSHI et al. 1983), although others have reported males to be more susceptible than females (CADMAN et al. 1965; HAJDU et al. 1977). The tumors were found

most often in the earlier adult years: 55 tumors (75%) occurred in patients
under 50 years of age, 40 (55%) under 40 years, and 15 (21%) under age 20,
with an average age of 37 years (Table 4). In the series of CADMAN et al.
(1965), 75% were under the age of 40, and in the series of 345 cases by
ENZINGER WEISS (1988b), 90% of the affected patients were under 50 years
of age, and 72% were under 40 years, with an average of 31, and 27 years,
respectively.

It is known that the tumors usually arise from the soft tissues in the
vicinity of large joints and appear intimately related to tendons or tendon
sheaths. Despite their name, they are only rarely found definitely within
joint cavities. In our series, most synovial sarcomas were located on the
extremities with 48 (72%) on the lower extremities and 15 (22%) on the
upper extremities (Table 5). The single most common site was the thigh (24
cases including the groin and the lowermost portion of the thigh), followed
by the knee region (nine cases). Synovial sarcomas accounted for 22%
among all of the 41 soft tissue sarcomas arising from the knee regions.
Furthermore, the peripheral portions of the extremities were not uncom-
monly affected by the tumors (lower leg and foot ten, and forearm and hand
six). Other rare sites included the neck in two cases and the chest wall in
one, although the Armed Forces Institute of Pathology (AFIP) series contained a greater number of cases in unusual locations (ROTH et al. 1975;
SHMOOKLER et al. 1982).

4.5 Malignant Schwannoma

A total of 63 patients had malignant schwannoma, including ten cases of
malignant triton tumors and four desmoplastic melanomas, with the tumor
being ranked fifth in frequency and comprising 6.3% in our series (Table 3).
There was a slight female preponderance with 28 men and 35 women
(TSUNEYOSHI and ENJOJI 1979). The male predominance in other studies
showing a high percentage of patients with neurofibromatosis of von
Recklinghausen is considered to be the result of a male bias in the latter
disease (GUCCION and ENZINGER 1979). The tumors may occur at any age;
49 (74%) patients were, however, in their third to sixth decades of life, with
the mean age of 42 (median 43) years (Table 4).

The tumors were attached anatomically to major nerve trunks in 24
(38%) of the 63 cases; 23 tumors were located in the lower extremities
(34%), 15 (24%) in the upper extremities, eight (13%) in the trunk; seven
(11%) in the head and neck, five in the retroperitoneum, and four in the
mediastinum (Table 5). Of the 63 tumors, 25 (40%) developed in association
with neurofibromatosis of von Recklinghausen, including nine cases with a
tumor closely connected anatomically to grossly discernible peripheral

nerves. A total of 38 cases were unassociated with neurofibromatosis, in which 15 had a close anatomic relation to discernible nerves.

4.6 Rhabdomyosarcoma

There were 54 cases of rhabdomyosarcoma comprising 5.4% in our adult series of soft tissue sarcomas and ranked sixth in frequency (Table 3), although in our entire series 108 rhabdomyosarcomas accounted for 9.7% and constituted the third largest group following MFH and liposarcoma. In 114 soft tissue sarcomas occurring in patients under 15 years of age, nearly a half (47%) of the cases were rhabdomyosarcomas (Table 4). There was a male predominance with 34 men and 20 women and a ratio of 1.7:1 in the adult cases (Table 3). The 54 cases of this tumor were grouped into three histologic types: 20 embryonal, 33 alveolar, and one pleomorphic. As has already been well established, the average age was different between the embryonal and alveolar types. In our entire series, the embryonal type occurred most often in the first decade with a mean age of 11 (median 5) years, and the alveolar type in the second and third decades with a mean age of 23 (median 22) years. Only one patient with pleomorphic rhabdomyosarcoma was 17 years old.

The head and neck were involved most often in both the embryonal and alveolar types, and the lower extremities and trunk were also frequently affected by these tumors. The soft tissues around the genitourinary tracts were preferential sites of embryonal rhabdomyosarcoma particularly in infants and children, while most rhabdomyosarcomas located in the upper extremities were of the alveolar type.

4.7 Fibrosarcoma

Forty-one cases of fibrosarcoma, excluding 17 cases of congenital or infantile forms, constituted a smaller group and comprised 4.1% in this series (Table 3) (IWASAKI and ENJOJI 1979). The apparent decline in the incidence of fibrosarcoma over the years is considered mainly to be due to the introduction of malignant fibrous histiocytoma as a specified tumor entity in addition to the separation of desmoid and other fibromatoses as non-metastasizing specific entities. Twenty-eight cases (68% of patients with adult fibrosarcoma) were found in the fourth through sixth decades, with a mean age of 46 (median 48) years (Table 4). The tumor occurred in both sexes with equal frequency (20 men and 21 women). Eighteen (44%) adult fibrosarcomas occurred on the trunk, nine (22%) in the upper extremities, seven (17%) in the head and neck, and six (15%) in the lower extremities (Table 5).

4.8 Extraskeletal Chondrosarcoma

Extraskeletal chondrosarcoma comprised 3.5% of this series (Table 3), consisting of 24 cases of myxoid chondrosarcoma (chordoid sarcoma), four of mesenchymal chondrosarcoma, and seven of dedifferentiated chondrosarcoma, with an average ages of 45, 23, and 45 years, respectively. Thirteen (54%) of the 24 extraskeletal myxoid chondrosarcoma were located in the extremities, with the most common sites found in the thigh and knee regions (eight cases) (TSUNEYOSHI et al. 1981). The number of the other two variants of extraskeletal chondrosarcoma were too small to evaluate.

4.9 Angiosarcoma

Thirty-two cases of angiosarcoma in this series included two cases of angiosarcoma associated with lymphedema (lymphangiosarcoma) arising in the upper arm and the foot, respectively (Table 3). The angiosarcomas not associated with lymphedema occurred in patients over 50 years of age in 23 cases (77%), with a mean age of 57 (median 64) years. The most frequent primary site of angiosarcoma was the head and neck (50%), particularly in the skin or superficial soft tissue of the scalp and forehead (Table 5).

4.10 Other Specified Sarcomas

The remaining sarcomas fell into 11 categories exclusive of unclassified sarcoma, and have been tabulated in Table 3 to show their relative frequency. Alveolar soft part sarcoma showed a marked female preponderance. Malignant neuroepithelioma, epithelioid sarcoma, alveolar soft part sarcoma, and extraskeletal Ewing's sarcoma were tumors of young adults or adolescents, with a median age of 18, 27, 24, and 20 years, respectively (Table 4). Malignant mesothelioma was principally seen in patients over 40, with a median age of 56 years. Most malignant hemangiopericytomas and clear cell sarcomas occurred in young and middle-aged adults, with a median age of 42 and 39 years, respectively.

Approximately one third of the malignant hemangiopericytomas and over half the alveolar soft part sarcomas were located in the extremities, expecially in the thigh and buttocks (Table 5). The retroperitoneum was the second most common site of malignant hemangiopericytoma and accounted for 23% of the cases. The site of occurrence of clear cell sarcoma was somewhat similar to epithelioid sarcoma in that distal portions of the extremities were a common site of origin. Eighty percent of clear cell sarcomas arose, however, in the lower extremities as contrasted with the predilection of epithelioid sarcomas for the hand and forearm. Malignant neuroepithelioma and extraskeletal Ewing's sarcoma affected the lower extremities in half of the cases and the trunk in 29% and 38% of the cases, respectively (HASHIMOTO et al. 1983). The similarities in the distribution of age and location between the two entities, as well as the common cytogenetic abnormality of both tumors, which was a reciprocal 11:22 chromosomal translocation (AURIAS et al. 1983; TURC-CAREL et al. 1983; WHANG-PENG et al. 1984), suggest a histogenetic overlap between the two tumors.

The other rare tumor groups were extraskeletal osteosarcoma, malignant mesenchymoma, malignant rhabdoid tumor of the soft parts and Kaposi's sarcoma, but here the numbers were too small to provide a meaningful statistical assessment.

5 Unclassified Sarcoma

Seventy-five sarcomas with an unclassifiable microscopic picture constituted a a rather large but diverse group in this series and included 7.5% of all soft tissue sarcomas (Table 3). These sarcomas occurred more often in patients in their fifth through eighth decades of life, although there was a more even distribution among every decade as compared to the specified sarcomas (Table 4). The anatomic locations of the tumors were also more evenly distributed than the more specified sarcomas, albeit the lower extremities were the most commonly affected (Table 5).

6 Conclusion

In addition to refined conventional light microscopy, modern ancillary methods of histochemistry, immunohistochemistry, and electron microscopy have improved the accuracy of the histologic diagnosis of soft tissue sarcomas. As WEISS and ENZINGER (1978) first stated, and as has been recently supported by the largest series of soft tissue sarcomas in adults from the Commission on Cancer of the American College of Surgeons, our data were based on a total of 1002 cases of soft tissue sarcomas which indicated that MFH was encountered most frequently and accounted for over one fourth of adult soft tissue sarcomas. Other common sarcomas in adults were liposarcoma, leiomyosarcoma, synovial sarcoma, malignant schwannoma, rhabdomyosarcoma, and fibrosarcoma, in the order of frequency, although rhabdomyosarcoma constituted the third largest group in our entire series including childhood sarcomas. However, a fair number of soft tissue sarcomas remained unclassifiable, constituting 7.5% in this series.

Malignant fibrous histiocytoma, leiomyosarcoma, angiosarcoma, and mesothelioma principally affected patients of late adult life, while synovial sarcoma, malignant schwannoma, fibrosarcoma, and clear cell sarcoma were more frequent in young or middle-aged adults. Malignant neuroepithelioma, extraskeletal Ewing's sarcoma, epithelioid sarcoma, and alveolar soft part sarcoma were tumors in adolescents and young adults as well as children.

The thigh and buttocks of the low extremities were the most common sites for all soft tissue malignancies in adults and for MFH as well. The next most frequent sites were the retroperitoneum and mesentery, which are sites particularly known for leiomyosarcoma and liposarcoma. Each tumor type had one or more of its own sites of notable predilection. Most liposarcomas, for instance, were found on the thigh, buttocks, and retroperitoneum, while synovial sarcomas predominantly occurred in the lower extremities in more than 70% of the cases. The distal portions of the extremities were also common sites of origin in both clear cell sarcoma and epithelioid sarcoma.

References

Agnarsson BA, Baldursson G, Benediktsdottir KR, Hrafnkelsson J (1991) Tumours in Iceland. 14. Malignant tumours of soft tissues. Histological classification and epidemiological considerations. Acta Pathol Microbiol Immunol Scand [A] 99: 443–448
Aurias A, Rimbaut C, Buffe D, Dubousset J, Mazabraud A (1983) Chromosomal translocations in Ewing's sarcoma. N Engl J Med 309: 496–497
Boring CC, Squires TS, Tong T (1991) Cancer statistics, 1991. CA 41: 19–36
Brumini R (1982) Cancer in Brazil. Histopathological data 1976–80. Dataprev, Rio de Janeiro
Cadman NL, Soule EH, Kelly PJ (1965) Synovial sarcoma: an analysis of 134 tumors. Cancer 18: 613–627
Costa J, Wesley RA, Glatstein E, Rosenberg SA (1984) The grading of soft tissue sarcomas. Results of a clinicopathologic correlation in a series of 163 cases. Cancer 53: 530–541
Crawford M, Chung EB, Leffall LD Jr, White JE (1970) Soft part sarcomas in negroes. Cancer 26: 503–512
Cutler SJ, Young JL Jr (1975) Third national cancer survey: incidence data. Natl Cancer Inst Monogr 41: 1–454
Dahl I, Angervall L (1974) Cutaneous and subcutaneous leiomyosarcoma: a clinicopathologic study of 47 patients. Pathol Eur 9: 307–315
Das Gupta TK (1983) Principles of classification and diagnosis. In: Das Gupta TK (ed) Tumors of the soft tissues. Appleton-Century-Crofts, Norwalk, pp 1–183
Eilber FR (1984) Soft tissue sarcomas of the extremity. Year Book Medical Publishers, Chicago, pp 1–41 (Current problems in cancer, 1984)
Enjoji M, Hashimoto H (1984) Dagnosis of soft tissue sarcomas. Pathol Res Pract 178: 215–226
Enjoji M, Hashimoto H, Tsunyoshi M, Iwasaki H (1980) Malignant fibrous histiocytoma. A clinicopathologica study of 130 cases. Acta Pathol Jpn 30: 727–741
Enzinger FM, Weiss SW (1988a) Malignant fibrohistiocytic tumors. In: Enzinger FM, Weiss SW (eds) Soft tissue tumors, 2nd edn. Mosby, St Louis, pp 269–300
Enzinger FM, Weiss SW (1988b) Synovial sarcoma. In: Enzinger FM, Weiss SW (eds) Soft tissue tumors, 2nd edn. Mosby, St Louis, pp 659–688

Ferrell HW, Frable WJ (1972) Soft part sarcomas revisited. Review and comparison of a second series. Cancer 30: 475–480

Fields JP, Helwig EB (1981) Leiomyosarcoma of the skin and subcutaneous tissue. Cancer 47: 156–169

Fisher C (1989) Pathology of soft tissue sarcomas. In: Pinedo HM, Verweij J (eds) Treatment of soft tissue sarcomas. Kluwer Academic, Boston, pp 1–21

Fletcher CDM (1990) Introduction. In: Fletcher CDM, McKee PH (eds) Pathobiology of soft tissue tumours. Churchill, Edinburgh, pp 1–7

Gaillard W, Chung EB, White JE, Leffall LD Jr (1974) Diagnosis and management of soft tissue sarcomas. Am Surg 40: 60–71

Guccion JG, Enzinger FM (1979) Malignant schwannoma associated with von Recklinghausen's neurofibromatosis. Virchows Arch [A] 383: 43–57

Hajdu SI (1979) History and classification of soft tissue tumors. In: Pathology of soft tissue tumors. Lea and Febiger, Philadelphia, pp 1–55

Hajdu SI, Shiu MH, Fortner JG (1977) Tenosynovial sarcoma. A clinicopathological study of 136 cases. Cancer 39: 1201–1217

Hare HF, Cerny MJ (1963) Soft tissue sarcoma. A review of 200 cases. Cancer 16: 1332–1337

Hashimoto H, Enjoji M (1982) Liposarcoma. A clinicopathologic subtyping of 52 cases. Acta Pathol Jpn 32: 933–948

Hashimoto H, Enjoji M, Nakajima T, Kiryu H, Daimaru Y (1983) Malignant neuroepithelioma (peripheral neuroblastoma). A clinicopathologic study of 15 cases. Am J Surg Pathol 7: 309–318

Hashimoto H, Tsuneyoshi M, Enjoji M (1985) Malignant smooth muscle tumors of the retro-peritoneum and mesentery: a clinicopathologic analysis of 44 cases. J Surg Oncol 28: 177–186

Hashimoto H, Daimaru Y, Tsuneyoshi M, Enjoji M (1986) Leiomyosarcoma of the external soft tissues. A clinicopathologic, immunohistochemical, and electron microscopic study. Cancer 57: 2077–2088

Horn RC Jr (1963) Sarcomas of soft tissues. J Am Med Assoc 183: 511–515

Iwasaki H, Enjoji M (1979) Infantile and adult fibrosarcomas of the soft tissues. Acta Pathol Jpn 29: 377–388

Japanese Society of Pathology (1984–1988) Annual of the pathological autopsy cases in Japan, vol 26–30 (in Japanese)

Kyriakos M (1990) Tumors and tumorlike conditions of the soft tissue. In: Kissane JM (ed) Anderson's pathology, 9th edn. Mosby, St Louis, pp 1838–1928

Lawrence W Jr, Donegan WL, Natarajan N, Mettlin C, Beart R, Winchester D (1987) Adult soft tissue sarcomas. A pattern of care survey of the American College of Surgeons. Ann Surg 205: 349–359

Lieberman Z, Ackerman LV (1954) Principles in management of soft tissue sarcomas. A clinical and pathologic review of one hundred cases. Surgery 35: 350–365

Myhre-Jensen O, Kaae S, Madsen EH, Sneppen O (1983) Histopathological grading in soft-tissue tumours. Relation to survival in 261 surgically treated patients. Acta Pathol Microbiol Immunol Scand [A] 91: 145–150

Myhre-Jensen O, Hogh J, Ostgaard SE, Nordentoft M, Sneppen O (1991) Histopathological grading of soft tissue tumours. Prognostic significance in a prospective study of 278 consecutive cases. J Pathol 163: 19–24

Rantakokko V, Ekfors TO (1979) Sarcomas of the soft tissues in the extremities and limb girdles. Analysis of 240 cases diagnosed in Finland in 1960–1969. Acta Chir Scand 145: 385–394

Roth JA, Enzinger FM, Tannenbaum M (1975) Synovial sarcoma of the neck: a followup study of 24 cases. Cancer 35: 1243–1253

Russell WO, Cohen J, Enzinger FM, Hajdu SI, Heise H, Martin RG, Meissner W, Miller WT, Schnitz RL, Suit HD (1977) A clinical and pathological staging system for soft tissue sarcomas. Cancer 40: 1562–1570

Shmookler BM, Enzinger FM (1983) Liposarcoma occurring in children. An analysis of 17 cases and review of the literature. Cancer 52: 567–574

Shmookler BM, Enzinger FM, Brannon RB (1982) Orofacial synovial sarcoma. A clinico-pathologic study of 11 new cases and review of the literature. Cancer 50: 269–276

Stout AP (1953) Tumors of the soft tissues. In: Atlas of tumor pathology, Fasc 5, Armed Forces Institute of Pathology, Washington DC

Suit HD, Russell WO, Martin RG (1975) Sarcoma of soft tissue: clinical and histopathologic parameters and response to treatment. Cancer 35: 1478–1483

Torosian MH, Friedrich C, Godbold J, Hajdu SI, Brennan MF (1988) Soft-tissue sarcoma: initial characteristics and prognostic factors in patients with and without metastatic disease. Semin Surg Oncol 4: 13–19

Trojani M, Contesso G, Coindre JM, Rouesse J, Bui NB, de Mascarel A, Goussot JF, David M, Bonichon F, Lagarde C (1984) Soft-tissue sarcomas of adults; study of pathological prognostic variables and definition of a histopathological grading system. Int J Cancer 33: 37–42

Tsujimoto M, Aozasa K, Ueda T, Morimura Y, Komatsubara Y, Doi T (1988) Multivariate analysis for histologic prognostic factors in soft tissue sarcomas. Cancer 62: 994–998

Tsuneyoshi M, Enjoji M (1979) Primary malignant peripheral nerve tumors (malignant schwannomas). A clinicopathologic and electron microscopic study. Acta Pathol Jpn 29: 363–375

Tsuneyoshi M, Enjoji M, Iwasaki H, Shinohara N (1981) Extraskeletal myxoid chondrosarcoma. A clinicopathologic and electron microscopic study. Acta Pathol Jpn 31: 439–447

Tsuneyoshi M, Yokoyama K, Enjoji M (1983) Synovial sarcoma. A clinicopathologic and ultrastructural study of 42 cases. Acta Pathol Jpn 33: 23–36

Turc-Carel C, Philip I, Berger M-P, Philip T, Lenoir GM (1983) Chromosomal translocations in Ewing's sarcoma. N Engl J Med 309: 497–498

Weiss SW, Enzinger FM (1978) Malignant fibrous histiocytoma. An analysis of 200 cases. Cancer 41: 2250–2266

Whang-Peng J, Triche TJ, Knutsen T, Miser J, Douglass EC, Israel MA (1984) Chromosome translocation in peripheral neuroepithelioma. N Engl J Med 311: 584–585

Wile AG, Evans HL, Romsdahl MM (1981) Leiomyosarcoma of soft tissue: a clinicopathologic study. Cancer 48: 1022–1032

Clinical Management of Soft Tissue Sarcomas

J. Treuner and M. Morgan

1 Introduction

The histological heterogeneity and the variable clinical manifestations of malignant soft tissue tumours calls for a variable therapeutic approach. The essential strategy for treatment is based on a number of factors: histology, site, tumour size, local invasiveness, systemic spread and the age at diagnosis. The tumour characteristics at diagnosis are to a certain extent interrelated and not entirely independent of one another, e.g., tumour size and primary site, tumour invasiveness and histology which is also related to site and age. In addition to the tumour characteristics, there are a number of important prognostic factors which influence the type of therapy and the outcome. The dynamic prognostic factors take into account the individual chemo- and radiosensitivity of the tumour, the physical and the psychological tolerance to treatment as well as the quality of the diagnostic procedure and the treatment. The aim of therapy in each case is to ensure a relapse-free survival and avoid mutilating surgery or loss of function of a part of the body. This goal can be achieved in many situations but not in all. The potential threat of the cancer has always priority over the functional, cosmetic aspects.

Current Topics in Pathology
Volume 89, Eds. D. Harms/D. Schmidt
© Springer-Verlag Berlin Heidelberg 1995

2 General Principles of Diagnosis

As a result of the variable biology of the tumour there are a number of basic principles which must be adhered to in the diagnosis and clinical management of soft tissue sarcomas. Every swelling not due to trauma or inflammation must be treated as malignant until proved otherwise. When this basic rule is observed, thoughtless management should be avoided.

Tumours which can be removed with a satisfactory margin without mutilating surgery should be primarily resected.

All tumour tissue must be histologically examined including immunocytochemistry. Today molecular biology is an important part of the pretherapeutic investigation.

Any suspicious malignant lesion must be documented radiologically before surgical resection to determine the exact limits and extension of the tumour.

When a definitive diagnosis of malignancy is confirmed, a systemic examination is necessary to look for metastatic tumour (lung, lymph nodes, skeleton, bone marrow, liver, and CNS).

Following disease staging, a multidisciplinary approach involving oncologist, radiotherapist and surgeon is essential for planning a therapeutic strategy.

3 Concept of Treatment

The diagnostic procedure is a part of the treatment, particularly in the case of primary resectable tumours. The three modalities of treatment, viz. surgery, chemotherapy and radiotherapy, can then be coordinated following histological confirmation and accurate disease staging. Before planning a therapeutic strategy the following questions need to be asked. Has the primary tumour been completely resected or is it possible to do so without mutilating the patient? Is the tumour localised or disseminated? Is the histological subtype of the tumour chemotherapy sensitive? When the tumour is primarily resectable without mutilating surgery, the question of adjuvant chemotherapy arises. This depends on the histology and the potential to metastasise. In the case of a non-resectable tumour, the most important question is whether the histological subtype is sensitive to chemotherapy. The more sensitive the tumour is to chemotherapy, the less likely is the need for radical surgery. In contrast, when a malignant tumour, either primary or metastatic, is not sensitive to cytostatics, surgical intervention must play a dominant role even to the extent of mutilation. Therefore the resectability of a malignant tumour and its sensitivity to chemotherapy are the main points to consider when planning the initial therapy. The age of the patient, primary site and local extension are the factors influencing tumour resectability. The expected response to chemotherapy, on the other hand, depends on histology, the size of the tumour, the way in which the treatment is administered and how well it is tolerated.

3.1 Treatment-Related Histological Aspects

The histology identifies the biological behaviour of the tumour with respect to proliferation, capacity to metastasise and the sensitivity to chemo- and radiotherapy. A careful histological examination of the surgical specimen from the second-look operation is essential, with particular emphasis on the resection margins and the viability of the tumour cells. Histological grading and DNA index provide additional evidence of malignancy. The associated cytogenetic and molecular-biological findings appear to provide further information about prognosis (see the chapter by Triche, this volume). Specific histological types correlate with certain primary sites, particular age group and likelihood of lymph node involvement and metastases. Soft tisue sarcomas in children and teenagers can be grouped according to sensitivity to chemotherapy:

1. Chemotherapy-sensitive soft tissue sarcomas: rhabdomyosarcoma (RMS), extraosseous Ewing sarcoma (EES)/peripheral neuroectodermal tumour (PNET), synovial sarcoma (SS) and undifferentiated sarcoma (US)
2. Moderately or rarely chemosensitive soft tissue sarcomas: epithelioid sarcoma, clear cell sarcoma, malignant fibrous histiocytoma, haemangio-sarcoma, leiomyosarcoma, fibrosarcoma, liposarcoma and neurofibro-sarcoma. (In CWS-86 leiomyosarcoma was included in the chemotherapy sensitive group but in subsequent studies this is no longer the case.)

There is no significant difference in outcome between the histological subtypes when the method of treatment and the qualitative influences are excluded. Therefore it can be concluded that the use of multimodal therapy in the management of soft tissue sarcomas has been adequately established.

The results of the German Cooperative Soft Tissue Sarcoma studies (CWS-81 and CWS-86) are shown in Tables 1–3. Protocol patients (PP) were treated according to the standard protocol. Non-protocol patients (NP) showed some deviation from the therapy regimen. There was no significant difference in survival between the various histological types in the group of chemotherapy sensitive sarcomas (group 1). The synovial sarcomas tended to have a better prognosis although this could be explained by the higher proportion of stage I and II patients compared with other histological subtypes.

The survival rate for patients with tumours not usually sensitive to chemotherapy (group 2) registered in the CWS studies is shown in Table 4

Table 1. Distribution of group 1 (soft tissue sarcomas sensitive to CT). CWS-81/86, PP, stages I–III

	n	DFS (%)	Survival (%)	Observation time (months)
RMS	264	67	73	52
SS	37	82	83	55
EES/PNET	35	36	60	26
US	5	40	40	16
LMS	10	77	88	44
Group 1	356	65	72	50

Table 2. Distribution by stage, CWS-81/86, PP, group 1

	RMS	SS	EES/PNET	US	LMS	Total
I	51	16	6	0	4	78
II	53	15	7	0	2	79
III	160	6	22	5	4	199
	264	37	35	5	10	356

Table 3. Survival rate according to stage. CWS-81/86, PP, group 1, stages I–III

	RMS (%)	SS (%)	EES/PNET (%)	US (%)	LMS (%)	Total (%)
I	96	82	83	0	67	91
II	83	100	100	0	100	87
III	62	50	44	40	100	59

and Fig. 1 compares the overall survival between the two histological groups. Table 5 shows the distribution according to stage of the various histological subtypes not sensitive to chemotherapy.

4 Stage and Prognosis

The tumour stage at diagnosis has been considered to have an appreciable influence on the prognosis. This concept of staging a tumour is not precisely defined. There are various systems used to describe the pre- and postoperative tumour extension. The most widely used is the post-surgical grouping system devised by the Intergroup Rhabdomyosarcoma Study (IRS):

Stage I   Localised disease completely resected
Stage II   Grossly resected with microscopic residual disease

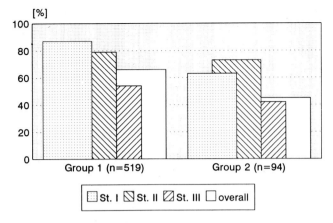

Fig. 1. Survival rate of histologic group 1 vs. group 2, CWS-81/86, PP + NP (no adults, no secondary tumours)

Table 4. Survival rate, group 2, stages I–III, CWS-81/86, PP + NP

	n	Survival rate (%)
Fibrosarcoma	20	49
Neurofibrosarcoma	22	43
Malignant fibrous histiocytoma	10	89
Liposarcoma	7	50
Haemangiosarcoma	3	– (1 lost, 2 dead)
Clear cell sarcoma	4	– (4 CCR)
Other	28	65

Table 5. Distribution of histology group 2 by stage, CWS-81/86

	I	II	III	Total
Fibrosarcoma	7	7	6	20
Neurofibrosarcoma	10	3	9	22
Malignant fibrous histiocytoma	6	2	2	10
Liposarcoma	3	2	2	7
Haemangiosarcoma	1	1	1	3
Clear cell sarcoma	4	0	0	4
Other	7	6	15	28
	38	21	35	94

Stage III   Incomplete resection with macroscopic residual disease or biopsy
            only

Stage IV   Disseminated disease.

From a prognostic point of view this system separates stages I and II considered together as a group from stages III and IV. The tumour size, local extension with respect to infiltration of neighbouring organs or tissue and the primary site are important considerations for the initial resectability of the tumour. An alternative method of describing the tumour characteristics is the preoperative TNM classification proposed by UICC.

T1 No Mo	Tumour limited to organ or tissue of origin
T2 No Mo	Tumour invades contiguous organs or tissues
T1/2 N1 Mo	T1 or T2 with lymph node involvement
T1/2 No/1 M1	T1 or T2, No or N1 with distant metastasis

There is also a postoperative TNM classification which takes into consideration the quality of the surgical resection. It appears that the preoperative TNM classification is more appropriate than either the postoperative one or the IRS grouping system when correlating the characteristics of the tumour with prognosis. From our own experience there is a significant difference with respect to survival between T1 and T2 and Ta versus Tb for localised rhabdomyosarcoma treated according to the protocol when all stages (I–III) are analysed together as a group (Tables 6 and 7). When the influence of T1/T2 is analysed according to individual stage (IRS system), this trend is present only in stages I and II, but not observed in stage III. In contrast, the tumour size <5 cm (a) or >5 cm (b) remains an essential prognostic factor in all stages, particularly in stage III. The local invasiveness of the primary tumour, regardless of the way in which it is described, has an appreciable influence on prognosis and, as a result, on the intensity of the therapy used. In conclusion, the T classification is prognostically significant for localised, resectable disease, but in the case of primary unresectable tumours, only the tumour size a or b has prognostic relevance.

Table 6. T1 vs. T2, CWS-81/86, RMS, PP, stages I–III

	CWS-81		CWS-86	
	n	DFS^a (%)	n	DFS^b (%)
T1	58	84	63	79
T2	76	52	67	55

$^a p < 0.001$
$^b p = 0.029$

Table 7. Ta vs. Tb, CWS-81/86, RMS, stages I–III

	CWS-81		CWS-86	
	n	DFS^a (%)	n	DFS^b (%)
Ta	74	81	76	79
Tb	56	47	54	47

$^a p < 0.001$
$^b p = 0.007$

4.1 Primary Site and Prognosis

Soft tissue sarcomas are manifested in all regions of the body and, dependent on age group, certain sites predominant. In children and teenagers, the distribution of the primary sites for histological groups 1 and 2 are illustrated in Figs. 2 and 3. In adults, however, most soft tissue sarcomas are located in the extremity. In order to be able to compare the analysis of the various national clinical trials and determine the prognostic factors, it was necessary to reach an agreement on the precise definition of primary sites. As a result of an international workshop in which the main study groups took part, seven categories were clearly defined:

Orbit
Head/neck non-parameningeal
Head/neck parameningeal

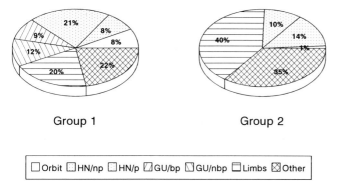

Group 1   Group 2

☐ Orbit ☐ HN/np ☐ HN/p ⧄ GU/bp ⬡ GU/nbp ☐ Limbs ⊠ Other

Fig. 2. Distribution of primary sites, histologic group 1 vs. group 2, CWS-81/86, PP + NP

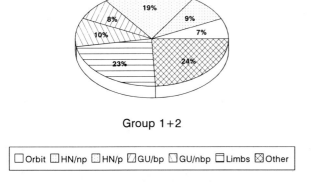

Group 1+2

☐ Orbit ☐ HN/np ☐ HN/p ⧄ GU/bp ⬡ GU/nbp ☐ Limbs ⊠ Other

Fig. 3. Distribution of primary sites, histologic group 1 + 2, CWS-81/86, PP + NP

Genitourinary non-bladder/prostate
Genitourinary bladder/prostate
Extremity
Other

These seven categories are prognostically different and require a different therapeutic approach. Table 8 shows the survival rate in the CWS studies for chemotherapy-sensitive tumours analysed according to the primary site. The survival data for patients with tumours not usually sensitive to chemotherapy are shown in the subsequent Table 9.

As an example of the variations in the clinical management of soft tissue sarcomas, the orbital and paratesticular RMS have been considered. Tumours in these two primary sites have a similar chance of being cured, but the treatment strategy differs (Table 10). The survival rate is similar in the two groups although the distribution of primary stage is quite different. With one exception, all the paratesticular RMS were stage I or II and

Table 8. Survival rate according to localisation. CWS-81/86, PP, group 1, stages I–III

	n	Survival rate (%)
Orbit	33	86
Head/neck – non-parameningeal	28	79
Head/neck – parameningeal	75	50
Urogenital – bladder and prostate	30	76
Urogenital – non-bladder and prostate	48	100
Limbs	63	78
Other	79	61

Table 9. Survival rate according to localisation. CWS-81/86, PP, group 2, stages I–III

	n	Survival rate (%)
Limbs	20	47
Head/neck	11	41
Other	17	45

Table 10. RMS, Orbit vs. paratesticular, CWS-81/86, PP + NP

	I	II	III	I–III Survival rate (%)	I–III Observation time (months)
Orbit	3	10	30	89	46
Paratesticular	39	7	1	100	61

treated by surgery and chemotherapy. In contrast, the orbital RMS were predominantly stage III and in most cases treated with chemotherapy and radiotherapy without radical surgical intervention. It is of interest that in both groups the tumour diameter was similar. Further it can be concluded that those soft tissue sarcomas which are chemo- and radiotherapy sensitive can be treated with the same degree of success as those which can be primarily totally resected and that a surgical approach to resect the tumour is preferable when this does not cause mutilation. However, there are exceptions to this general rule as seen in extremity tumours (Fig. 4) of specific histological subtypes, alveolar RMS, synovial sarcoma and probably also peripheral neuroectodermal tumours. Although these tumours may be primarily resectable (stage I), the chance of survival is worse for those who do not receive additional radiotherapy. It is therefore necessary to distinguish between favourable and unfavourable histology when planning treatment for stage I disease.

4.1.1 Chemotherapy and Prognosis

The response to chemotherapy at a defined stage of treatment is a prognostic factor for chemosensitive sarcomas. From the CWS-81 data, the degree of tumour regression at weeks 7–9 after the first VACA cycle was a long-term independent prognostic factor in unresectable RMS (Table 11). This information was used in planning the follow-up study CWS-86. This response/time factor was incorporated into the overall concept. In addition, the radiotherapy protocol was altered. Radiation was administered earlier in the treatment at weeks 10–13 for good and poor responders instead of at weeks 16–20. The dose for good responders (>2/3) was reduced to 32 Gy, while poor responders received 48 Gy. The results of the CWS-86 study show that

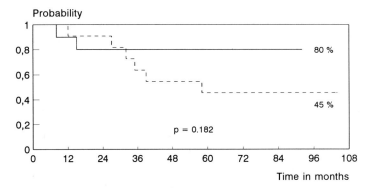

Fig. 4. Survival of extremity tumours, irradiated (*solid line*, n = 12) vs. non-irradiated (*broken line*, n = 10). CWS-81/86, group 1, stage I, PP + NP

Table 11. RMS, stage III, response, CWS-81, PP

	n	Survival rate (%)
Complete response	18	82
Good response	24	58
Poor response	26	49
No response	8	38

this time–response–prognosis factor is no longer relevant. This has been a consequence of risk-adapted therapy.

Further questions arise about the role of chemotherapy in the entire concept of the treatment:

– What are the most effective cytotoxics and in which combination?
– What is the optimal duration of chemotherapy?
– What are the immediate and long-term side effects?
– What is the role of bone marrow transplant in primary disseminated sarcomas?

These questions can only be dealt with in brief.

5 Cytostatics

Combination chemotherapy rather than monotherapy must be considered when referring to the primary response rate (BAUM et al. 1981; CRIST et al. 1987; GHAVIMI et al. 1981; KINGSTON et al. 1983; MAURER et al. 1978). The best response rates are achieved with regimens comprising ifosfamide, actinomycin-D, vincristine or adriamycin (TREUNER et al. 1989, 1991).

The same applies to ifosfamide/etoposide (VP-16)/vincristine or cisplatin/ etoposide/adriamycin combinations, both of which are very effective. Following a comparison of the two German trials, the substitution of cyclo-phosphamide (CWS-81) by ifosfamide (CWS-86) produced no long-term benefit in patients in favourable risk categories although the initial response rate was higher with the ifosfamide-containing regimen. It is not possible to comment on the primary response rate of the chemotherapy combinations used in the most common soft tissue sarcomas in adults as cytostatics are in most situations used as adjuvant therapy.

The response rate of the different cytostatics available before and after 1970 is shown: (a) before 1970: vincristine 59%, actinomycin 42%, cyclo-phosphamide 54%, dacarbazine 11%, adriamycin 31%; (b) after 1970:

cisplatin 15%, VP-16 10%–15%, methotrexate 10%, ifosfamide 58%, melphalan 30%.

The response to combination chemotherapy is clearly better: VAC + adriamycin 90%, CDDP + VP-16 50%, IVA 90%, ifosfamide + CDDP 68%.

As standard therapy, VAC or IVA is appropriate. However, when there is a high risk of relapse or in the relapse situation, additional adriamycin and cisplatin or etoposide should be administered.

5.1 Duration of Chemotherapy

The duration of chemotherapy depends on the initial risk group and varies between 20 and 104 weeks in the different studies. During the last few years, there has been a tendency to administer more intensive treatment over a shorter time period. When the various clinical trials are compared, the reduction in duration of therapy has not affected the possibility of achieving a cure. More recently, however, there has been a suspicion that the benefits achieved from the intensification of treatment, namely the reduced duration, have been forfeited as the overall results could not be improved. The reduction of therapy-induced long-term side effects as a consequence of a shorter period of treatment must also be considered in this type of analysis.

6 Risk Grouping System

The concept of grouping the chemotherapy-sensitive soft tissue sarcomas into defined risk categories was introduced into the current German clinical trial CWS-91. From the CWS-81 and -86 data, it appeared that patients could be divided into three risk groups (A, B, C). This was based on a combination of the post-surgical stage and primary site. Patients with primary unresectable tumours in risk groups B and C are stratified into a low- or high-risk category, dependent on the initial response to chemotherapy, tumour size and local extension. A retrospective analysis of RMS in the two previous trials showed the results given in Table 12 when the risk grouping system was considered. When group C patients are analysed according to the criteria response to chemotherapy, tumour size and extension at diagnosis, they can be divided into a favourable and an unfavourable group (Table 13). Group C included patients from CWS-81 who were treated with the VACA regimen and did not receive ifosfamide. This group had a

Table 12. Risk grouping of patients with RMS

	DFS rate CWS-81 (%)	EFS rate CWS-86 (%)
Group A	96	84
Group B	80	77
Group C	49	60
p	0.001	0.045

Table 13. Response to chemotherapy of group C patients

	DFS rate CWS-81 (%)	EFS rate CWS-86 (%)
Favourable group	92	77
Unfavourable group	41	66

favourable outcome with a better EFS than in the CWS-86 study. The risk groups are defined as follows:

Group A   All stage I patients excluding parameningeal, orbital and extremity tumours, alveolar RMS

Group B   Stage I parameningeal and extremity tumours
All stage II patients except orbit and alveolar RMS
Stage III genitourinary non-bladder/prostate

Group C   Stage III patients excluding genitourinary non-bladder/prostate
Orbital RMS. Alveolar RMS.

All stage III patients in risk groups B and C are subsequently stratified into a low- or high-risk category based on the preoperative TNM classification and response to chemotherapy.

Low-risk group   T1a any response
T1b good response (>2/3)
T2a good response (>2/3)

High-risk group   T1b poor response
T2a poor response
T2b any response
All N1

The parameters describing tumour invasiveness, T1/T2 and tumour size, a/b refer to the situation at diagnosis. For all stage III patients, the chemotherapy response is evaluated at week 12 of therapy. The subsequent treatment modalities surgery, chemotherapy, radiotherapy are determined by stratifying into low- or high-risk groups.

7 Bone Marrow Transplantation for Disseminated Soft Tissue Sarcoma

The results of therapy for stage IV RMS is unsatisfactory in the various national studies. Only 10%–20% of these patients survive long term in spite of intensive chemotherapy. The question that remains is whether ablative chemotherapy with autologous or allogeneic bone marrow rescue can improve the prognosis in this group of patients (MISER 1990; EMMINGER and EMMINGER-SCHMIDMEIER 1991). So far the limited experience with bone marrow transplant in stage IV patients does not appear to improve the outcome. However, an important point to consider is that the transplant was not part of the initial therapy, but carried out in most situations following relapse. In the future the transplant will be performed in first remission to determine prospectively the benefit of this form of treatment.

8 Conclusion

In summarising the current state of knowledge, the following conclusions can be made:

1. Primary surgical resection should be attempted provided it does not cause mutilation.
2. All patients with a high-grade chemotherapy-sensitive sarcoma should receive preoperative or adjuvant chemotherapy.
3. Radiotherapy is given to all patients whose primary tumour is completely resected but have unfavourable histology and to patients who have residual tumour following surgery and initial chemotherapy.
4. The intensity of the various treatment modalities depends on the risk group.

References

Baum ES et al. (1981) Phase II study in cisdichlorodiamine-platinum in refactory childhood cancer: Children's Cancer Study Group Report. Cancer Treat Rep 65: 815–822

Crist WM et al. (1987) Intensive chemotherapy including cisplatin with or without etoposide for children with soft tissue sarcoma. Med Pediatr Oncol 15: 51–57

Emminger W, Emminger-Schmidmeier W (1991) High dose melphalan, etoposide ± carboplatin (MEC) combined with 12-gray fractionated total-body irradiation in children with generalized solid tumors. Pediatr Hematol Oncol 8: 13–22

Ghavimi F et al. (1981) Multidisciplinary treatment of embryonal rhabdomyosarcoma in children: a progress report. Natl Cancer Inst Monogr 56: 111–120

Kingston JE, Mc Elwain TJ, Malpas JS (1983) Childhood rhabdomyosarcoma: experience of Children's Solid Tumour Group (CSTG). Br J Cancer 48: 195–207

Maurer HM et al. (1978) The intergroup rhabdomyosarcoma study. Natl Cancer Inst Monogr
    56: 61–68
Miser J (1990) Autologous bone marrow transplantation for the treatment of sarcomas. In:
    Johnson FL, Pochedly C (eds) Bone marrow transplantation in children. Greenwood, New
    York, pp 289–298
Treuner J, Koscielniak E, Keim M (1989) Comparison of the rates of response to ifosfamide
    and cyclophosphamide in primary unresectable rhabdomyosarcomas. Cancer Chemother
    Pharmacol 24: 48–50
Treuner J, Flamant F, Carli M (1991) Results of treatment of rhabdomyosarcoma in the
    European Studies. In: Maurer, Ruymann, Pochedly (eds) Rhabdomyosarcoma and related
    tumors in children and adolescents. CRC Press, Boca Raton, pp 227–241

Soft Tissue Sarcomas
in the Kiel Pediatric Tumor Registry

D. Harms

1 Introduction

The Kiel Pediatric Tumor Registry (KPTR) was set up in 1977 as the (morphological) Central Tumor Registry of the German Society of Pediatric Oncology. The principle functions of this registry are: (a) to collect and evaluate tumor specimens; (b) to provide consultation on and classification and grading of tumors; (c) to publish aquired knowledge and new data; and (d) to function as a reference center in cooperative therapy study.

Over the years the registry has received a large number of tumor specimens (for detail see Harms et al. 1991). Until 1991 the files contained 15 282 specimens of different malignant and benign tumors including tumor-like lesions. Up to now 1687 cases of soft tissue malignancies have been collected, and these are the basis of this evaluation.

The majority of soft tissue tumors can be diagnosed with confidence using conventional light microscopy. In a significant number of cases, however, the tumors are too undifferentiated to allow a clear definition of their histogenesis, and other tumors of unknown histogenesis may be difficult to classify.

The development of new immunohistochemical techniques has increased the capabilities for precise diagnosis, and the proportion of unclassifiable cases has decreased considerably. Regarding the files of the Kiel Pediatric Tumor Registry, the percentage of unclassified malignant soft tissue tumors decreased from 17.6% (42/238) in 1982 to 4.5% in 1989 (50/1112) and to 3.9% (66/1687) in 1991 after reevaluation of the material employing immunohistochemistry if necessary and if block material was available in unclear cases.

Current Topics in Pathology
Volume 89, Eds. D. Harms/D. Schmidt
© Springer-Verlag Berlin Heidelberg 1995

The most useful immunohistochemical stains for the diagnosis and differential diagnosis of soft tissue tumors are against intermediate filaments (particularly desmin, vimentin, and cytokeratins), myoglobin, muscle-specific actin, so-called neural markers, such as neuron-specific enolase (NSE), leu 7, protein S-100, and chromogranin A; furthermore, reactions with antibodies against epithelial membrane antigen (EMA) and panleukocytic antigen. This list is not complete. There may be need for additional stainings in special cases.

2 General Overview of Soft Tissue Sarcomas in Childhood and Adolescence

A total of 1687 malignant soft tissue tumors has been collected at the Kiel Pediatric Tumor Registry. The relative incidence, age and sex distribution are shown in Table 1. Rhabdomyosarcoma (RMS) was by far the most frequent type of soft tissue sarcoma (766 cases = 45.4%), followed by malignant peripheral neuroectodermal tumor (MPNT; synonym: peripheral neuroepithelioma) with 17.8% of the cases. Next in frequency were malignant schwannoma (6.8%), synovial sarcoma (6.2%), extraosseous Ewing's sarcoma (5.0%), leiomyosarcoma (4.3%), and fibrosarcoma (2.3%). All

Table 1. Malignant soft tissue tumors in childhood and adolescence. Frequency of tumor types, age and sex distribution. (Data from the Kiel Pediatric Tumor Registry 1991)

Tumor type	Age (years)					Total		Sex
	0–1 (n)	1–5 (n)	5–10 (n)	10–15 (n)	>15 (n)	(n)	(%)	M/F
Rhabdomyosarcoma, embryonal	51	214	141	80	55	541	32.07	339/202
Rhabdomyosarcoma, alveolar	10	36	58	56	55	215	12.74	116/99
Rhabdomyosarcoma, pleomorphic	0	4	1	0	5	10	0.59	5/5
MPNT	8	31	43	76	143	301	17.84	172/129
Malignant schwannoma	11	5	17	39	42	114	6.76	53/61
Synovial sarcoma	2	6	14	34	48	104	6.16	57/47
Extraosseous Ewing's sarcoma	2	4	13	30	35	84	4.98	42/42
Leiomyosarcoma	9	9	13	16	25	72	4.27	42/30
Fibrosarcoma	16	6	4	9	3	38	2.25	25/13
Malignant fibrous histiocytoma	0	0	9	7	13	29	1.72	18/11
Liposarcoma	0	3	5	10	9	27	1.60	16/11
Malignant rhabdoid tumor, extrarenal	14	7	1	0	1	23	1.36	15/8
Malignant vascular tumors	0	2	5	11	4	22	1.30	12/10
Epithelioid sarcoma	0	2	3	6	5	16	0.95	13/3
Alveolar soft part sarcoma	0	1	3	4	5	13	0.77	6/7
Clear cell sarcoma, soft tissue	0	0	2	6	4	12	0.71	5/7
Unclassified	11	9	10	15	21	66	3.91	30/36
	134	339	342	399	473	1687		966/721

other tumor types occurred only rarely, comprising together only 142 cases (8.4%); 66 cases (3.9%) remained unclassified.

The overall male-to-female ratio was 966:721 = 1.3:1. There was a distinctive predominance of male patients with RMS (male-to-female ratio of 1.5:1 or 3:2), whereas patients with non-rhabdomyosarcomatous tumors (non-RMS) showed only a slight male predominance (1.2:1).

Most RMS occurred in the first 5 years of life (315 cases = 41.1% of RMS). In contrast, the majority of non-RMS were diagnosed in children more than 10 years old and in adolescence (621 cases = 67.4%) (Fig. 1).

The ratio of RMS to non-RMS was highest in the age group 1–5 years (3.0:1). With increasing age the proportion RMS to non-RMS decreases significantly (Fig. 2). In children of 5–10 years the proportion is 1.4:1, in the age group 10–15 years 0.5:1, and in adolescense the proportion is only 0.3:1. It is noteworthy that in infants below 1 year the relative frequency of non-RMS was slightly higher than the frequency of RMS.

3 Relative Incidence, Age and Sex Distribution of RMS Subtypes

Three main subtypes of RMS are distinguished for this statistical evaluation: embryonal, alveolar, and pleomorphic RMS. Cases of botryoid RMS, which is the fourth classic subtype in the conventional RMS classification proposed by HORN and ENTERLINE (1958), is documented in the embryonal RMS (eRMS) group since they are basically true eRMS and differ from classic

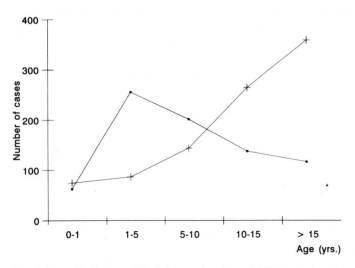

Fig. 1. Age distribution of RMS (*squares*) and non-RMS (*crosses*) at time of diagnosis. Highest incidence of RMS (all types) in the age group 1–5 years. Distinctive increase of non-RMS with increasing age

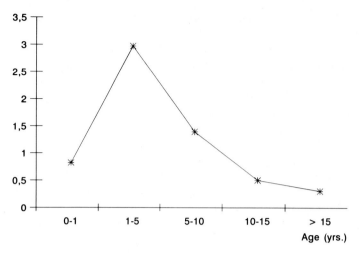

Fig. 2. The proportion of RMS ($n = 766$) to non-RMS ($n = 921$) is highest ($2.99:1$) in the age group 1–5 years at time of diagnosis. With increasing age the RMS:non-RMS proportion decreases significantly

eRMS only in the characteristic grape-like growth pattern. Cases of spindle cell RMS (CAVAZZANA et al. 1992) (synonym: type A RMS in the classification of PALMER et al. 1983) are variants of eRMS and therefore listed as eRMS too.

RMS presenting with an alveolar pattern were classified as alveolar RMS (aRMS) (RIOPELLE and THÉRIAULT 1956; ENZINGER and SHIRAKI 1969) independent of the quantity of alveolar foci. Thus, even RMS exhibiting very small foci with an alveolar pattern were considered to be aRMS (HARMS et al. 1985), and, consequently, predominantly "embryonal" RMS with alveolar foci were classified in accordance with the National Cancer Institute (NCI) classification (TSOKOS et al. 1984) as aRMS. Moreover, the solid variant of aRMS (TSOKOS et al. 1984, 1992), which displays the same histological and cytological patterns except the formation of alveolar spaces and shows the same (unfavorable) biological behavior as classic RMS, was included in the group of RMS (HARMS et al. 1985; D. Harms, this volume). "True" mixed ("composite") alveolar/embryonal RMS are, in our personal experience and in accordance with data from cytogenetic and molecular biological studies (T.J. Triche, this volume) extremely rare.

Overall, our material contains 766 cases of RMS (45.4% of all soft tissue sarcomas in childhood and adolescence) (Table 1): 541 cases belong to the embryonal category, 215 tumors are aRMS, and only ten RMS are classified as pleomorphic RMS. The percentual distributions of the RMS categories can be calculated as 70.6%, 28.1%, and 1.3%, respectively.

Thus, in practice, only two basic types, eRMS and aRMS, have to be considered, since pleomorphic RMS is a very rare tumor not only in childhood but also in adults (MOLENAAR et al. 1985).

The age distribution of eRMS and aRMS is summarized in Table 2 and in Fig. 3. About half of the eRMS occurred in the first 5 years of life (49.0%) and approximately a quarter in the second quinquennium (26.1%). Thus, 75.1% of all eRMS were diagnosed in children up to 10 years of age. By contrast, cases with aRMS are distributed almost equally among the different age groups except the age group 0–5 years which contains a slightly lower number of cases. But, importantly, aRMS can also occur in young children and even in the first year of life (ten cases).

The proportion of eRMS to aRMS is quite variable in the different age groups (Fig. 4). In the first 5 years of life the eRMS to aRMS ratio is the highest (5.8:1; 5.1:1 in the first year and 5.9:1 in the age group 1–5 years). With increasing age the ratio decreases significantly, and in adolescents older than 15 years cases of eRMS and aRMS are distributed equally.

Table 2. Age distribution of RMS with regard to eRMS and aRMS

Age group (years)	eRMS + aRMS		eRMS		aRMS		Proportion eRMs:aRMS	aRMS per age group (%)
	(n)	(%)	(n)	(%)	(n)	(%)		
0–1	61	8.1	51	9.4	10	4.7	5.1 ⎫ 5.8	16.4 ⎫ 14.8
1–5	250	33.1	214	39.6	36	16.7	5.9 ⎭	14.4 ⎭
5–10	199	26.3	141	26.1	58	27.0	2.4	29.1
10–15	136	18.0	80	14.8	56	26.0	1.4	41.2
>15	110	14.6	55	10.2	55	25.6	1.0	50.0
	756		541		215		2.5	28.4

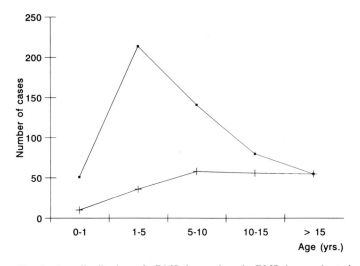

Fig. 3. Age distribution of aRMS (*crosses*) and eRMS (*squares*) at time of diagnosis. The incidence of aRMS is nearly constant in older children, while the incidence of eRMS decreases distinctly with increasing age following a maximum in the age group 1–5 years

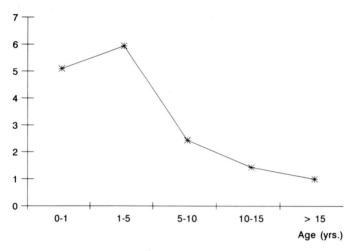

Fig. 4. The proportion of eRMS ($n = 541$) to aRMS ($n = 215$) decreases with increasing age at time of diagnosis

With regard to Fig. 3, the relative incidence of aRMS remains almost unchanged with increasing age, whereas the incidence of eRMS decreases considerably. Thus, the clinical impression that aRMS occurs more frequently in older children essentially depends on a decreased number of eRMS and only to a minor degree on an increased number of alveolar tumors.

Rhabdomyosarcomas occur more frequently in male than in female patients. The overall male to female distribution of RMS is 1.5:1 in our material and thus almost identical with data from the Intergroup Rhabdomyosarcoma Study (IRS) published by MAURER et al. (1977). Interestingly enough, eRMS and aRMS do not differ only in age distribution but also in sex distribution: the male to female ratio is significantly higher ($\chi^2 = 4.86$) in eRMS (1.68:1) than in aRMS (1.17:1) (Table 3).

4 Relative Incidence, Age and Sex Distribution of Soft Tissue Sarcomas Other Than RMS (Non-RMS)

The group of non-RMS includes 921 cases (54.6% of all cases).

Malignant (primitive) peripheral neuroectodermal tumor (MPNT) (synonym: peripheral neuroepithelioma) was by far the most frequent non-RMS tumor type making up 301 cases (17.8% of all cases; 32.7% of non-RMS). The male to female ratio is 1.3:1 158 cases occurred in children below 15 years with a maximum in the age group 10–15 years (76 cases). A comparably high number of patients (143) were more than 15 years old. Thus, 47.5% of MPNT were found in adolescence and in young adults. Concerning the partially selected material of soft tissue sarcomas in patients

Table 3. Sex distribution of eRMS and aRMS. Embryonal RMS shows a significantly higher proportion of male patients than aRMS

	Total (n)	Male (n)	Female (n)	Male:female	
eRMS	541	339	202	1.68:1	$\chi^2 = 4.86$
aRMS	215	116	99	1.17:1	
	756	455	301	1.51:1	

more than 15 years old (473 cases), MPNT encompass 30.2% of the cases, while RMS (all types) account for only 24.3% in this age group.

The relatively high percentage of MPNT even in childhood (13.0% of the childhood soft tissue malignancies) needs a brief commentary since its relative incidence is much lower in other series, e.g., 4.4% in the material presented by Hashimoto (this volume):

1. There may be some selection of MPNT because the Kiel Pediatric Tumor Registry is the pathology referral center of the Cooperative Soft Tissue Sarcoma Study (CWS) and the Cooperative Ewing's Sarcoma Study (CESS) of the German Society of Pediatric Oncology and Hematology (GPOH).

2. It is possible that a considerable number of MPNT primarily located in bone were categorized as soft tissue malignancies since such tumors can extend into the surrounding soft tissues and, therefore, present as a large soft tissue mass clinically. Thus, it can be impossible to decide whether the MPNT originated in the bones or in the soft tissue. The same is true for osseous and extraosseous Ewing's sarcoma. But, in practice, the majority of MPNT occur primarily in soft tissue while classic Ewing's sarcomas develop predominantly in the bone.

3. Many likely "Ewing's sarcomas" (classic and atypical) are indeed MPNT when studied by electron microscopy and modern immunohistochemistry. The morphological diagnosis of Ewing's sarcoma is a diagnosis of exclusion (MISER et al. 1989). Consequently, sarcomas displaying Ewing's cytology by conventional light microscopy but expressing neural markers, e.g., NSE, protein S-100, and Leu7, should be categorized by definition as MPNT and not as classic Ewing's sarcoma. Since immunohistochemical reactions have been performed regularly in our laboratory, the percentage of MPNT has increased considerably.

4. It is a question of definition whether the presence of Homer-Wright rosettes is mandatory for the diagnosis of MPNT (HASHIMOTO et al. 1983; LLOMBART-BOSCH et al. 1989) or not (ISRAEL et al. 1989; SCHMIDT et al. 1985, 1991a; HARMS and SCHMIDT 1993a). In our opinion pseudorosettes are, of course, useful diagnostic criteria of MPNT but not absolutely necessary in otherwise typical cases displaying the expression of at least

two so-called neural markers (SCHMIDT et al. 1991a; D. Schmidt, this volume).

Thus, the comparably high percentage of MPNT in our material can be explained without difficulty. By the way, in spite of a close histogenetic relationship between MPNT and Ewing's sarcoma both tumor (sub)types should be distinguished and categorized as different entities since the prognosis of MPNT in our definition is significantly more unfavorable than the prognosis of typical Ewing's sarcoma (SCHMIDT et al. 1991a).

Next in frequency, but by far much rarer than MPNT, is *malignant schwannoma* (114 cases), which accounts for 6.8% of all soft tissue sarcomas (12.4% of non-RMS). Most cases occurred in the age groups 10–15 years and more than 15 years (39 and 42 cases, respectively). But, on the other hand, 11 cases were observed in infants below 1 year of life (8.2% of infantile soft tissue malignancies).

Malignant schwannoma of infancy is quite similar to infantile fibrosarcoma (CHUNG and ENZINGER 1976) by conventional light microscopy, but can be distinguished from the latter by electron microscopy and, more importantly, by immunohistochemistry. Thus, malignant "fibrosarcoma-like" schwannoma of infancy ("infantile malignant schwannoma") should express protein S-100, while infantile fibrosarcoma, by definition, has to be completely protein S-100 negative. Infantile malignant schwannomas are usually well differentiated, in contrast to malignant schwannomas in older children which usually show fully malignant biological behavior (GUCCION and ENZINGER 1979; ENZINGER and WEISS 1988), whereas most infantile malignant schwannomas present as locally aggressive tumors with low metastatic potential, thus being similar to infantile fibrosarcoma not only morphologically but also biologically.

There were 104 cases of *synovial sarcoma* (6.2% of all cases; 11.3% of non-RMS); it occurred predominantly in older children and adolescents. According to a recently published series of our files (SCHMIDT et al. 1991b), 60% of the cases were biphasic presenting with epithelioid differentiation (solid groups of epithelioid cells and gland-like structures) *and* a fibrosarcoma-like spindle-cellular component which in most cases prevailed quantitatively. But, on the other hand, some biphasic tumors displayed, at least focally, a very distinctive epithelioid adenocarcinoma-like differentiation.

The identification of monophasic fibroblastic synovial sarcoma and its distinction from other spindle-cellular tumors, e.g., fibrosarcoma, malignant schwannoma, leiomyosarcoma, can be very difficult by conventional light microscopy (EVANS 1980). In such cases electron microscopy and immunohistochemistry can be very helpful (MIETTINEN et al. 1983; ABENOZA et al. 1986; FISCHER 1986; ORDÓNEZ et al. 1990; SCHMIDT et al. 1991b). In our experience (SCHMIDT et al. 1991b; SCHMIDT and HARMS 1991), groups of polygonal cells displaying coexpression of cytokeratins and vimentin, the so-called transitional cells, are the diagnostic hallmark of such questionable cases since these cells represent an early epithelioid differentiation.

Extraosseous Ewing's sarcoma (EOS) accounts for 84 cases (5.0% of all cases; 9.1% of non-RMS). Thëage distribution shows a predilection of older children and adolescents. Deducting cases of adolescents more than 15 years old, our files contain 49 cases of EOS. Thus, the relative incidence (4.0%) of EOS is in the same range as in the IRS material (5%; NEWTON et al. 1988) and in the Japanese series (4.4%) published by H. Hashimoto (this volume).

It is worth mentioning that our material contains 72 cases of *leiomyosarcoma* (4.3% of all cases; 7.8% of non-RMS). The existence of leiomyosarcoma in childhood is controversial in the literature. In Japan, childhood leiomyosarcoma virtually does not occur (H. Hashimoto, this volume), but in other countries some well-documented cases have been published, and most recently SWANSON et al. (1991) reported on six of their own cases (with an additional review of the literature). Thus, the existence, in principal, of childhood leiomyosarcoma has been proven. But, in practice, it may be very difficult to identify leiomyosarcoma since the immunuhistochemical expression of desmin and actin can be weak or even absent (generally, RMS show more intensively positive reactions than leiomyomatous tumors).

Leiomyosarcomas have to be distinguished mainly from the leiomyomatous (spindle-cellular) subtype of embryonal RMS (CAVAZZANA et al. 1992; LEUSCHNER et al. 1992; I. Leuschner, this volume), which is located mainly in the paratesticular site, and, equally importantly, from infantile myofibromatosis (CHUNG and ENZINGER 1981). Small cellular biopsies of myofibromatosis displaying no "zonal phenomenon" may be indistinguishable from well-differentiated leiomyosarcoma. Thus, we cannot exclude with certainty that some cases of leiomyosarcoma observed in infancy are indeed myofibromatoses, but, nevertheless, most cases manifest in older children, i.e., in age groups in which myofibromatosis is very rare. Thus, leiomyosarcoma of childhood is certainly rare, but can indeed occur.

Fibrosarcoma, of course, needs some critical commentary too – 38 cases have been collected in the Kiel Pediatric Tumor Registry (2.3% of all cases; 4.1% of non-RMS). Obviously, and in accordance with data from the literature (see ENZINGER and WEISS 1988; KATENKAMP and STILLER 1990; CHUNG et al. 1991), fibrosarcoma is a rare tumor. The same is true for congenital and infantile (juvenile) fibrosarcoma (STOUT 1962; CHUNG and ENZINGER 1976), which has to be distinguished mainly from cellular variants of infantile fibromatosis. Our material contains 16 cases of infantile fibrosarcoma in infants below 1 year of age (42.1% of all fibrosarcomas; 11.9% of all soft tissue malignancies in infants). Thus, despite the rarity of fibrosarcoma, this tumor shows a predilection for the very young age groups.

Fibrosarcoma is a tumor of fibroblasts and displays "no other evidence of cellular differentiation" (ENZINGER and WEISS 1988) except collagen production. Owing to the development of modern diagnostic techniques including immunohistochemistry and cytogenetics it has become evident that tumors containing fibroblast-like cells can show various other lineages of differentiation. Such tumors are, by definition, not bona fide fibrosarcomas. Briefly, the relative incidence of fibrosarcoma will decrease with increasing investigation of a given specimen (HARMS and SCHMIDT 1993b), and the rarity of fibrosarcoma in infancy, childhood, and adolescents in our files reflects this development. Consequently, we have categorized fibrosarcoma of childhood as a seemingly common but in fact rare tumor ("overdiagnosed" tumor) (HARMS and SCHMIDT 1993b).

All *other soft tissue tumors* are very rare in the pediatric age groups. They include *malignant fibrous histiocytoma (MFH)* and *liposarcoma*, the most frequent soft tissue sarcomas of the adult (29 and 27 cases, respectively).

Among the various subtypes of *MFH*, only angiomatoid MFH (ENZINGER 1979) exhibits a predilection for childhood and adolescence. The median age is 13 years (ENZINGER 1979). This quite distinctive low-grade malignancy, showing hemorrhagic pseudocysts and a very prominent mononuclear inflammatory infiltrate at the periphery, has been observed three times in our registry. According to FLETCHER (1991), angiomatoid MFH should be separately reclassified as a low-grade myosarcoma ("angiomatoid myo-sarcoma") since most tumors, in contrast to other MFH subtypes, express desmin intermediate filaments.

Liposarcoma is extremely rare in younger children (SWANSON and DEHNER 1991). In this age group most tumors resembling liposarcoma are indeed benign lipoblastomas or lipoblastomatoses (ENZINGER and WEISS 1988) which contain immature adipocytes and lipoblasts at different stages of maturation but do not exhibit significant cellular atypia.

Among the remaining tumors, *malignant rhabdoid tumor of the soft tissue* (23 cases), *malignant vascular tumors*, including epithelioid and spindle-cell hemangioendothelioma (22 cases), *epithelioid sarcoma* (16 cases), *alveolar soft part sarcoma* (13 cases), and *clear cell sarcoma* of the soft tissue (12 cases) are mentioned only briefly. Most tumors were diagnosed in older children and in adolescence, except malignant (extrarenal) rhabdoid tumor which shows distinctive predominance in the very young age groups: 14/23 (60.1%) cases occurred in the first year of life and 21/23 (91.3%) in children below 5 years.

Since malignant rhabdoid tumors (MRT) belong to the prognostically most unfavorable tumors of childhood, whether they are located in the kidney or in the soft tissue, a short commentary on this highly characteristic "new" malignancy of uncertain histogenesis is necessary. MRT was first described as rhabdomyosarcomatoid nephroblastoma (BECKWITH and PALMER 1978), then designated as malignant rhabdoid tumor of the kidney (HAAS et al. 1981). Tumors of analogous histology have occasionally been observed in the soft tissues, and smaller series of soft tissue MRT have been published by TSUNEYOSHI et al. (1985), SOTELO-AVILA et al. (1986), SCHMIDT et al. (1989), and TSOKOS et al. (1989).

The diagnosis of MRT can be established only in cases which fully exhibit the characteristic histological, cytological, and immunohistological patterns since many malignant tumors of "known" histogenesis can mimic the appearance of MRT (WEEKS et al. 1989a,b, 1991). Such tumors, termed "pseudo-rhabdoid" tumors (WEEKS et al. 1986), have to be distinguished from "true" MRT. True MRT, renal and extrarenal, exhibit medium-sized to large, round or polygonal cells with large vesicular nuclei, distinct nuclear membranes, prominent, often centrally located nucleoli and frequently possess hyaline spherical inclusions in an eosinophilic glassy cytoplasm (HAAS et al. 1981; SCHMIDT et al. 1982, 1989; WEEKS et al. 1989a,b).

It is noteworthy that our series of 23 extrarenal MRT shows an identical distribution of age (predominance of infancy) and sex (male predominance) to renal MRT (see WEEKS et al. 1989b), and one case was associated with medulloblastoma (SCHMIDT et al. 1989), an association which is very characteristic for renal MRT. This case bears witness to the fact that extrarenal MRT can be interpreted as an analogous soft tissue counterpart of renal MRT.

5 Conclusions

The spectrum of soft tissue malignancies in childhood and adolescence differs considerably from that in the adult. Above all, the most frequent sarcomas of the adults, MFH, liposarcoma, and leiomyosarcoma, occur only rarely in childhood. In contrast, in childhood and adolescence RMS are by far the most frequent sarcomas accounting for 45.4% of all soft tissue sarcomas collected in the Kiel Pediatric Tumor Registry and for 53.6% of the cases younger than 15 years. Thus, for practical reason, the childhood soft tissue malignancies can indeed be subdivided into two main categories: RMS and sarcomas other than RMS (non-RMS).

On the other hand, the proportion RMS to non-RMS is by no means constant in the younger age groups. According to our data the RMS to non-RMS proportion is highest in the first 5 years of life then decreases substantially, so that in children older than 10 years the number of non-RMS cases exceeds that of RMS (all RMS types taken together), and in adolescents (more than 15 years old) approximately two thirds of the tumors are non-RMS.

Regarding RMS, two main categories have to be distinguished: embryonal (including botryoid and the spindle-cellular subtypes) and alveolar (including the solid variant). These two basic RMS types account for 98.7% of all RMS. In contrast, our files contain only ten cases (1.3%) of pleomorphic RMS. Thus, our data confirm reports from the literature (MOLENAAR et al. 1985; ENZINGER and WEISS 1988; NEWTON et al. 1988) that pleomorphic RMS is a very rare tumor which can be neglected in a statistical evaluation.

Embryonal and alveolar RMS (eRMs and aRMS) account for 70.6% and 28.1%, respectively, of our cases, which where treated predominantly in the (German) Cooperative Soft Tissue Sarcoma Study (CWS). These data are in remarkable concordance with data from the Intergroup Rhabdomyosarcoma Study (IRS): from a total of 1319 RMS, 73.2% were eRMS and 26.0% aRMS (NEWTON et al. 1988).

While eRMS shows a predominance in younger age groups, below 10 years of life, the relative incidence of aRMS is nearly constant in childhood and adolescence. Thus, the decreasing ratio of eRMS to aRMS with increasing age is mainly due to a decrease of eRMS rather than an increase of cases with aRMS. Similar data were also published by the IRS (HAYS et al. 1982; RUYMANN and GRUFFERMAN 1991).

Since in comparison to eRMS the prognosis of aRMS is more unfavorable, it is very important to recognize and distinguish aRMS from other RMS types, and it was one of the main objectives of the International Childhood Soft Tissue Sarcoma Pathology Classification Study (NEWTON et al. 1989) to define aRMS by histological criteria permitting an exact and reproducible diagnosis (W.A. Newton, this volume).

Malignant peripheral neuroectodermal tumor (MPNT; peripheral neuroepithelioma) was by far the most frequent non-RMS soft tissue malignancy in our files. At first sight the high percentage of MPNT in our files may be surprising. But, owing to the examination of a large series of small, round, and blue cell tumors with modern methods, especially immunohistochemistry, it was possible to develop criteria which are typical for this Ewing's sarcoma-related entity and which permit the distinction from classic Ewing's sarcoma as well as from other malignancies (including neuroblastoma) (SCHMIDT et al. 1985, 1991a). Thus, the increase of MPNT numbers is the consequence of sampling, looking, and learning.

The large material of the Kiel Pediatric Tumor Registry offers the opportunity to study and to reevaluate tumor specimens with modern methodology and to get more experience with uncommon tumors and tumor variants. Unclear cases or cases with unusual follow up and discrepancies with regard to the primary diagnoses are discussed by the Cooperative Soft Tissue Sarcoma Study Pathologist's Panel. The "control function" of such a panel is highly appreciated since it gives more certainty for the individual diagnoses and for statistical evaluation.

In conclusion, we consider the Kiel Pediatric Tumor Registry to be a "living organism" with open eyes and ears for new developments. Nothing is unchangeable – this is also applicable in soft tissue tumor pathology.

References

Abenoza P, Manivel JC, Swanson PE, Wick MR (1986) Synovial sarcoma: Ultrastructural study and immunohistochemical analysis by a combined peroxidase-antiperoxidase/avidinbiotin-peroxidase complex procedure. Hum Pathol 17: 1107–1115

Beckwith JB, Palmer NF (1978) Histopathology and prognosis of Wilms' tumor. Results from the first National Wilms' Tumor Study. Cancer 41: 1937–1948

Cavazzana AO, Schmidt D, Ninfo V, Harms D, Tollot M, Carli M, Treuner J, Betto R, Salviati G (1992) Spindle cell rhabdomyosarcoma. A prognostically favorable variant of rhabdomyosarcoma. Am J Surg Pathol 16: 229–235

Chung EB, Enzinger FM (1976) Infantile fibrosarcoma. Cancer 38: 729–739

Chung EB, Enzinger FM (1981) Infantile myofibromatosis. Cancer 48: 1807–1818

Chung EB, Cavazzana AO, Fassina AS, Ninfo V (1991) Fibrous and fibrohistiocytic tumors and tumorlike lesions. In: Ninfo V, Chung EB, Cavazzana AO (eds) Tumors and tumorlike lesions of soft tissue. Churchill Livingstone, New York, pp 11–66

Enzinger FM (1979) Angiomatoid malignant fibrous histiocytoma. A distinct fibrohistiocytic tumor of children and young adults simulating a vascular neoplasm. Cancer 44: 2147–2157

Enzinger FM, Shiraki M (1969) Alveolar rhabdomyosarcoma. An analysis of 110 cases. Cancer 24: 18–31

Enzinger FM, Weiss SW (1988) Soft tissue tumors, 2nd edn. Mosby, St Louis

Evans HL (1980) Synovial sarcoma. A Study of 23 biphasic and 17 probable monophasic examples. Pathol Ann 15/II: 309–331

Fisher C (1986) Synovial sarcoma: ultrastructural and immunohistochemical features of epithelial differentiation in monophasic and biphasic tumors. Hum Pathol 17: 996–1008

Fletcher CDM (1991) Angiomatoid "malignant fibrous histiocytoma": an immunohistochemical study indicative of myoid differentiation. Hum Pathol 22: 563–568

Guccion JG, Enzinger FM (1979) Malignant schwannoma associated with von Recklinghausen's neurofibromatosis. Virchows Arch [A] 383: 43–57

Haas JE, Palmer NF, Weinberg AG, Beckwith JB (1981) Ultrastructure of malignant rhabdoid tumor of the kidney. A distinctive renal tumor of children. Hum Pathol 12: 646–657

Harms D, Schmidt D (1993a) Critical commentary to "Cytogenetics of Askin's tumor". Pathol Res Pract 189: 242–244

Harms D, Schmidt D (1993b) Rare tumors in childhood: pathological aspects. Experience of the Kiel Pediatric Tumor Registry. Med Pediatr Oncol 21: 239–248

Harms D, Schmidt, Treuner J (1985) Soft-tissue sarcomas in childhood. A study of 262 cases including 169 cases of rhabdomyosarcoma. Z Kinderchir 40: 140–145

Harms D, Schmidt D, Jürgens H (1991) Therapiestudien aus der pädiatrischen Onkologie. Pathologe 12: 175–181

Hashimoto H, Enjoji M, Nakajima T, Kiryu H, Daimaru Y (1983) Malignant neuroepithelioma (peripheral neuroblastoma). A clinicopathologic study of 15 cases. Am J Surg Pathol 7: 309–318

Hays DM, Soule EH, Lawrence W Jr, Gehan EA, Maurer HM, Donaldson M, Raney RB, Tefft M (1982) Extremity lesions in the Intergroup Rhabdomyosarcoma Study (IRS-I): a preliminary report. Cancer 48: 1–8

Horn RC Jr, Enterline HT (1958) Rhabdomyosarcoma: a clinicopathological study of 39 cases. Cancer 11: 181–199

Israel MA, Miser JS, Triche TJ, Kinsella T (1989) Neuroepithelial tumors. In: Pizzo PA, Poplack DG (eds) Principles and practice of pediatric oncology. Lippincott, Philadelphia, pp 623–634

Katenkämp D, Stiller D (1990) Weichgewebstumoren. Pathologie, histologische Diagnostik und Differentialdiagnose. Barth, Leipzig

Leuschner I, Schmidt D, Newton WA, Harms D (1992) Spindle cell subtype of embryonal rhabdomyosarcoma (RMS) in childhood. J Cancer Res Clin Oncol 118[Suppl]: R97

Llombart-Bosch A, Terrier-Lacombe J, Peydro-Olaya A, Contesso G (1989) Peripheral neuroectodermal sarcoma of soft tissue (peripheral neuroepithelioma): a pathologic study of ten cases with differential diagnosis regarding other small, round-cell sarcomas. Hum Pathol 20:273–280

Maurer HM, Moon T, Donaldson M, Fernandez C, Gehan EA, Hammond D, Hays DM, Lawrence W Jr, Newton W, Ragab B, Soule EH, Sutow WW, Tefft M (1977) The Intergroup Rhabdomyosarcoma Study. A preliminary report. Cancer 40: 2015–2026

Miettinen M, Lehto VP, Virtanen I (1983) Monophasic synovial sarcoma of spindle-cell type. Epithelial differentiation as revealed by ultrastructural features, content of perkeratin and binding of peanut agglutinin. Virchows Arch [B] 44: 187–199

Miser JS, Triche TJ, Pritchard DJ, Kinsella T (1989) Ewing's sarcoma and the nonrhabdomyosarcoma soft tissue sarcomas of childhood. In: Pizzo PA, Poplack DG (eds) Principles and practice of pediatric oncology. Lippincott, Philadelphia, pp 659–688

Molenaar WM, Oosterhuis AM, Ramaekers FCS (1985) The rarity of rhabdomyosarcomas in the adult. A morphologic and immunohistochemical study. Pathol Res Pract 180: 400–404

Newton WA Jr, Soule EH, Hamoudi AB, Reiman HM, Shimada H, Beltangady M, Maurer H (1988) Histopathology of childhood sarcomas, Intergroup Rhabdomyosarcoma Studies I and II: Clinicopathologic correlation. J Clin Oncol 6: 67–75

Newton W, Triche T, Marsden H, Ninfo V, Harms D, Gehan E, Maurer H (1989) International Childhood Soft Tissue Sarcoma Pathology Classification Study: design and implementation utilizing Intergroup Rhabdomyosarcoma Study II clinical and pathology data. Med Pediatr Oncol 17: 308

Ordónez NG, Mahfouz SM, Mackay B (1990) Synovial sarcoma: an immunohistochemical and ultrastructural study. Hum Pathol 21: 733–749

Palmer NF, Foulkes WA, Sachs N, Newton WA (1983) Rhabdomyosarcoma: a cytological classification of prognostic significance. Proc Am Soc Clin Oncol 2: 229

Riopelle JL, Thériault (1956) Sur une forme méconnue de sarcome des parties molles: le rhabdomyosarcome alvéolaire. Ann Anat Pathol 1: 88–111

Ruymann FB, Grufferman S (1991) Introduction and epidemiology of soft tissue sarcomas. In: Maurer HM, Ruymann FB, Pochedly C (eds) Rhabdomyosarcoma and related tumors in children and adolescents. CRC Press, Boca Raton, pp 3–18

Schmidt D, Harms D (1991) Tumors in synovial tissue. In: Ninfo V, Chung EB, Cavazzana AO (eds) Tumors and tumorlike lesions of soft tissue. Churchill Livingstone, New York, pp 179–194

Schmidt D, Harms D, Zieger G (1982) Malignant rhabdoid tumor of the kidney. Histopathology, ultrastructure and comments on differential diagnosis. Virchows Arch [A] 398: 101–108

Schmidt D, Harms D, Burdach S (1985) Malignant peripheral neuroectodermal tumours of childhood and adolescence. Virchows Arch [A] 406: 351–365

Schmidt D, Leuschner I, Harms D, Sprenger E, Schäfer HJ (1989) Malignant rhabdoid tumor. A morphological and flow cytometric study. Pathol Res Pract 184: 202–210

Schmidt D, Herrmann C, Jürgens H, Harms D (1991a) Malignant peripheral neuroectodermal tumor and its necessary distinction from Ewing's sarcoma. A report from the Kiel Pediatric Tumor Registry. Cancer 68: 2251–2259

Schmidt D, Thum P, Harms D, Treuner J (1991b) Synovial sarcoma in children and adolescents. A report from the Kiel Pediatric Tumor Registry. Cancer 67: 1667–1672

Sotelo-Avila C, Gonzalez-Crussi F, de Mello D, Vogler C, Gooch WM III, Gale G, Pena R (1986) Renal and extrarenal rhabdoid tumors in children: a clinicopathologic study of 14 patients. Sem Diagnostic Pathol 3: 151–163

Stout AP (1962) Fibrosarcoma in infants and children. Cancer 15: 1028–1040

Swanson PE, Dehner LP (1991) Pathology of soft tissue sarcomas in children and adolescents. In: Maurer HM, Ruyman FB, Pochedly C (eds) Rhabdomyosarcoma and related tumors in children and adolescents. CRC Press, Boca Raton, pp 385–420

Swanson PE, Wick MR, Dehner LP (1991) Leiomyosarcoma of somatic soft tissues in childhood: an immunohistochemical analysis of six cases with ultrastructural correlation. Hum Pathol 22: 569–577

Tsokos M, Miser A, Pizzo P, Triche T (1984) Histologic and cytologic characteristics of poor prognosis childhood rhabdomyosarcoma. Lab Invest 50: 61A

Tsokos M, Kouraklis G, Chandra RS, Bhagavan BS, Triche TJ (1989) Malignant rhabdoid tumor of the kidney and soft tissues. Arch Pathol Lab Med 113: 115–120

Tsokos M, Webber BL, Parham DM, Wesley RA, Miser A, Miser JS, Etcubanas E, Kinsella T, Grayson J, Glatstein E, Pizzo PA, Triche TJ (1992) Rhabdomyosarcoma. A new classification scheme related to prognosis. Arch Pathol Lab Med 116: 847–855

Tsuneyoshi M, Daimaru Y, Hashimoto H, Enjoji M (1985) Malignant soft tissue neoplasms with the histologic features of renal rhabdoid tumors: an ultrastructural and immunohistochemical study. Hum Pathol 16: 1235–1242

Weeks DA, Beckwith JB, Mierau GW (1986) "Pseudo-rhabdoid" tumors of kidney. Lab Invesst 54: 10P

Weeks DA, Beckwith JB, Mierau GW (1989a) Rhabdoid tumor. An entity or a phenotype? Arch Pathol Lab Med 113: 113–114

Weeks DA, Beckwith JB, Mierau GW, Luckey DW (1989b) Rhabdoid tumor of kidney. A report of 111 cases from the National Wilms' Tumor Study Pathology Center. Am J Surg Pathol 13: 439–458

Weeks DA, Beckwith JB, Mierau GW, Zuppan CW (1991) Renal neoplasms mimicking rhabdoid tumor of kidney. A report from the National Wilms' Tumor Study Pathology Center. Am J Surg Pathol 15: 1042–1054

Molecular Biological Aspects of Soft Tissue Tumors

T.J. TRICHE

1 Introduction

Soft tissue sarcomas of childhood as a group represent a particularly fascinating group of human malignancies. Recent advances in our understanding of the genetic basis of malignancy have focused on specific genetic lesions that are apparently etiologic or at least represent significant risk factors for the development of these tumors. Further, immunophenotypic analyses have led to the identification of tumor-specific (or at least tumor-associated) antibodies useful for diagnosis in this group of tumors. Alternatively, gene cloning has led to the creation of DNA probes or assays useful for diagnosis or estimation of prognosis. The discussion to follow will summarize a host of useful new laboratory information that bears on the diagnosis and clinical management of these patients, particularly where said information has affected patient management or our under-

Current Topics in Pathology
Volume 89, Eds. D. Harms/D. Schmidt
© Springer-Verlag Berlin Heidelberg 1995

standing of the underlying disease process and its impact on prognosis and treatment.

The tumors to be discussed are some of the common soft tissue tumors of children and young adults. It is important to remember that each of these tumors displays a peak age incidence in patients less than 20 years of age, but virtually all occur in young adults also; examples in patients in their 30s and even 40s are well documented. The specific topics and tumors to be discussed in this chapter include:

– Non-specific genetic alterations in sarcomas
– Rhabdomyosarcoma
– Extra-osseous Ewing's sarcoma and related neuroectodermal tumors
– Polyphenotypic tumors (malignant ectomesenchymoma, etc.)
– Intra-abdominal desmoplastic small round cell tumor
– Clear cell sarcoma/melanoma of soft parts
– Synoviosarcoma

2 Nonspecific Genetic Alterations in Sarcomas

The widespread awareness of the retinoblastoma-associated tumor-suppressor gene RB and the extraordinary frequency of abnormalities of the p53 tumor-suppressor gene in human malignancy have overshadowed an important point: genetic alterations in both of these genes are more frequent in sarcomas as a whole (i.e., about 50%) than virtually any other tumor system (with the exception of RB abnormalities in retinoblastoma). For this reason, a general discussion of these two genes and the more recently described mdm2 gene, which appears to function (or dysfunction) in concert with p53, is warranted.

2.1 RB1

The retinoblastoma gene, RB1, encodes a phosphoprotein intimately involved in the control of cell cycle, and therefore proliferation (COOPER and WHYTE 1989; DOWDY et al. 1993; EWEN et al. 1993; KATO et al. 1993). In retinoblastoma, the gene is frequently mutated, if not deleted (CAVENEE et al. 1983; DRYJA et al. 1984; FRIEND et al. 1986). In fact, like all tumor suppressors, both copies normally present in the human genome (one per copy of chromosome 13) must be lost or inactivated for loss of function that leads to uncontrolled proliferation, the hall mark of neoplasia. In retinoblastoma, one copy of the gene is lost in the germ line (i.e., from one parent) in familial retinoblastoma; the subsequent loss of the remaining

allele results in malignancy (FUNG et al. 1987). Why retinal cells are particularly susceptible in early childhood is unknown, but the effect of RB1 loss
is generalizable to other tumors as well (BRACHMAN et al. 1991; GOODRICH et
al. 1992; HABER et al. 1991; HENSEL et al. 1990; MURAKAMI et al. 1991;
STRATTON et al. 1989). In fact, the high frequency of second malignancies in
these patients, particularly in irradiated fields, is strongly associated with
mutation of RB1 in the second tumor's cells (BRACHMAN et al. 1991). The
most common of these second malignancies is osteosarcoma, and RB1
mutation or loss in both alleles is common in osteosarcoma, whether as a
second malignancy or sporadic (FRIEND et al. 1986; TOGUCHIDA et al. 1988;
WEICHSELBAUM et al. 1988). None the less, only about 50% of osteosarcomas demonstrate RB1 abnormalities, and many tumors such as rhabdomyosarcoma show no abnormality of RB1 (DE CHIARA et al. 1993). These
findings suggest that detection of RB abnormalities in most childhood soft
tissue sarcomas will likely be of little clinical value.

2.2 p53

The other tumor suppressor gene to evoke widespread attention is p53.
Unlike RB1, p53, which is also an integral component in the control of the
cell cycle, is reportedly mutated in over half of all human malignancy, as
opposed to the restricted distribution of RB1 abnormalities (LEVINE et al.
1991). Many of the tumors under discussion here, including Ewing's sarcoma and rhabdomyosarcoma, show mutation of the p53 gene. In tumors
with p53 mutations, like RB1, one allele is commonly lost or mutated,
sometimes even in the germline, prior to loss of function of the second
allele. When a mutated p53 allele is inherited (the Li-Fraumeni syndrome),
patients are inordinately prone to develop malignancies of diverse type,
including breast carcinoma, adrenal cortical carcinoma, brain tumors, and of
course sarcomas, including osteosarcoma (MALKIN et al. 1990, 1992;
SRIVASTAVA et al. 1990). At this point, p53 mutations appear to be even
more common in osteosarcoma than RB1 (MILLER et al. 1990; WADAYAMA et
al. 1993).
    Detection of p53 mutations, in contrast to RB, has been widely believed
to be of considerable importance in predicting the clinical behavior of a
variety of adult malignancies, as well as detecting children (and adults)
prone to high incidence of malignancy due to inherited abnormalities of p53
(the Li-Fraumeni syndrome). The methodology of doing so has been the
subject of a voluminous literature that will not be exhaustively reviewed
here. Suffice it to say that three major approaches have been adopted: (a)
direct detection of mutation (DNA sequencing); (b) indirect detection
(using gel electrophoresis methods such as single-strand confirmation poly-
morphism, SSCP, or differential gradient gel electrophoresis, DGGE); or

(c) detection of increased amounts of the p53 protein that occurs when the p53 gene is mutated by immunocytochemistry. Examples of each are shown in the first three figures; an abnormal band detected by SSCP (Fig. 1) is subsequently sequenced and a mutation is confirmed (Fig. 2). The corresponding appearance by immunohistochemistry is seen in Fig. 3.

2.3 mdm2

Despite the high incidence of mutational inactivation of RB1 and p53, there remains a significant percentage of cases lacking any known abnormality of either. This observation has clearly indicated that, while loss of either or both of these genes clearly contributes to malignancy, they are not alone sufficient to explain it. Clearly, multiple abnormalities of genes important in regulation of cell growth, infiltration, and vascular dissemination are neces-

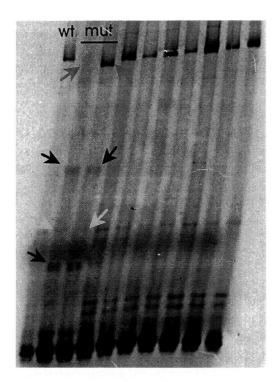

Fig. 1. Indirect detection of *p53* mutation by SSCP. Nine rhabdomyosarcoma tumor samples and a normal control (cDNA from mRNA) were electrophoresed simultaneously. Note that all lanes except 2 and 3 (*medium gray arrows*) appear identical, indicating that only these two are seemingly mutated. Both high-molecular (*double black arrows*) and low-molecular (*single black arrow*) weight bands are aberrant

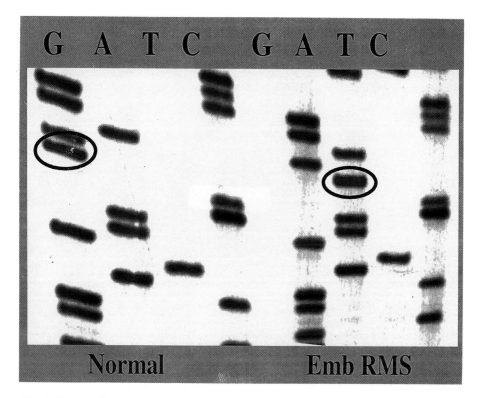

Fig. 2. Direct *p53* mutation analysis by reverse transcription–polymerase chain reaction (RT-PCR) sequencing. DNA sequencing gels generated from cDNA products of the same RT-PCR reaction used in Fig. 1, compared with known wild type *p53* (*left lane*) readily detect even single base mutations, as seen here. In this case, from an embryonal RMS, the normal coding triplet (read from the bottom up) of CGG (*left circle*) is replaced by CAG (*right circle*), resulting in the substitution of an abnormal glutamine (Gln) in lieu of the normal arginine (Arg) at this position. The resultant mutant *p53* protein is functionally abnormal

sary for the development of the full-blown malignant phenotype (FEARON and VOGELSTEIN 1990). p53 is the single most commonly mutated gene in this cascade, and one would assume that tumors lacking either p53 abnormalities might demonstrate genetic abnormality of another, possibly functionally related gene. This appears to be the case.

The original observation that certain murine sarcomas are associated with amplification of a gene or gene cluster (as chromosomal fragments, double minutes, or dms) led to the search for a human homologue of this gene, termed mdm2 (for murine double minute) (FAKHARZADEH et al. 1991; OLINER et al. 1992). Preliminary studies of human sarcomas, most commonly osteosarcoma, have shown a very high incidence of amplification and over-expression of the human mdm2 gene (OLINER et al. 1992). Notably, these cases are commonly those lacking p53 or RB1 abnormalities. However, some cases may have abnormalities of both p53 and mdm2, and a

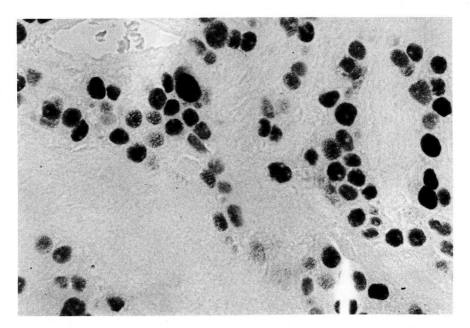

Fig. 3 Mutant *p53* detection by immunohistochemistry. The nuclei of these tumor cells show a heterogeneous speckled reaction product in some but not all cells. The abnormally increased amount, as opposed to distinction between wild type versus mutant p53 protein, is the basis for this analysis. Little protein is normally present, and is normally localized to nuclei only, a fact that is typical of transcription factors such as p53 in general

small percentage lack either (KOVAR et al. 1993; LADANYI et al. 1993a; WABER et al. 1993).

2.4 Implications for Prognosis and Treatment

The most intriguing clinical aspect of the genetic abnormalities discussed above and in the literature is their potential association with clinical behavior. Generally speaking, these defects likely contribute to loss of cellular control mechanisms and therefore increasingly aggressive clinical behavior. Screening for these abnormalities may prove to be a useful prognostic determinant in these tumors; screening of cancer prone families for mutation in RB1 or p53 may identify family members at inordinate risk of developing malignancy. Several methods for doing so, such as SSCP and DGGE, are in use and will likely be applied to tumor samples in the foreseeable future (FREBOURG et al. 1992; KNUDSON 1993; MALKIN et al. 1990). However, a note of caution is in order; it will require prospective study of large patient populations otherwise treated similarly to determine the real clinical utility of these observations (FREBOURG and FRIEND 1993). At the moment, initial retrospective findings are encouraging.

Clearly, a better understanding of which genetic alterations predispose to which cancers, as well as how these alterations contribute to the clinical aggressiveness of the resultant tumors, will be mandatory before clinical acceptance of these data. That is not yet the case, but almost certainly will become a part of the cancer patient (and family?) workup in the future.

3 Rhabdomyosarcoma

Rhabdomyosarcoma (RMS) accounts for 50% of the soft tissue sarcomas in children and adolescents, and a high percentage of such sarcomas in young adults as well (HARMS and SCHMIDT 1986). The clinically important issues in this disease are (a) determination of whether the tumor in question is a rhabdomyosarcoma, and (b) the existence of two forms with vastly different prognoses; embryonal RMS currently is curable in about 80% of cases, while alveolar RMS is less than 40% curable, by current therapy (CRIST et al. 1990; NEWTON et al. 1988). It is, therefore, of some clinical value to correctly discriminate the two. Conventional histology is not universally successful, due to conflicting criteria for categorization and the presence of ambiguous tissue patterns that defy classification (TSOKOS et al. 1992). However, if a specific genetic lesion connotes a particular clinical behavior, detection of this abnormality could obviate the problematic histopathology issues. Fortunately, such class-specific lesions appear to have been detected in these two major categories and they promise to become useful diagnostic tools in the foreseeable future.

3.1 Myogenesis Regulatory Genes

In connection with the first issue, it is important to note that the elementary diagnosis of RMS is often disputed; up to 17% of cases in past Intergroup Rhabdomyosarcoma Study studies (IRS I and II) have lacked demonstrable morphologic evidence of myogenic differentiation (NEWTON et al. 1988). This is clearly a rather crude and insensitive means of detecting rhabdo-myogenesis; immunohistochemical detection of muscle-specific gene expression such as myoglobin, muscle myosin, and muscle actin is a far superior method of doing so, and has become common practice over the past decade (PARHAM 1993; PARHAM et al. 1991). Since these genes are expressed sequentially with muscle differentiation, detection of the earliest such gene could be useful for diagnosis.

In the past several years, the development biology of muscle differentiation has been deduced in remarkable detail, and the critical first steps in myogenesis have been delineated. MyoD1 is a critical controlling gene in rhabdomyogenesis, both normal and neoplastic (OLSON 1990). Consequently, current diagnostic efforts have focused on detecting MyoD1 in suspected RMS (DIAS et al. 1990). However, recent data show that MyoD is not singular in its function in myogenesis; it may be replaced by Myf5 and possibly myogenin (JAN and JAN 1993; TADSCOTT and WIENTRAUB 1991; WEINTRAUB et al. 1991; WRIGHT et al. 1989). Our own experience clearly shows that some bona fide rhabdomyosarcomas express on MyoD1 but do express Myf5 and/or myogenin (SORENSEN et al., submitted for publication).

Although highly informative when positive, problems with available monoclonal antibodies which generally do not work on paraffin sections have limited their utility in practice. Development of antibodies that work on routine specimens (Fig. 4), more widespread availability of fresh tissue, or alternative methods of detecting myogenic transcription factor expression, such as polymerase chain reaction (PCR) of mRNA (Fig. 5) will likely circumvent this problem.

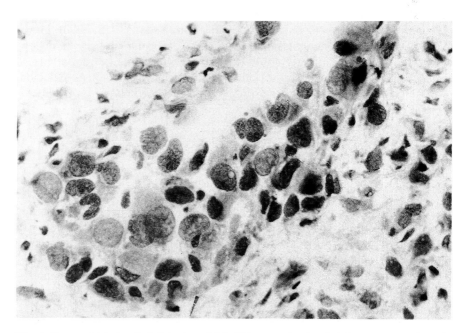

Fig. 4. Immunohistochemical detection of MyoD1 expression by rhabdomyosarcoma (RMS). Nuclei most of the tumor cells in this nest of alveolar RMS cells are stained positively with this affinity-purified polyclonal MyoD1 antibody. Heterogeneity is typical in immunohistochemistry of transcription factors, as noted above, as is nuclear localization. Surrounding stromal cells are negative, providing a built-in negative control

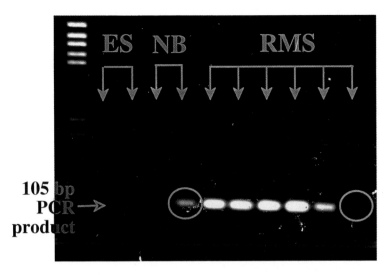

Fig. 5. PCR analysis of MyoD1 expression by rhabdomyosarcoma (RMS). Six RMS (as indicated *on the right*) were analyzed in parallel with two neuroblastomas (*NB*) and two Ewing's sarcomas (*ES*). cDNA was prepared from mRNA by reverse transcription–polymerase chain reaction (RT-PCR) and amplified with MyoD1 specific PCR primers. Genomic MyoD1 was not amplified as the primers were chosen from two different exons, thus precluding amplification of genomic DNA, due to the large intervening intron. The presence of bands of the expected 105 bp size (*arrow* and *legend*) in five of six RMS is specific. The absence in one of six is now known to be typical, as other myogenic transcription factors such as myf5 or myogenin may substitute for MyoD in rhabdomyogenic tumors. The positive reaction in one of two neuroblastomas is highly unusual, and suggests either polyphenotypism or aberrant gene expression

3.2 Embryonal RMS and Chromosome 11p Loss of Heterozygosity

Diagnosis of the embryonal type of RMS (ERMS), by far the most common, is generally the most straightforward, due to typical histology and cytology. However, confirmation of the diagnosis would be helpful, and should be forthcoming with the identification of a presumed tumor suppressor gene on the short arm of chromosome 11, at 11p15.5. This locus routinely shows loss of heterozygosity (LOH) in ERMS Tumors (NEWSHAM et al. 1994; SCRABLE et al. 1989); LOH, or loss of one allele, is typical of loss of function genes such as tumor suppressors, where loss of both copies is necessary to observe biologic effect, unlike dominant oncogenes, where activation of either copy leads to biologic activity. Interestingly, this locus is also implicated in a second Wilms' tumor gene, and is also abnormal in hepatoblastoma, another embryonal tumor that can occur in the Beckwith-Wiedemann syndrome, which is linked to development of Wilms' tumor (KOUFOS et al. 1985, 1989). In aggregate, these observations strongly suggest that one or more loci in this region are implicated in the genesis of ERMS. With identification and characterization, this ERMS locus will be a useful diagnostic tool, just as p53 and RB1 have been (vide supra).

3.3 Alveolar RMS and the t(2;13) Translocation

In contrast to ERMS, where no consistent chromosomal abnormality has been observed, alveolar RMS (ARMS) shows a t(2;13) or variant t(1;13) in well over 50% of cases, strongly suggesting a tumor-specific locus on chromosome 13, at the breakpoint (13q14) (BARR et al. 1991; DEL CIN et al. 1991; TURC-CAREL et al. 1986; VALENTINE et al. 1989; WHANG-PENG et al. 1992). Though seemingly close to the RB1 breakpoint observed in retinoblastoma, the ARMS breakpoint is distal to RB1, which is not involved (SHAPIRO et al. 1992). Two groups have cloned and characterized this breakpoint; a new member of the Fork head family of transcription factors, termed FKHR by GALILI et al. (1993) and ALV by SHAPIRO et al. (1993) is involved from chromosome 13, and is fused with the PAX3 gene on chromosome 2. A PCR-based test to identify this translocation for diagnostic purposes is already available (SHAPIRO et al., USCAP, San Francisco, March, 1994) and is illustrated in Fig. 6.

3.4 Relevance for Prognosis and Treatment

Once characterized, methods to detect the suppressor locus on 11p15.5 in ERMS, coupled with the newly available assay for the PAX3/FKHR(ALV) fusion gene in ARMS, similar to those used to detect BCR/ABL in chronic myelogenous leukemia (CML) and EWS/FLI1 in Ewing's, will undoubtedly become routine diagnostic tools. Once this occurs, there should be no

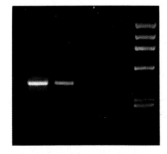

Fig. 6. Diagnosis of alveolar rhabdomyosarcoma (RMS) by t(2;13) (*pax3/alv*). Reverse transcription–polymerase chain reaction (RT-PCR) of cDNA extracted from alveolar RMS tumors and a control cell line yields a positive reaction product only in the presence of a chromosomal translocation fusing the PAX3 gene from chromosome 2 with the ALV (FKHR) gene from chromosome 13, as the PCR primers are chosen from each and can therefore amplify only if the chimeric gene is present. The majority of alveolar RMS cases, and certainly all with this translocation, should react positively with this assay, based on preliminary data

reason to routinely miscategorize ERMS and ARMS, or even RMS versus non-RMS. Perhaps as many as 10% of soft tissue sarcomas are currently misdiagnosed, and 15%–20% of RMS may be incorrectly subcategorized. The clinical implication of correctly distinguishing these patients from one another at diagnosis, and thereby treating low- and high-risk patients uniformly and appropriately, should not be overlooked. Certainly, this is the necessary prerequisite for identifying particular prognostic subgroups within this disease, where individual tumor types vary from greater than 95% to less than 25% survival (Tsokos et al. 1992).

4 Extra-osseous Ewing's Sarcoma

Several lines of investigation over the past decade have demonstrated that osseous Ewing's sarcoma is simply the most common and least differentiated peripheral primitive neuroectodermal tumor (pPNET) (Cavazzana et al. 1987; Kudo 1989; Lipinski et al. 1987; Perez-Atayde et al. 1985; Schmidt et al. 1985). Numerous clinicopathologic entities (Askin tumor [Askin et al. 1979], adult neuroblastoma [Mackay et al. 1976]) originally thought to be unrelated are in fact simply variants of the same basic neuroectodermal tumor system (Linnoila et al. 1986). This is also true of the small round cell tumor of soft tissue first described by Angervall and Enzinger (1975), later to be recognized as extra-osseous Ewing's sarcoma (Shimada et al. 1988). Several studies have documented neuroectodermal features in these tumors, such as neural gene expression, neural ultrastructure, and even the Ewing's sarcoma in bone-associated t(11;22) translocation (Casorzo et al. 1989; Kudo 1989; Ladanyi et al. 1990; Mierau 1985; Shimada et al. 1988; Stuart et al. 1986). In the face of such evidence, there is widespread acceptance that extra-osseous Ewing's sarcoma is simply ESB in soft tissue or, to use current terminology, a soft tissue PNET.

The intrinsic problem in all these tumors has been positive identification. Diagnosis until recently has been a process of successive exclusion of unrelated tumors with similar phenotype (the "small round cell tumor" problem). Fortunately, several unique features of great diagnostic utility have now been described in the Ewing's family of neuroectodermal tumors (Triche 1993).

4.1 MIC2 Gene Expression

Although the previously noted neuroectodermal immunophenotype of Ewing's sarcoma occurs even in the absence of demonstrable neural morphology, it can be used for nonspecific tumor diagnosis using appropriate antibodies such as neuron-specific enolase (NSE), neurofilament protein, neural cell adhesion molecule (NCAM), and numerous others, none of which is unique to Ewing's sarcoma (USHIGOME et al. 1989). The lack of HLA Class I antigen expression (e.g., β_2-microglobulin) by neuroblastoma, but its abundant expression by Ewing's sarcoma has been useful in distinguishing metastatic neuroblastoma in bone from primary Ewing's sarcoma, to name only one example (DONNER et al. 1985). However, there is still a highly subjective element in the diagnosis of Ewing's sarcoma using these tissue-specific (as opposed to tumor-specific) markers.

The first relatively unique antigen expressed by Ewing's sarcoma to be detected is the MIC2 gene and its glycoprotein product, p30–32 (FELLINGER et al. 1991a). This protein is not truly a tumor-specific antigen, as it is normally expressed as a component of the T cell receptor complex. For unknown reasons, it is highly expressed among sarcomas and childhood tumors only in the Ewing's family of tumors (Ewing's sarcoma, peripheral neuroepithelioma, PNET of bone, Askin tumor, adult neuroblastoma, "metastatic neuroblastoma with regressed primary" in adolescents and adults, and probably others as well). Best of all, antibodies against MIC2, such as HBA71 and 12E7 work well on routine paraffin-embedded, formalin-fixed tissues (FELLINGER et al. 1991b). This has allowed even retrospective positive diagnosis of Ewing's tumors, and has rapidly become the diagnostic method of choice (AMBROS et al. 1991; FELLINGER et al. 1991a, 1992; GARIN-CHESA et al. 1991). The only caveat is the rare but documented expression of MIC2 in a small percentage of other tumors; even T cell lymphoma of bone (which is uniformly MIC2+) can present a differential diagnostic problem. Thus, a true tumor marker is still needed for absolute confirmation.

4.2 t(11;22) Translocation and the Ewing's Sarcoma Fusion Gene

It has been known since the mid-1980s that the Ewing's family of tumors all share a common chromosomal translocation in over 90% of cases (AURIAS et al. 1983; TURC-CAREL et al. 1983, 1988). The t(11;22) translocation joins the long arm of chromosome 11 with the long arm of 22, forming a (q24;q12.1) translocation. The high incidence of this abnormality in Ewing's sarcoma, and apparently no other tumor, has long suggested that it is etiologic to the disease. Unfortunately, conventional cytogenetic analysis requires at least 2 weeks for completion, and is not successful in all tumors. A more time-sensitive and convenient method of detecting this abnormality would, therefore, be of great diagnostic, and clinical, utility.

Fortunately, the translocation breakpoint in Ewing's family tumors has recently been cloned (ZUCMAN et al. 1992). The fusion creates a gene composed of the 5' (upstream) portion of the newly identified gene EWS on chromosome 22 with a 3' portion of the human FLI-1 genen from chromosome 11. FLI-1, a member of the ets family of oncogenes, is not normally expressed in nonhematopoietic tissues, unlike EWS, which is ubiquitously expressed; the fusion results in constitutive expression of the fusion gene product, EWS/FLI-1, presumably since the chimeric gene expression is under the control of EWS (KLEMSZ et al. 1993).

As a result, numerous approaches to diagnosis based on the presence of this tumor-specific structural abnormality have now become possible, including Southern analysis of rearrangement in the EWSR1 and/or FLI-1 region, Northern analysis of EWSR1/FLI-1 expression, PCR amplification of the mRNA message, and fluorescent in situ hybridization (FISH) analysis (DESMAZE et al. 1992; LADANYI et al. 1993b; SORENSEN et al. 1993; ZUCMAN et al. 1992). Each of these methods has its advantages, as well as disadvantages. PCR analysis of mRNA (with sequence confirmation if necessary) is probably the most clinically useful (Fig. 7), although inexplicable failures are to be expected and a negative result is *not* proof of negativity; only 85%

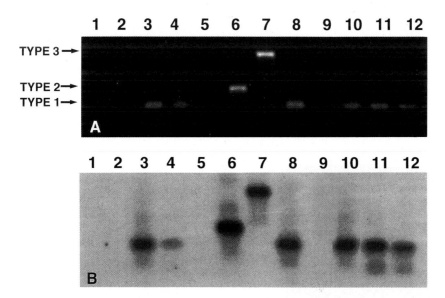

Fig. 7. Reverse transcription–polymerase chain reaction (RT-PCR) detection of EWS/FLI-1 fusion gene in Ewing's sarcoma/peripheral primitive neuroectodermal tumor (pPNET). A series of ten tumors (*lanes 3–12*) plus negative controls were analyzed by PT-PCR for the Ewing's EWS/FLI-1 fusion gene, using primers for EWS (5') and FLI-1 (3') (*upper panel*). Eight of ten of the tumors were positive (only lanes 5 and 9 are negative), although at least three variant fusion gene products, termed type 1, 2, or 3 (*labeled*) are detected, differing in the number of intervening nucleotides and therefore final molecular weight of the resultant protein. Other variants of EWS/FLI-1 have also been documented, but all are specific for Ewing's sarcoma or at least fusion of the EWS gene with FLI-1. The results in the *upper panel* were confirmed by Southern blotting using an EWS/FLI-1 probe; the reactivity seen in the lower panel of the blot from the gel shown in the upper panel is confirmation of the identity of the PCR products seen in the upper panel.

of tumors are PCR-positive (SORENSEN et al. 1993; ZUCMAN et al. 1993b). Another 10% show an alternative fusion gene that is functionally identical (SORENSEN et al. 1994; ZUCMAN et al. 1993b). Alternatively, the translocation can be detected by use of EWS-specific-labeled probes for FISH. An example of a typical t(11;22) involving EWS on chromosome 22 and FLI-1 on chromosome 11 is illustrated in Fig. 8. Ultimately, rearrangement of EWS is the lowest common denominator, as it is perturbed in all known cases of Ewing's sarcoma and related pPNETs. Detection of this rearrangement by Southern blot analysis with EWS-specific probes is thus the ultimate proof, albeit time-consuming and difficult compared to the FISH and PCR. Nonetheless, when they are negative, ambiguous, and conflicting, Southern analysis is mandatory. An example of a positive result is illustrated in Fig. 9.

4.3 Diagnosis by Immunocytochemistry and/or Breakpoint Analysis

As a consequence of the above laboratory advances, it is now possible to positively diagnose Ewing's sarcoma and its several relatives with great certainty. The very existence of so many eponyms (e.g., Ewing's sarcoma, Askin tumor) is indicative of the confusion that has historically plagued the diagnosis of these tumors. At present, this problem is largely obviated by the routine use of MIC2 antibodies in diagnosis. In the near future, diagnosis will increasingly focus on detection of the Ewing's sarcoma chimeric gene or its product. Both PCR-based detection of the transcript and direct visualization of the translocation of interphase cells are timely and diag-

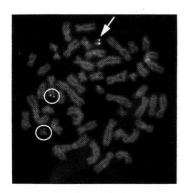

Fig. 8. Fluorescent in situ hybridization (FISH) detection of EWS/FLI-1 fusion. This metaphase spread from a peripheral primitive neuroectodermal tumor (pPNET) clearly shows a bright fluorescent signal (*arrow*) involving a derivative chromosome 22. In the original color photograph, this is seen to be a fusion of red and green signals. The normal EWS gene probe is poorly seen in the *lower left circle* on the normal chromosome 22; the normal FLI-1 gene, (brighter) is seen on the distal short end of the normal chromosome 11 (*upper circle*). In actual practice, these probes are applied to interphase cells, such as those obtained from tumor touch preparations, fine-needle aspirations, or cytology preparations

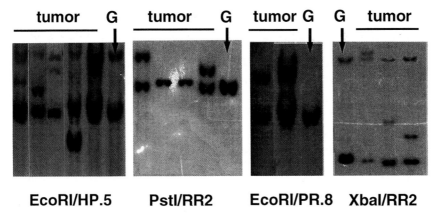

EcoRI/HP.5   PstI/RR2   EcoRI/PR.8   XbaI/RR2

Fig. 9. Rearrangement of Ewing's/sarcoma/peripheral primitive neuroectodermal tumor (pPNET) EWS gene by Southern analysis. Because PCR analyses may fail iatrogenically, and because FISH results on interphase nuclei may be ambiguous in some cases, absolute confirmation of rearrangement of the EWS gene can be sought by Southern blot analysis of genomic DNA extracted from the tumor. This illustration shows a variety of tumor DNA digested with three different restriction enzymes (EcoR1, Pst1, and Xbal), electrophoresed, and hybridized with three different genomic probes for EWS (HP.5, RR@, and PR.8). Note that tumor DNA is clearly distinguishable from normal germline DNA (*labeled "G" in each blot*) in the majority of cases (tumor lanes 2 and 3 in the Pst1/RR2 blot being a notable exception). However, with a combination of restriction enzymes and probes, all tumors studied to date will show rearrangement of EWS, one way or another

nostic; both can be performed within a day of biopsy, and, therefore, are concurrent with routine diagnostic evaluation. Both have a low probability (~10%) of false negatives, and the underlying reason for this has recently been explicated.

It should be noted that most of the bona fide cases lacking an EWS/FLI-1 fusion gene will show an alternative variant, EWS/ERG, fusion gene, as recently described (TAPSCOTT and WIENTRAUB 1991). These cases also lack the typical t(11;22) translocation by cytogenetic analysis; instead, a t(21;22) is found. Interestingly, chromosome 21 is the site of ERG, precisely at the observed breakpoint, as expected. This is notworthy, as this alternative fusion event uses that same portion of EWS (5'), but deletes the native RNA binding region as with FLI-1 fusion events. In this case, ERG, which is also a member of the large family of ETS oncogenes (LIPINSKI et al. 1987), is utilized instead. This obviously implicates a common oncogenetic mechanism in the development of Ewing's tumors, in each case fusing the 5' portion of EWS with downstream member of the ETS family of genes.

4.4 Future Treatment Implications

Needless to say, the truly exciting prospect will be the development of treatment strategies based on inactivation of this chimeric gene, much as current efforts are focused on controlling expression of the similar tumor-specific translocation bcr/abl in CML. This presumes the fusion gene is etiologic to the disease, a fact that has not yet been demonstrated, although it appears likely, just as BCR/ABL has been demonstrated etiologic of CML. If true, Ewing's tumors in the largest sense will be ideal targets for future gene therapy protocols.

5 Biphenotypic Tumors (Myogenic and Neurogenic)

Conventional pathologic diagnostic criteria for diagnosis of tumors assumes a cluster of morphologic features in one or another tissue type and, therefore, tumor type. This clustering is not always mutually exclusive, however. Tumors that clearly show simultaneous rhabdomyogenic and neurogenic differentiation, even in single tumor cells, are well-documented. Further, some tumors show no differentiation at presentation but develop unequivocal terminal myogenic and/or neurogenic differentiation after chemotherapy. An example in a chest wall tumor (initially thought to be an Askin tumor) is illustrated in Fig. 10, where prior to therapy the usual undifferentiated pPNET appearance of this chest wall tumor is evident (panel A); after polychemotherapy, the resection specimen showed unequivocal evidence of terminal myogenic differentiation (panel B top) coexistent with persistent undifferentiated tumor cells (panel B bottom). Although cytogenetic analysis was unsuccessful (as is the case in 30% or more of cases), molecular genetic analysis showed unequivocal evidence of the typical Ewing's tumor fusion gene, EWS/FLI-1 (Fig. 11), although in this case EWS was fused with ERG, not FLI-1, as recently described for upwards of 10% of cases (SORENSEN et al. 1994; ZUCMAN et al. 1993b).

Historically, malignancies such as these were referred to as "malignant ectomesenchymoma" and were thought to occur almost exclusively in head and neck and sacrococcygeal areas, sites of known neural crest cell accumulation during embryogenesis that gives rise to both neural and somatic

$\longrightarrow$

Fig. 10a,b. Histoligc appearance of biphenotypic sarcoma. **a** Appearance at presentation. The hematoxylin and eosin (H&E) appearance of this chest wall tumor at the time of first biopsy was indistinguishable from a typical peripheral primitive neuroectodermal tumor (PNET) or Askin tumor. Blastic, undifferentiated cells with intervening smaller dark cells predominated. No atypical cells or variable phenotype (e.g., spindle cells) were identified, although electron microscopy *did* reveal single tumor cells with mixed neural and myogenic differentiation. This was of course not visible at the light microscopic level. **b** Appearance after polychemotherapy. After several courses of intensive polychemotherapy, the chest wall was resected. The resection specimen showed residual disease, but two patterns were present: persistent pPNET or undifferentiated small round tumor cells (*top*) and separate foci of terminally differentiated neoplastic rhabdomyoblasts (*bottom*). This in vivo differentiation documents the latent myogenic potential of the tumor

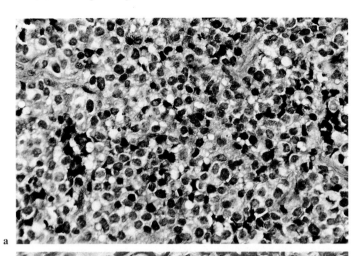

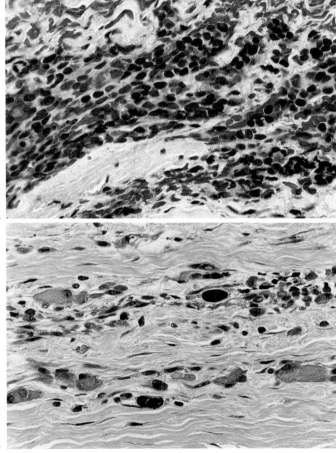

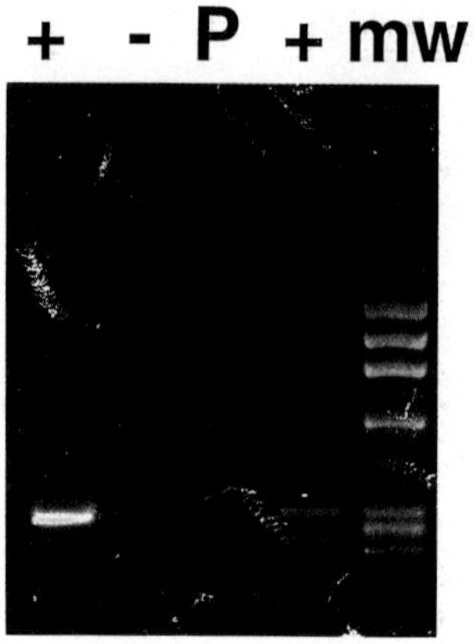

Fig. 11. Reverse transcription–polymerase chain reaction (RT-PCR) of *ews/erg* fusion gene. RT-PCR of tumor tissue from the resection specimen of this patient clearly showed an EWS/FLI-1 fusion gene. This recently reported variant (see text) is functionally identical to the more common EWS/FLI-1, and confirms the impression of peripheral primitive neuroecto-dermal tumor (pPNET) noted on the tumor at presentation. Thus, simultaneous neurogenic and rhabdomyogenic phenotype is expression is present in this primitive small round cell tumor; whether this should be termed a primitive malignant ectomesenchymoma or an other diagnosis is correct remains to be determined

tissues, such as muscle (Cozzutto et al. 1982; Holimon and Rosenblum 1971; Karcioglu et al. 1977; Kawamoto et al. 1987; Kodet et al. 1986; Naka et al. 1975; Schmidt et al. 1988; Shuangshoti and Chutchavaree 1980; Shuangshoti et al. 1984; Sirikulchayanonta and Wongwaisayawan 1984). However, the poorly differentiated tumors under discussion here occur anywhere in the body, and appropriate nomenclature is not yet established. We have routinely referred to them as polyphenotypic tumors, especially since melanogenesis and even chondrogenesis can be found as well. We view them as the undifferentiated and far more common counterpart to the relatively rare and highly differentiated, but historically well-recognized, malignant ectomesenchymoma (Hachitanda et al. 1991).

5.1 Treatment Implications

The real issue with these unusual tumors, of course, is appropriate treatment. Our observations to date would suggest that they have a poor prognosis and are not successfully treated on less aggressive chemotherapy regimens. Whether treated as RMS or Ewing's sarcoma/PNET, they should be recognized as very aggressive tumors, at least in the absence of intensified therapy. Specific therapy, particularly whether oriented towards rhabdomyosarcoma or pPNET, is currently a matter of some controversy.

6 Other Sarcomas with Unique Known Molecular Genetic Abnormalities

Three additional tumors merit at least a brief discussion, as they have recently been shown to harbor unique and, therefore, possibly diagnostic molecular genetic abnormalities.

6.1 Intra-abdominal Desmoplastic Small Round Cell Tumor

This tumor, first described by GERALD and ROSAI (1989), has achieved a degree of notoriety due to its unique histologic appearance and enigmatic character. Cytologically similar in most cases to extra-osseous Ewing's sarcoma and other small round cell tumors (as the name implies), the tumor is nonetheless notable for its occurrence in somewhat older patients, within the abdominal cavity, and with a striking desmoplastic response by the surrounding soft tissue (GERALD et al. 1991; ORDONEZ et al. 1993).

Given the appearance of this tumor and its known propensity for multi-phenotypic differentiation (ASANO et al. 1993; GONZALEZ-CRUSSI et al. 1990; YACHNIS et al. 1992), it is superficially tempting to consider it within the spectrum of Ewing's sarcoma/pPNET. However, since this group is defined by abnormality of EWS and has no known abnormality of the short arm of chromosome 11, the recent cytogenetic observations of two groups effectively precludes this conclusion (BIEGEL et al. 1993; SAWYER et al. 1992). These tumors appear to display a recurring t(11;22), but at (p13;q12). It has now been demonstrated to fuse EWS with the WT1 gene. (Cancer Res 54: 2837–2840, 1994). Thus, this tumor can be successfully distinguished from the erstwhile similar extra-osseous Ewing's sarcoma and pPNETs, as well as biphenotypic tumors as discussed above, by this distinction. This may become increasingly relevant as more cases of intra-abdominal desmoplastic small round cell tumor (IADSRCT) are encountered that lack the characteristic desmoplasia, thus rendering them otherwise largely indistinguishable from intra-abdominal extra-osseous Ewing's sarcoma or other small round cell tumors (ORDONEZ et al. 1993).

6.2 Clear Cell Sarcoma (Melanoma of Soft Parts)

Recent work on this now well recognized tumor (CHUNGA and ENZINGER 1983; SARA et al. 1990) has demonstrated a recurring cytogenetic abnormality, a t(12;22)(q13;q12) that appears unique to this tumor (MROZEK et al. 1993; PEULVÉ et al. 1991; REEVES et al. 1992). These findings would seem to set this tumor apart from all other tumors, including melanoma, with which it has more recently been identified (as indicated by the change in name from clear cell sarcoma of tendon sheath and aponeuroses to melanoma of soft parts). However, a striking recent observation suggests at least some degree of commonality with the Ewing's sarcoma and pPNET family, as this is the only other known tumor with translocation through the EWS gene. In this case, however, EWS is fused with a non-ETS family gene, ATF (ZUCMAN et al. 1993a). Further, though the resultant tumor resembles Ewing's sarcoma, it is actually distinct from it, with demonstrable melano-cytic differentiation. It is known that both pPNETs and melanoma share some overlapping neural crest phenotype, but this relationship would cer-tainly never have been suspected in the absence of a common translocation involving EWS, the Ewing's sarcoma gene. The etiologic, nosologic, and prognostic implications of this finding await further study, but warrant con-tinued interest on the reader's part.

6.3 Synovial Sarcoma

Synovial sarcoma is included in this discussion not because of any known or suspected relationship to other tumors under discussion here, but rather due to its unique cytogenetic abnormality found in a very high percentage of cases (BRIDGE et al. 1988; GILGENKRANTZ et al. 1990; GRIFFIN and EMANUEL 1987; NOGUERA et al. 1988; REEVES et al. 1989; SHENG et al. 1987). Like the Ewing's sarcoma family of tumors, which are now largely defined by their recurring EWS translocation, cloning of the (X;18) breakpoint will likely define this tumor in the future (DE LEEUW et al. 1993; GILGENKRANTZ et al. 1990; KNIGHT et al. 1992; LEE et al. 1993). This, too, is an area where rapid developments in the human genome project will likely resolve the issue in the very near future. With this information, appropriate molecular genetic diagnostic tests will render issues such as histopathologic diagnosis of "monophasic" synoviosarcoma irrelevant.

7 Summary

In the preceding, the reader has hopefully developed an appreciation of the major malignant tumors to be encountered in somatic soft tissues in children, adolescents, and young adults. In aggregate, this group of tumors accounts for about 20% of cancer in this age group. Importantly, they are curable tumors when nonmetastatic at presentation, but therapy appropriate to prognosis and tumor responsiveness is highly dependent on precise diag-nosis. The historical morphologic methods alone will not suffice for this purpose, but the anticipated rapid advent of molecular genetic diagnostic and prognostic methods should. Useful, practical, and rapid genetic tests, available in the same time frame as the routine histopathologic evaluation of these tumors, are likely to forever change the diagnosis and management of these tumors, individually and as a group.

Acknowledgements. The author wishes to acknowledge the invaluable assistance and support of the many individuals who performed the work illustrated in this chapter while working in his laboratory. Specifically, Dr. Dolores Lopez-Terrada contributed Figs. 1, 2, and 8. Dr. Chien-Koh Shieh prepared the MyoD antibody used in Fig. 4 and the primers used in Fig. 5. Dr. Chris Biggs performed the MyoD analysis shown in Fig. 5. Ms. Xian Liu, a research specialist in my laboratory, prepared most of the PCR analyses. Dr. Poul Sorensen performed the Southern analysis for EWS rearrangement shown in Fig. 9. I thank each of them for their contributions. Finally, Lourdes Cruz performed the arduous editing and finishing work on the manuscript, for which I am grateful.

References

Ambros IM, Ambros PF, Strehl S, Kovar H, Gadner H, Salzer-Kuntschik M (1991) MIC2 is a specific marker for Ewing's sarcoma and peripheral primitive neuroectodermal tumors. Cancer 67: 1886

Angervall L, Enzinger F (1975) Extraskeletal neoplasm resembling Ewing's sarcoma. Cancer 36: 240

Asano T, Fukuda Y, Fukunaga Y, Yamamoto M, Yokoyama M, Yamanaka N (1993) Intra-abdominal desmoplastic small cell tumor in an adolescent suggesting a neurogenic origin. Case report. Acta Pathol Jpn 43: 275

Askin FB, Rosai J, Sibley RK, Dehner LP, McAlister WH (1979) Malignant small cell tumor of the thoracopulmonary region in childhood. Cancer 43: 2438

Aurias A, Rimbaut C, Buffe D, Dubousset J, Mazabraud A (1983) Chromosomal translocations in Ewing's sarcoma. N Engl J Med 309: 496

Barr FG, Biegel JA, Bellinger B, Womer RB, Emanuel BS (1991) Molecular and cytogenetic analysis of chromosomal arms 2q and 13q in alveolar rhabdomyosarcoma. Genes Chrom Cancer 3: 153

Biegel JA, Conard K, Brooks JJ (1993) Translocation (11;22)(p13;q12): Primary change in intra-abdominal desmoplastic small round cell tumor. Genes Chrom Cancer 7: 119

Brachman DG, Hallahan DE, Beckett MA, Yandell DW, Weichselbaum RR (1991) p53 gene mutations and abnormal retinoblastoma protein in radiation-induced human sarcomas. Cancer Res 51: 6393

Bridge JA, Bridge RS, Borek DA, Shaffer B, Norris CW (1988) Translocation t(x;18) in orofacial synovial sarcoma. Cancer 62: 935

Casorzo L, Fessia L, Sapino A, Ponzio G, Bussolati G (1989) Extraskeletal Ewing's tumor with translocation t(11;22) in a patient with Down syndrome. Cancer Genet Cytogenet 37: 79

Cavazzana AO, Miser JS, Jefferson J, Triche TJ (1987) Experimental evidence for a neural origin of Ewing's sarcoma of bone. Am J Pathol 127: 507

Cavenee WK, Dryja TP, Phillips RA, Benedict WF, Godbout R, Gallie BL, Murphree AL, Strong LC, White RL (1983) Expression of recessive alleles by chromosomal mechanisms in retinoblastoma. Nature 305: 779

Chung EB, Enzinger FM (1983) Malignant melanoma of soft parts. Am J Surg Pathol 7: 405

Cooper JA, Whyte P (1989) RB and the cell cycle: entrance or exit? Cell 58: 1009

Cozzutto C, Comelli A, Bandelloni R (1982) Ectomesenchymoma. Report of two cases. Virchows Arch [A], 398: 185

Crist WM, Garnsey L, Beltangady MS, Gehan E, Ruymann F, Webber B, Hays DM, Wharam M, Maurer HM (1990) Prognosis in children with rhabdomyosarcoma: a report of the Intergroup Rhabdomyosarcoma Studies I and II. Intergroup Rhabdomyosarcoma Committee. J Clin Oncol 8: 443

De Chiara A, T'Ang A, Triche TJ (1993) Expression of the retinoblastoma susceptibility gene in childhood rhabdomyosarcomas. J Natl Cancer Inst 85: 152

de Leeuw B, Suijkerbuijk RF, Balemans M, Sinke RJ, de Jong B, Molenaar WM, Meloni AM, Sandberg AA, Geraghty M, Hofker M et al. (1993) Sublocalization of the synovial sarcoma-associated t(X;18) chromosomal breakpoint in Xp11.2 using cosmid cloning and fluorescence in situ hybridization. Oncogene 8: 1457

Del Cin P, Brock P, Aly MS, Casteels-Van Daele M, De Wever I, Van Damme B, Van den Berghe H (1991) A variant 2;13 translocation in rhabdomyosarcoma. Cancer Genet Cytogenet 54: 1

Desmaze C, Zucman J, Delattre O, Thomas G, Aurias A (1992) Unicolor and bicolor in situ hybridization in the diagnosis of peripheral neuroepithelioma and related tumors. Genes Chrom Cancer 5: 30

Dias P, Parham DM, Shapiro DN, Webber BL, Houghton PJ (1990) Myogenic regulatory protein (MyoD1) expression in childhood solid tumors: diagnostic utility in rhabdomyosarcoma. Am J Pathol 137: 1283

Donner L, Triche TJ, Israel MA, Seeger RC, Reynolds CP (1985) In: Evans AE, D'Angio GJ, Seeger RC (eds) Advances in neuroblastoma research. Liss, New York

Dowdy SF, Hinds PW, Louie K, Reed SI, Arnold A, Weinberg RA (1993) Physical interaction of the retinoblastoma protein with human D cyclins. Cell 73: 499

Downing JR, Head D, Parham DM, Shapiro DN (1994) A multiplex RT-PCR assay for the diagnosis of alveolar rhabdomyosarcoma and Ewing's sarcoma. Lab Invest 70: 147

Dryja TP, Cavenee W, White R, Rapaport JM, Petersen R, Albert DM, Bruns GA (1984) Homozygosity of chromosome 13 in retinoblastoma. N Engl J Med 310: 550

Ewen ME, Sluss HK, Sherr CJ, Matsushime H, Kato J, Livingston DM (1993) Functional interactions of the retinolastoma protein with mammalian D-type cyclins. Cell 73: 487

Fakharzadeh SS, Trusko SP, George DL (1991) Tumorigenic potential associated with enhanced expression of a gene that is amplified in a mouse tumor cell line. EMBO J 10: 1565

Fearon ER, Vogelstein B (1990) A genetic model for colorectal tumorigenesis. Cell 61: 759

Fellinger EJ, Garin-Chesa P, Su SL, DeAngelis P, Lane JM, Rettig WJ (1991a) Biochemical and genetic characterization of the HBA71 Ewing's sarcoma cell surface antigen. Cancer Res 51: 336

Fellinger EJ, Garin-Chesa P, Triche TJ, Huvos AG, Rettig WJ (1991b) Immunohistochemical analysis of Ewing's sarcoma cell surface antigen p30/32M1C2. Am J Pathol 139: 317

Fellinger EJ, Garin-Chesa P, Glasser DB, Huvos AG, Rettig WJ (1992) Comparison of cell surface antigen HBA71 (p30/32^{MIC2}), neuron-specific enolase, and vimentin in the immunohistochemical analysis of Ewing's sarcoma of bone. Am J Surg Pathol 16: 746

Frebourg T, Friend SH (1993) The importance of p53 gene alterations in human cancer: is there more than circumstantial evidence? Commentary. J Natl Cancer Inst 85: 1554

Frebourg T, Kassel J, Lam KT, Gryka MA, Barbier N, Andersen TI, Borresen A-L, Friend SH (1992) Germ-line mutations of the p53 tumor suppressor gene in patients with high risk for cancer inactivate the p53 protein. Proc Natl Acad Sci USA 89: 6413

Friend SH, Bernards R, Rogelj S, Weinberg RA, Rapaport JM, Albert DM, Dryja TP (1986) A human DNA segment with properties of the gene that predisposes to retinoblastoma and osteosarcoma. Nature 323: 643

Fung YK, Murphree AL, T'Ang A, Qian J, Hinrichs SH, Benedict WF (1987) Structural evidence for the authenticity of the human retinoblastoma gene. Science 236: 1657

Galili N, Davis RJ, Fredericks WJ, Mukhopadhyay S, Rauscher F3, Emanuel BS, Rovera G, Barr FG (1993) Fusion of a fork head domain gene to PAX3 in the solid tumour alveolar rhabdomyosarcoma. Nat Genet 5: 230

Garin-Chesa P, Fellinger EJ, Huvos AG, Beresford HR, Melamed MR, Triche TJ, Rettig WJ (1991) Immunohistochemical analysis of neural cell adhesion molecules: differential expression in small round cell tumors of childhood and adolescence. Am J Pathol 139: 275

Gerald WL, Rosai J (1989) Case 2. Desmoplastic small cell tumor with divergent differentiation. Pediatr Pathol 9: 177

Gerald WL, Miller HK, Battifora H, Miettinen M, Silva EG, Rosai J (1991) Intra-abdominal desmoplastic small round-cell tumor. report of 19 cases of a distinctive type of high-grade polyphenotypic malignancy affecting young individuals (see comments). Am J Surg Pathol 15: 499

Gilgenkrantz S, Chery M, Teboul M, Mujica P, Leotard B, Gregoire MJ, Boman F, Duprez A, Hanauer A (1990) Sublocalisation of the x breakpoint in the translocation (x;18)(p11.2;q11.2) primary change in synovial sarcomas. Oncogene 5: 1063

Gonzalez-Crussi F, Crawford SE, Sun C-CJ (1990) Intraabdominal desmoplastic small-cell tumors with divergent differentiation. Observations of three cases of childhood. Am J Surg Pathol 14: 633

Goodrich DW, Chen Y, Scully P, Lee W-H (1992) Expression of the retinoblastoma gene product in bladder carcinoma cells associates with a low frequency of tumor formation. Cancer Res 52: 1968

Griffin CA, Emanuel BS (1987) Translocation (x;18) in a synovial sarcoma (letter). Cancer Genet Cytogenet 26: 181

Haber DA, Housman DE (1991) Rate-limiting steps: the genetics of pediatric cancers. Cell 64: 5

Hachitanda Y, Aoyama C, Triche T, Shimada H (1991) The most primitive form of ectomesenchymoma: an immunohistochemically and ultrastructurally identified entity. Lab Invest 64: 5

Harms D, Schmidt D (1986) Classification of solid tumors in children – the Kiel Pediatric Tumor Registry. Monogr Paediatr 18: 1

Hensel CH, Hsieh C-L, Gazdar AF, Johnson BE, Sakaguchi AY, Nalor, SL, Lee W-H, Lee EY-HP (1990) Altered structure and expression of the human retinoblastoma susceptibility gene in small cell lung cancer. Cancer Res 50: 3067

Holimon JL, Rosenblum WI (1971) Gangliorhabdomyosarcoma: a tumor of ectomesenchyme. Case report. J Neurosurg 34: 417

Jan YN, Jan LY (1993) HLH proteins, fly neurogenesis, and vertebrate myogenesis. Cell 75: 827

Karcioglu Z, Someren A, Mathes SJ (1977) Ectomesenchymoma. A malignant tumor of migratory neural crest (ectomesemchyme) remnants showing ganglionic, Schwannian, melanocytic, and rhabdomyoblastic differentiation. Cancer 39: 2486

Kato J-Y, Matsushime H, Hiebert SW, Ewen ME, Sherr CJ (1993) Direct Binding of Cyclin D to the Retinoblastoma Gene Product (pRb) and pRb Phosphorylation by the Cyclin D-dependent Kinase CDK4. Genes Dev 7: 331

Kawamoto EH, Weidner N, Agostini RM Jr, Jaffe R (1987) Malignant ectomesenchymoma of soft tissue. Report of two cases and review of the literature. Cancer 59: 1791

Knight JC, Reeves BR, Kearney L, Monaco AP, Lehrach H, Cooper CS (1992) Localization of the synovial sarcoma t(X;18)(p11.2;q11.2) breakpoint by fluorescence in situ hybridization. Hum Mol Genet 1: 633

Knudson AG (1993) All in the (cancer) family. Nature Genet 5: 103–104

Kodet R, Kasthuri N, Marsden HB, Coad NA, Raafat F (1986) Gangliorhabdomyosarcoma: a histopathological and immunohistochemical study of three cases. Histopathology 10: 181

Koufos A, Hansen MF, Copeland NG, Jenkins NA, Lampkin BC, Cavenee WK (1985) Loss of heterozygosity in three embryonal tumours suggests a common pathogenetic mechanism. Nature 316: 330

Koufos A, Grundy P, Morgan K, Aleck KA, Hadro T, Lampkin BC, Kalbakji A, Cavenee WK (1989) Familial Wiedemann-Beckwith syndrome and a second Wilms tumor locus both map to 11p15.5. Am J Hum Genet 44: 711

Kovar H, Auinger A, Jug G, Aryee D, Zoubek A, Salzer-Kuntschik M, Gadner H (1993) Narrow spectrum of infrequent p53 mutations and absence of MDM2 amplification in Ewing tumours. Oncogene 8: 2683

Kudo M (1989) Neuroectodermal differentiation in "extraskeletal Ewing's sarcoma". Acta Pathol Jpn 39: 795

Ladanyi M, Heinemann FS, Huvos AG, Rao PH, Chen QG, Jhanwar SC (1990) Neural differentiation in small round cell tumors of bone and soft tissue with the translocation t(11;22)(q24;q12): an immunohistochemical study of 11 cases. Hum Pathol 21: 1245

Ladanyi M, Cha C, Lewis R, Jhanwar SC, Huvos AG, Healey JH (1993a) MDM2 gene amplification in metastatic osteosarcoma. Cancer Res 53: 16

Ladanyi M, Lewis R, Garin-Chesa P, Rettig WJ, Huvos AG, Healey JH, Jhanwar SC (1993b) EWS rearrangement in Ewing's sarcoma and peripheral neuroectodermal tumor. Molecular detection and correlation with cytogenetic analysis with MIC2 expression. Diagn Mol Pathol 2: 141

Ladanyi M, Gerald W (1994) Fusion of the EWS and WT1 genes in the desmoplastic small round cell tumor. Cancer Res 54: 2837

Lautenberger JA, Burdett LA, Gunnell MA, Qi S, Watson DK, O'Brien SJ, Papas TS (1992) Genomic dispersal of the ets gene family during metazean evolution. Oncogene 7: 1713

Lee W, Han K, Harris CP, Shim S, Kim S, Meisner LF (1993) Use of FISH to detect chromosomal translocations and deletions. Analysis of chromosome rearrangement in synovial sarcoma cells from paraffin-embedded specimens. Am J Pathol 143: 15

Levine AJ, Momand J, Finlay CA (1991) The p53 tumour suppressor gene. Nature 351: 453

Linnoila RI, Tsokos M, Triche TJ, Chandra RS (1986) Evidence for neural origin and PAS positive variants of the malignant small cell tumor of thoracopulmonary region ("Askin tumor"). Am J Surg Pathol 10: 124

Lipinski M, Braham K, Philip I, Wiels J, Philip T, Goridis C, Lenoir GM, Tursz T (1987) Neuroectoderm-associated antigens on Ewing's sarcoma cell lines. Cancer Res 47: 183

Mackay B, Luna MA, Butler JJ (1976) Adult neuroblastoma. Electron microscopic observations in nine cases. Cancer 37: 1334

Malkin D, Li FP, Strong LC, Fraumeni JF Jr, Nelson CE, Kim DH, Kassel J, Gryka MA, Bischoff FZ, Tainsky MA, Friend SH (1990) Germ line p53 mutations in a familial syndrome of breast cancer, sarcomas, and other neoplasms. Science 250: 1233

Malkin D, Jolly KW, Barbier N, Look AT, Friend SH, Gebhardt MC, Andersen TI, Borresen A-L, Li FP, Garber J, Strong LC (1992) Germline mutations of the p53 tumor-suppressor gene in children and young adults with second malignant neoplasms. N Engl J Med 326: 1309

May WA, Gishizky ML, Lessnick SL, Lunsford LB, Lewis BC, Delattre O, Zucman J, Thomas G, Denny CT (1993) Ewing sarcoma 11;22 translocation produces a chimeric transcription factor that requires the DNA-binding domain encoded by FLI-1 for transformation. Proc Natl Acad Sci USA 90: 5752

Mierau GW (1985) Extraskeletal Ewing's sarcoma (peripheral neuroepithelioma). Ultrastruct Pathol 9: 91

Miller CW, Aslo A, Tasy C, Slamon D, Ishizaki K, Toguchida J, Yamamuro T, Lampkin B, Koeffler HP (1990) Frequency and structure of p53 rearrangements in human osteosarcoma. Cancer Res 50: 7950

Mrozek K, Karakousis CP, Perez-Mesa C, Bloomfield CD (1993) Translocation t(11;22) (q13;q12.2–12.3) in a clear cell sarcoma of tendons and aponeuroses. Genes Chrom Cancer 6: 249

Murakami Y, Hayashi K, Hirohashi S, Sekiya T (1991) Aberrations of the tumor suppressor p53 and retinoblastoma genes in human hepatocellular carcinomas. Cancer Res 51: 5520

Naka A, Matsumoto S, Shirai T, Ito T (1975) Ganglioneuroblastoma associated with malignant mesenchymoma. Cancer 36: 1050

Newsham I, Daub D, Besnard-Guerin C, Cavenee WE (1994) Molecular sublocalization and characterization of the 11;22 translocation breakpoint in a malignant rhabdoid tumor. Genomics (in press)

Newton WJ, Soule EH, Hamoudi AB, Reiman HM, Shimada H, Beltangady M, Maurer H (1988) Histopathology of childhood sarcomas, Intergroup Rhabdomyosarcoma Studies I and II: clinicopathologic correlation. J Clin Oncol 6: 67

Noguera R, Lopz GC, Gil R, Carda C, Pellin A, Llombart BA (1988) Translocation (x;18) in a synovial sarcoma: a new case (letter). Cancer Genet Cytogenet 33: 311

Oliner JD, Kinzler KW, Meltzer PS, George DL, Vogelstein B (1992) Amplification of a gene encoding a p53-associated protein in human sarcomas (see comments). Nature 358: 80

Olson EN (1990) MyoD family: a paradigm for development? Genes Dev 4: 1454

Ordonez NG, El-Naggar AK, Ro JY, Silva EG, Mackay B (1993) Intra-abdominal desmoplastic small cell tumor: a light microscopic, immunocytochemical, ultrastructural, and flow cytometric study. Hum Pathol 24: 850

Parham DM (1993) Immunohistochemistry of childhood sarcomas: old and new markers. Mod Pathol 6: 113

Parham DM, Webber B, Holt H, Williams WK, Maurer H (1991) Immunohistochemical study of childhood rhabdomyosarcomas and related neoplasms. Results of an Intergroup Rhabdomyosarcoma Study Project. Cancer 3072

Perez-Atayde AR, Grier H, Weinstein H, Delorey M, Leslie N, Vawter G (1985) Neuroectodermal differentiation in bone tumors presenting as Ewing's sarcoma. In: SIOP, XVIII meeting. Venice, Italy

Peulvé P, Michot C, Vannier J-P, Tron P, Hemet J (1991) Clear Cell Sarcoma with t(12;22) (q13–14;q12). Genes Chrom Cancer 3: 400

Reeves BR, Smith S, Fisher C, Warren W, Knight J, Martin C, Chan AM-L, Gusterson BA, Westbury G, Cooper CS (1989) Analysis of a specific chromosomal translocation, t(X;18), found in human synovial sarcomas. Cancer Cells 7: 69

Reeves BR, Fletcher CDM, Gusterson BA (1992) Translocation t(12;22)(q13;q13) is a nonrandom rearrangement in clear cell sarcoma. Cancer Genet Cytogenet 64: 101

Sara AS, Evans HL, Benjamin RS (1990) Malignant melanoma of soft parts (clear cell sarcoma). Cancer 65: 367

Sawyer JR, Tryka AF, Lewis JM (1992) A novel reciprocal chromosome translocation t((11;22) (p13;q12) in an intraabdominal desmoplastic small round-cell tumor. Am J Surg Pathol 16: 411

Schmidt D, Mackay B, Osborne BM, Jaffe N (1982) Recurring congenital lesion of the cheek. Ultrastruct Pathol 3: 85

Schmidt D, Harms D, Burdach S (1985) Malignant peripheral neuroectodermal tumours of childhood and adolescence. Virchows Arch (Pathol Anat) 406: 351

Scrable H, Witte D, Shimada H, Seemayer T, Wang-Wuu S, Soukup S, Koufus A, Houghton P, Lampkin B, Cavenee W (1989) Molecular differential pathology of rhabdomyosarcoma. Genes Chrom Cancer 1: 23

Shapiro DN, Valentine MB, Sublett JE, Sinclair AE, Tereba AM, Scheffer H, Buys CHCM, Look AT (1992) Chromosomal sublocalization of the 2;13 translocation breakpoint in alveolar rhabdomyosarcoma. Genes Chrom Cancer 4: 241

Shapiro DN, Sublett JE, Li B, Downing JR, Naeve CW (1993) Fusion of PAX3 to a member of the forkhead family of transcription factors in human alveolar rhabdomyosarcoma. Cancer Res 53: 5108

Sheng WW, Soukup SW, Lange BJ (1987) Another synovial sarcoma with t(x;18)(letter). Cancer Genet Cytogenet 29: 179

Shimada H, Newton WJ, Soule EH, Qualman SJ, Aoyama C, Maurer HM (1988) Pathologic features of extraosseous Ewing's sarcoma: a report from the Intergroup Rhabdomyosarcoma Study. Hum Pathol 19: 442

Shuangshoti S, Chutchavaree A (1980) Parapharyngeal neoplasm of mixed mesenchymal and neuroepithelial origin. Arch Otolaryngol 106: 361

Shuangshoti S, Kasantikul V, Suwangool P, Chittmittrapap S (1984) Malignant neoplasm of mixed mesenchymal and neuroepithelial origin (ectomesenchymoma) of thigh. J Surg Oncol 27: 208

Sirikulchayanonta V, Wongwaisayawan S (1984) Malignant ectomesenchymoma (neoplasm of mixed mesenchymal and neuroepithelial origin) of wrist joint. J Med Assoc Thai 67: 356

Sorensen PHB, Liu XF, Thomas G, DeLattre O, Rowland JM, Biggs CA, Triche TJ (1993) Reverse transcriptase PCR amplification of EWS/FLI-1 fusion transcripts as a diagnostic test for peripheral primitive neuroectodermal tumors of childhood. Diag Mol Pathol 2: 147

Sorensen PHB, Lessnick SL, Lopez-Terrada D, Liu XF, Triche TJ, Denny CT (1994) A second Ewing's sarcoma translocation, t(21;22), fuses the EWS gene to another ETS-family transcription factor, ERG. Nature Genet 6: 146

Srivastava S, Zou ZQ, Pirollo K, Blattner W, Chang EH (1990) Germ-line transmission of a mutated p53 gene in a cancer-prone family with Li-Fraumeni syndrome (see comments). Nature 348: 747

Stratton MR, Williams S, Fisher C, Ball A, Westbury G, Gusterson BA, Fletcher CD, Knight JC, Fung YK, Reeves BR, Cooper CS (1989) Structural alterations of the RB1 gene in human soft tissue tumours. Br J Cancer 60: 202

Stuart HR, Wills EJ, Philips J, Langlands AO, Fox RM, Tattersall MH (1986) Extraskeletal Ewing's sarcoma: a clinical, morphological and ultrastructural analysis of five cases with a review of the literature. Eur J Cancer Clin Oncol 22: 393

Tapscott SJ, Wientraub H (1991) MyoD1 and the regulation of myogenesis by helix-loop-helix proteins. J Clin Invest 87: 1133

Toguchida J, Ishizaki K, Sasaki MS, Ikenaga M, Sugimoto M, Kotoura Y, Yamamuro T (1988) Chromosomal reorganization for the expression of recessive mutation of retinoblastoma susceptibility gene in the development of osteosarcoma. Cancer Res 48: 3939

Triche TJ (1993) Pathology of pediatric malignancies. In: Pizzo PA, Poplack DG (eds) Principles and practice of pediatric oncology, vol 2. Lippincott, Philadelphia

Tsokos M, Webber BL, Parham DM, Wesley RA, Miser A, Miser JS, Etcubanas E, Kinsella T, Grayson J, Glatstein E, Pizzo PA, Triche TJ (1992) Rhabdomyosarcoma. A new classification scheme related to prognosis. Arch Pathol Lab Med 116: 847

Turc-Carel C, Lizard-Nacol S, Justrabo E, Favrot M, Philip T, Tabone E (1986) Consistent chromosomal translocation in alveolar rhabdomyosarcoma. Cancer Genet Cytogenet 19: 361

Turc-Carel C, Aurias A, Mugneret F, Lizard S, Sidaner I, Volk C, Thiery JP, Olshwang S, Philip I, Berger MP (1988) Chromosomes in Ewing's sarcoma. I. An evaluation of 85 cases of remarkable consistency of t(11;22)(q24;q12). Cancer Genet Cytogenet 32: 229

Turc-Carel C, Philip I, Berger MP, Philip T, Lenoir GM (1983) Chromosomal translocation in Ewing's sarcoma. N Engl J Med 309: 497

Ushigome S, Shimoda T, Takaki K, Nikaido T, Takakuwa T, Ishikawa E, Spjut HJ (1989) Immunocytochemical and ultrastructural studies of the histogenesis of Ewing's sarcoma and putatively related tumors. Cancer 64: 52

Valentine M, Douglass EC, Look AT (1989) Closely linked loci on the long arm of chromosome 13 flank a specific 2;13 translocation breakpoint in childhood rhabdomyosarcoma. Cytogenet Cell Genet 52: 128

Waber PG, Chen J, Nisen PD (1993) Infrequency of MDM2 gene amplification in pediatric solid tumors and lack of association with p53 mutations in adult squamous cell carcinomas. Cancer Res 53: 6028

Wadayama B, Toguchida J, Yamaguchi T, Sasaki MS, Yamamuro T (1993) p53 expression and its relationship to DNA alterations in bone and soft tissue sarcomas. Br J Cancer 68: 1134

Weichselbaum RR, Beckett M, Diamond A (1988) Some retinoblastomas, osteosarcomas, and soft tissue sarcomas may share a common etiology. Proc Natl Acad Sci USA 85: 2106

Weintraub H, Davis R, Tapscott S, Thayer M, Krause M, Benezra R, Blackwell TK, Turner D, Rupp R, Hollenberg S, Zhuang Y, Lassar A (1991) The MyoD gene family: nodal point during specification of the muscle cell lineage. Science 251: 761

Whang-Peng J, Knutsen T, Thiel K, Horowitz ME, Triche TJ (1992) Cytogenetic studies in subgroups of rhabdomyosarcoma. Genes Chrom Cancer 5: 299

Wright WE, Sassoon DA, Lin VK (1989) Myogenin, a factor regulating myogenesis, has a domain homologous to MyoD. Cell 56: 607

Yachnis AT, Rorke LB, Biegel JA, Perilongo G, Zimmerman RA, Sutton LN (1992) Desmoplastic primitive neuroectodermal tumor with divergent differentiation. Am J Surg Pathol 16: 998

Zucman J, Delattre O, Desmaze C, Plougastel B, Joubert I, Melot T, Peter M, De Jong P, Rouleau G, Aurias A et al. (1992) Cloning and characterization of the Ewing's sarcoma and peripheral neuroepithelioma t(11;22) translocation breakpoints. Genes Chrom Cancer 5: 271

Zucman J, Delattre O, Desmaze C, Epstein AL, Stenman G, Speleman F, Fletchers CD, Aurias A, Thomas G (1993a) EWS and ATF-1 gene fusion induced by t(12;22) translocation in malignant melanoma of soft parts. Nat Genet 4: 341

Zucman J, Melot T, Desmaze C, Ghysdael J, Plougastel B, Peter M, Zucker JM, Triche TJ, Sheer D, Turc-Carel C, Ambros P, Combaret V, Lenoir G, Aurias A, Thomas G, Delattre O (1993b) Combinational generation of variable fusion proteins in the Ewing family of tumours. EMBO J 12: 4481

Characteristic Chromosome Abnormalities and Karyotype Profiles in Soft Tissue Tumors

C. Turc-Carel, F. Pedeutour, and E. Durieux

1 Introduction

Our purpose is to discuss the value of cytogenetic data which are of importance to the clinician and pathologist in the diagnosis, prognosis, and classification of soft tissue tumors. It is well known that "accurate classification of a given tumor is often not easy, so much that acknowledged international experts are still unable to pin a label on about 10% of sarcomas" (FLETCHER 1990). In this context, any new tumor marker is of paramount interest. Cytogenetic data have already provided support for histological grouping within some soft tissue tumor types (SANDBERG and TURC-CAREL 1987; MOLENAAR et al. 1989; FLETCHER et al. 1991). We will update the key cytogenetic data and give, when possible, molecular correlates, principally for peripheral primitive neuroectodermal tumor, adipose tissue tumor, rhabdomyosarcoma, and synovial sarcoma. But new data of potential importance are emerging on other soft tissue tumors, e.g., fibrohistiocytic tumors and clear cell sarcoma/malignant melanoma of the soft parts.

Clonal-consistent (nonrandom, recurrent) primary chromosome abnormalities associated with specific tumor types are potential markers of

Current Topics in Pathology
Volume 89, Eds. D. Harms/D. Schmidt
© Springer-Verlag Berlin Heidelberg 1995

diagnostic value at any step of the clinical outcome since they are present, usually unchanged, in the primary tumors as well as in recurrences and metastases (SANDBERG and TURC-CAREL 1987). Their reliability is directly related to their consistency and the frequency of their association with a defined tumor type. Secondary chromosome changes, observed in addition to the primary specific abnormalities, are related to tumor cell progression and cause the complex karyotypes often found in cancer. They may occur in a seemingly random fashion but, when nonrandom, they are candidates for prognostic markers.

2 Peripheral Neuroepithelioma and Askin's Tumor

Peripheral neuroepithelioma (PN) and the related small cell malignancy of the thoracopulmonary region, Askin's tumor (AT), are rare tumors which belong to the so-called peripheral primitive neuroectodermal tumors (PNETs). Included here is also the uncommon extraskeletal form of Ewing's sarcoma (ES). The difficulty in distinguishing these entities from the other members of the so-called small, round, blue cell tumors has engendered an abundant literature (TRICHE and ASKIN 1983), as well as the controversy which has so long surrounded their nosology (DEHNER 1986). In 1983, a consistent reciprocal translocation t(11;22)(q24;q12), not observed in neuroblastoma, was described in skeletal ES by two independent groups (AURIAS et al. 1983; TURC-CAREL et al. 1983). This finding, of paramount interest in the histopathological context mentioned above, was shortly followed by the description of a t(11;22)(q24;q12) in extraskeletal ES (BECROFT et al. 1984), in PN (WHANG-PENG et al. 1984) and in AT (DE CHADERAVIAN et al. 1984). The outstanding frequency of the association of the t(11;22) to ES was then demonstrated in 85 cases, mainly of the skeletal but also of the extraskeletal forms (TURC-CAREL et al. 1988b). Regarding PN and AT, the original finding has also been confirmed. About 30 cases (two thirds being PN, one third AT) have been reported since 1984 (GORMAN et al. 1991; CHRISTIANSEN et al. 1992; KEES et al. 1992, and references in it, ZUCMAN et al. 1992), In these two entities considered as a whole, the t(11;22)(q24;q12) has been observed in 60% of all cases. In 20%, the translocation is complex (other chromosomes involved with the 11 and 22), "variant" (another chromosome than the 11 is translocated with the 22), or incomplete with the presence of the only derivative 22. In the remaining 20%, no abnormalities were seen at the breakpoints 11q24 and 22q12. In addition, the t(11;22) has similarly been found in very rare osseous forms of primitive neuroectodermal tumors (KEES et al. 1992, and references in it). This brings up to 80% the frequency of the t(11;22) (simple, complex, variant, or incomplete) in PN and AT. In our opinion, this frequency is an underestimate due to the absolute number of cases without the translocation which have been described in cell lines established at a time when the diagnosis of the primary tumor of origin may not have been as accurate as later on. Nevertheless, the frequency and presentation of the t(11;22) in PN and AT are very reminiscent of the findings in Ewing's sarcoma (TURC-CAREL et al. 1988b). As in Ewing's sarcoma (FLETCHER et al. 1991; TURC-CAREL 1991), the t(11;22) should serve as a valuable diagnostic marker for PN and AT. The cytogenetic similarities between Ewing's sarcoma, PN, and AT present a strong argument for the hypothesis of a neural crest origin for Ewing's sarcoma. This hypothesis is further supported by immunohistological and in vitro culture observations (CAVAZZANA et al. 1987; LIPINSKI et al. 1987). But an even more compelling argument comes from very recent molecular data. The breakpoints of the translocation t(11;22)(q24;q12) have been cloned and characterized in both Ewing's sarcoma and PN (DELATTRE et al. 1992; ZUCMAN et al. 1992). In both diseases, the translocation results in the fusion of genes belonging to families not previously implicated in human carcinogenesis, the ETS family coding for DNA-binding proteins (the human homologue of the mouse FLI-1 gene, on chromosome 11) and the family coding for RNA-binding proteins (the "EWS" gene, on chromosome 22).

Alteration of genes at the chromosome 11 and 22 breakpoints was demonstrated in all 20 tumors and cell lines studied, regardless of the nature of the translocation (typical, or complex, or variant) and could even be observed in a tumor without cytogenetic involvement of the chromosomes 11 and 22, a situation which is reminiscent of the BCR-ABL gene fusion in chronic myeloid leukemia. Furthermore, no evidence was found for any specific difference in the position of the translocation breakpoints in Ewing's sarcoma and PN. This clearly confirms the cytogenetic inferences and makes it obvious that a very close relationship exists between Ewing's sarcoma (skeletal and extraskeletal) and the PNETs (of soft tissues and bone). To discuss further the significance of the cytogenetic and molecular data, whether they prove an identical specific cell of origin or only reflect an identical genetic basis for malignant transformation in any primitive neuroectodermal cell line (FLETCHER and MC KEE 1990) is here beyond our scope. We would stress that these data deserve to be viewed as a model of the importance of cytogenetically characterized solid tumors.

3 Fibrohistiocytic Tumors

3.1 Malignant Fibrous Histiocytoma

Malignant fibrous histiocytoma (MFH) is the most frequent soft tissue sarcoma of adulthood (ENZINGER and WEISS 1988). Despite its relatively frequent occurrence, the number of cases of MFH subjected to cytogenetic analysis is still quite limited (not over 50) (MANDAHL et al. 1988a, 1989a; BRIDGE et al. 1987; MOLENAAR et al. 1989; ÖRNDAL et al. 1992). The complexity of most karyotypes in MHF, with multiple numerical and structural chromosome abnormalities, often only partially identified or not identified at all, is such that recurrent primary changes have not yet been recognized in any of the different types of MFH. However, novel prognostic information has recently been suggested. The largest series has been published by MANDAHL et al. (1988a, 1989a). All tumors are of the storiform–pleomorphic and myxoid subtypes. The chromosome number is commonly in the hypotriploid range. Spectacular structural changes are encountered, such as ring chromosomes, telomeric associations, dicentric chromosomes, and the cytogenetic features of gene amplification (HSRs and dmins) together with more classical rearrangements such as unbalanced translocations or deletions. Although no common denominator change has been found, some chromosome bands are preferentially involved, particularly band 19p13. In almost all cases, the addition of unknown material to the 19p13 band gives rise to a 19p+ marker. Taking together the 22 cases of MFH with clonal aberrations from the MANDAHL et al. series, RYDHOLM et al. 1990 found that the presence of a 19p+ marker correlates with a higher relapse rate (local recurrence and distant metastasis) and that a covariation could be seen between the cytogenetic changes and the clinicopathological factors previously known to be of prognostic importance (storiform–pleomorphic histological subtype, high-grade, large tumors). Conversely, myxoid, low-grade, and small MFHs are characterized by a more simple cytogenetic profile with single supernumerary ring chromosome(s) (RYDHOLM et al. 1990; ÖRNDAL et al. 1992). However, occasionally very simple numerical and/or structural changes have been recorded in highly malignant pleomorphic MFHs (BRIDGE et al. 1987; MANDAHL et al. 1989c). Should these cytogenetic results be confirmed, clinicopathological correlations should be carefully carried out to confirm the clinical relevance of the cytogenetic data in identifying MFH subgroups of different prognosis. Amplification of the SAS gene, preferentially found in centrally located MFHs (not otherwise cytogenetically characterized) has been recently proposed as a potential prognostic marker (SMITH et al. 1992). It would be of importance to conduct both cytogenetic and molecular studies on the aggressive forms of MFH to define the reciprocal involvement of the SAS gene amplification and the 19p+ marker in the clinical behavior of these tumors.

3.2 Dermatofibrosarcoma Protuberans and Other Fibrohistiocytic Tumors

Very little is known about the chromosomal status of other subtypes of fibrohistiocytic tumors. The rare dermatofibrosarcoma protuberans (DFSP) (Darier Ferand tumor) is perhaps the best explored with ten cases published to date (BRIDGE et al. 1990a; MANDAHL et al. 1990; STEPHENSON et al. 1992a; ÖRNDAL et al. 1992; PEDEUTOUR et al. 1993, in press). All cases are characterized by a supernumerary ring chromosome. The ring is seen as a single cytogenetic change or with few additional numerical chromosome changes. In four cases the origin of the ring was unidentified. But we showed in all our five cases that the rings consistently contained chromosome 17 sequences that could be positively "painted" with specific chromosome 17 probes after in situ fluorescent hybridization to metaphase chromosomes (Fig. 1) (PEDEUTOUR et al. 1993, in press). This finding indicates the necessity to investigate the origin of the ring chromosomes also found in myxoid MFHs. Should they be different, the ring chromosome 17 would be proposed as a new characteristic chromosome marker to be used in distinguishing DFSP from other fibrohistiocytic tumors of low-grade malignancy.

Regarding cytogenetic data in fibrohistiocytic tumors other than MFH and DFSP, the only report we are aware of is of a plexiform fibrohistiocytic tumor (SMITH et al. 1990). It is noteworthy that this recently recognized soft tissue neoplasm (ENZINGER and ZHANG 1988) has a different pattern of chromosome changes than reported in MFH and DFSP, hence providing support for its unique histological identity within fibrohistiocytic tumors.

4 Adipose Tissue Tumors

Next to MFH, liposarcoma is the most common soft tissue sarcoma of adult life and ordinary benign lipoma the most frequent mesenchymal tumor (ENZINGER and WEISS 1988). Adipose tissue tumors have been the soft tissue

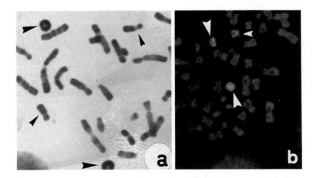

Fig. 1a,b. Ring chromosomes (*large arrowheads*) in a R-banded partial metaphase from a dermatofibrosarcoma protuberans (**a**). The rings are shown to contain chromosome 17 sequences after FISH painting with a probe specific to chromosome 17 (**b**). *Small arrowheads* point to normal chromosomes 17

tumors most extensively studied by cancer cytogeneticists. In less than 10 years, for the whole spectrum from the most malignant to the most truly benign tumor subtypes, cytogenetic data have been accumulated which correlate with histopathological forms. The newest molecular studies of the chromosomal changes bring additional support for such correlations.

4.1 Myxoid Liposarcoma and Pleomorphic Liposarcoma

Myxoid liposarcoma (MLPS) is characterized by a specific reciprocal translocation, t(12;16)(q13;q11)(Fig. 2), that was originally discovered in three

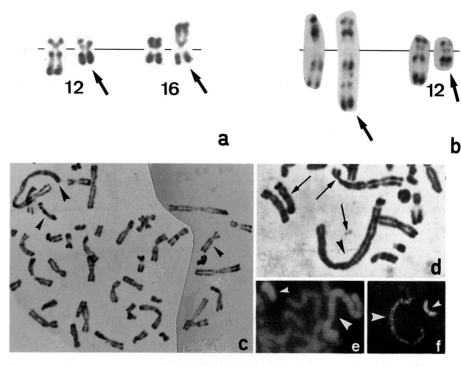

Fig. 2a–f. Characteristic chromosome abnormalities involving chromosome 12 in adipose tissue tumors. R-banded partial karyotypes showing (**a**) the translocation t(12;16)(q13;p11) in a myxoid liposarcoma, and (**b**) the translocation t(3;12)(q27;q14) in a benign lipoma. *Arrows* point to the derivative chromosomes. R-banded large marker chromosomes in **c** – a metaphase with an otherwise normal karyotype from a retroperitoneal lipoma-like well-differentiated liposarcoma and in **d** a partial metaphase with additional complex sructural abnormalities (*arrows*) from a lipoma-like well-differentiated liposarcoma of the thigh. The large markers are shown to contain chromosome 12 sequences after FISH painting with probes specific to this chromosome (**e** and **f**, respectively). The *large arrowheads* point to the large markers and the small ones to the normal chromosomes 12

independent cases (TURC-CAREL et al. 1986c). The number of MLPS cases published with chromosome data is now approaching 35. These consist of single case reports and small series of cases (KARAKOUSIS et al. 1987; see references in the following: ENEROTH et al. 1990; SHREEKANTAIAH et al. 1992; AMAN et al. 1992). The tumor karyotype was most often pseudo- or near diploid with the t(12;16) present as a single change in half the cases. The characteristic t(12;16) translocation is found in all but three of these 35 cases. Thus, the consistency of the t(12;16) is remarkably high (more than 90% of the published cases). As for the specificity of this translocation, it is outstanding in its association with the myxoid form of liposarcoma. We have used the t(12;16) marker to help in the diagnosis of myxoid undifferentiated tumors of soft tissue (unpublished observations). ENEROTH et al. (1990) were able to localize the breakpoints to subbands 12q13.3 and 16p11.2. This fine localization was confirmed by physical mapping and chromosomal breakpoint translocation mapping (CRAIG et al. 1992). The genetic rearrangement of the 12q13 breakpoint has been identified (AMAN et al. 1992). By testing candidate genes assumed to be involved in adipocyte differentation, a consistent rearrangement was detected in each of 11 t(12;16)-associated MLPS. The rearrangement involves the CHOP/GADD153 gene, a member of the CCAAT/enhancer binding protein (C/EBP) family. So far, the change appears highly specific for MLPS.

We have included in this section three cases of "mixed liposarcoma" with myxoid and round cell components (see AMAN et al. 1992). All were associated with the t(12;16) described in MLPS. Whether the t(12;16) characterizes both histological components or only the myxoid one would be of importance to determine keeping in mind the view that the round cell liposarcoma, if distinct from MLPS because of its aggressiveness, represents its poorly differentiated form (ENZINGER and WEISS 1988).

The chromosome picture of highly malignant pleomorphic liposarcoma (PLPS) is not yet as well drawn as in other forms of liposarcoma. Only around ten cases of PLPS have been reported. These cases appear distinctively characterized by very high chromosome number counts (70–200), multiple, complex structural rearrangements and translocated segments which, on most chromosomes, could not be identified (SREEKANTAIAH et al. 1992, and references in it; unpublished personal observations).

4.2 Well-Differentiated Liposarcoma/Atypical Lipoma

Of the four closely related histological forms of well-differentiated liposarcoma (WDLPS) distinguished by ENZINGER and WEISS (1988), the lipomalike WDLPS is the most common. It may be located in the subcutaneous tissue, muscle, or retroperitoneum. However, since the term "atypical lipoma" was introduced in 1975 by KINDBLOM, it has been employed synonymously for the subcutaneous and muscular forms of WDLPS to emphasize their favorable clinical course, while "retroperitoneal well-differentiated liposarcoma" refers to the more malignant form (EVANS et al. 1979). Therefore, the cytogenetic data pertinent to these adipose tissue tumors are recorded under one synonym or the other and are thus included in data on either lipomas or liposarcomas.

Although no individual characteristic chromosome changes, either numerical or structural, have been found in WDLPS/atypical lipoma, recurrent cytogenetic profiles, distinguishing them clearly from the other types of malignant or benign lipomatous tumors, could be deduced from the rather scarce investigations reported so far. Around 20 tumors have been reported under the rubric of WDLPS (KARAKOUSIS et al. 1987; SREEKANTAIAH et al. 1992; STEPHENSON et al. 1992b; PEDEUTOUR et al. 1993, 1994). They were located in the retroperitoneum or in the limbs and were from the lipoma-like or sclerosing subtypes when they were specified. Six tumors were reported under the name of atypical lipoma, principally by the group of F. Mitelman (for review see HEIM et al. 1988; SREEKANTAIAH et al. 1991a). Whereas the chromosome number is usually near-diploid the most striking cytogenetic features, seen in all cases except three, are ring chromosomes (1–5 copies), large markers with homogeneously stained regions (HSRs) or abnormally banded regions (ABRs) known to represent cytologic pictures of DNA sequence amplifications, and random telomeric associations which give rise to apparently multicentric giant markers. These abnormalities can be seen together within a single metaphase, in addition to more classical structural chromosome abnormalities (Fig. 2). By contrast, roughly an equal number of cases show a very simple karyotype with only supernumerary large marker(s) or ring chromosome(s) in an otherwise normal metaphase (Fig. 2). The non-retroperitoneal WDLPLS (non-rp-WDLPS)/atypical lipoma (AL) has a more favorable clinical outcome (mild tendency to recur locally, without distal metastases) as compared to the more aggressive behavior of the retroperitoneal WDLPS (rp-WDLPS) (high rate of recurrence in very large tumors that may be the cause of death) (ENZINGER and WEISS 1988). With this in mind, we compared the numbers of non-rp-WDLPS/AL and rp-WDLPS as to their cytogenetic profiles defined as "simple" (supernumerary ring or large marker chromosomes) or "complex" (with additional numerous other changes) (PEDEUTOUR et al. 1994).

We found that both subtypes are characterized by simple and complex profiles. Since the natural history and the proper diagnostic label for well-differentiated lipoma-like liposarcomas arising in the extremities is still controversial, it is of particular interest to note that, when WDLPS are considered on histological grounds and not anatomical location, they are defined by a common cytogenetic feature (rings or large markers) which distinguishes them from other lipomatous tumors. This concordance is substantiated by our finding that, in both non-rp-WDLPS and rp-WDLPS, chromosome 12 and an amplification of the MDM2 and/or SAS genes (see below) are consistently involved in the formation of the rings and the large markers, whether the rest of the karyotype is normal or not (PEDEUTOUR et al. 1993, 1994). However, non-rp-WDLPS/AL more frequently has an otherwise simple karyotypic profile than rp-WDLPS. These results must be confirmed with a larger number of cases. If so, they will give additional support to the clinical behavior–location-based subtyping. In addition, it would be necessary to learn, within each clinically based subtype (non-rp-WDLPS/AL and rp-WDLPS), whether a complex or a simple karyotype in addition to the ring(s) or large marker(s) correlates with a high or low rate of recurrence. It would confirm that caution should be exercised in using the term "atypical lipoma" as stated by ENZINGER and WEISS (1988).

As reported above, using in situ hybridization techniques with specific chromosome painting probes, we have observed the consistent involvement of chromosome 12 sequences in the generation of the supernumerary large markers (Fig. 2) as well as in the ring chromosome(s) in all of our six WDLPS cases characterized by these abnormalities. Molecular studies carried out on four of these cases showed amplification of genes located at the 12q13–14 region (data not shown) such as the MDM2 and SAS genes, recently shown to be amplified in liposarcoma (OLINER et al. 1989; SMITH et al. 1992). These results represent new information on the genetic content of the ring chromosomes found in cancer cells. Although the phenomenon of amplification of genes is well known in HSRs and ABRs of large markers, it was not suspected, to our knowledge, in ring chromosomes. Many questions have to be answered as to the role of the amplified sequences in the large markers and the ring chromosomes in the pathogenesis of WDLPS as compared to the content of ring chromosomes (not yet known to contain gene amplifications) encountered in: (a) other sarcomas of similar low and borderline malignancy such as the myxoid MFH and dermatofibrosarcoma protuberans; and (b) highly malignant pleomorphic MFH (see Sect. 3). Another question to be answered is: what is the underlying biological significance of the striking involvement of the same band 12q13 in distinctive chromosome changes in various distinctive histopathological forms of lipomatous tumors? It seems that the answer is in the nature of the genes in that region and of their rearrangement. The CHOP gene which is structurally rearranged in MLPS, as noted above, is not amplified, although other genes in very close proximity are amplified in WDLPS. These molecular data add to the uniqueness of these two very distinctive clinical and histopathological forms of liposarcoma: MLPS and WDLPS.

4.3 Lipomas and Rare Variant Forms

Single and multiple lipomas occur as superficial or deep-seated (inter- or intramuscular) tumors and constitute the most common mesenchymal tumor in humans. They cause few complaints or complications and usually present no difficulties in diagnosis (ENZINGER and WEISS 1988). Defining specific chromosome changes in this tumor appeared, thus, to be of little consequence. However, the nature of the cytogenetic data in lipoma, together with those in other benign tumors and liposarcoma, has created such interest that the number of lipomas studied cytogenetically is now up to 250 reported cases (for review of the literature, see SREEKANTAIAH et al. 1991b).

A reciprocal translocation involving chromosome region 12q13–14, as described in the first reports (HEIM et al. 1986; TURC-CAREL et al. 1986b), has been confirmed as the most consistent chromosome change in lipoma. The precise assignment of the breakpoint to 12q13, or q14 (the large majority of cases), or q15 has been disputed. Whether it represents interpretation differences or physically different breakpoints is the issue (TURC-CAREL et al. 1988c; SREEKANTAIAH et al. 1991b). The variable breakpoint hypothesis has received support from chromosomal mapping with probes from the 12q13–14 region (unpublished personal observations). Whether or not a molecular rearrangement occurs in the same gene (in spite of the observed variable chromosomal breakpoint) is still to be determined. The large series (MANDAHL et al. 1989c; SREEKANTAIAH et al. 1991b) agree on the cytogenetic subdivision of ordinary lipomas into three main subgroups characterized by: (a) a normal karyotype (about half of cases); (b) structural chromosome changes involving 12q13–14 (25%–30% of cases); (c) various structural abnormalities other than of chromosome 12 (the remaining cases), predominantly affecting specific regions, such as parts of chromosomes 6 and 13. Analyses of multiple tumors from the same patient (two to six tumors) have shown both similar (the majority of cases) and different karyotypic abnormalities (DAL CIN et al. 1988; HEIM et al. 1988; SREEKANTAIAH et al. 1991b; personal unpublished data), as found in other benign tumors occurring at multiple sites (NILBERT and HEIM 1990). The interest raised by the finding, in particular, of the nonrandom involvement of the region 12q13–15 derives from:

1. The concomitant observation of the recurrent involvement of the same chromosome region in the malignant counterpart of the benign lipoma, MLPS (see Sect. 4.1.1). Although malignant transformation of lipoma into MLPS is extremely rare [three cases recorded by HUVOS (1985) in a retrospect review of the literature going back to 1918], it has been asked whether or not these two lipomatous tumors shared a common pathogenetic molecular basis (TURC-CAREL et al. 1986b; MANDAHL et al. 1987).
2. The nonrandom involvement of the 12q13–15 region also observed in other different histopathological tumors, pleomorphic adenomas of the salivary glands, uterine leiomyomas, chondromas (for review, see SANDBERG 1990) raised the question of the rearrangement of a common gene involved in tissue-unspecific proliferation (MANDAHL et al. 1988c).

Regarding the first question, molecular studies indicate different primary events since the CHOP gene at 12q13 is involved in MLPS but not in lipoma, nor in the other benign entities (AMAN et al. 1992). Regarding the second question, there is not yet any answer since the molecular changes at 12q in these different tumors are still unknown.

In the very scarce cytogenetic reports of variants of the ordinary lipoma, fibrolipoma , angiolipoma, angiomyolipoma, it is of interest, however, to underline that, except for one angiomyolipoma case, none had the common changes observed in lipoma (SANDBERG et al. 1986; DE JONG et al. 1988; DEBIEC-RYCHTER et al. 1992; SREEKANTAIAH et al. 1991b). Noteworthy also is the common involvement of the band 8q12 in translocations (others than the 12q13–15) in two infantile lipoblastomas (SANDBERG et al. 1986; OHJIMI et al. 1992). Finally, we mention here that chromosome changes different from those seen in the above benign adipose tissue tumors have been recently described in a single case of hibernoma (DAL CIN et al. 1992b). Further additional studies of these rare variants are warranted to find and confirm that cytogenetic changes may correlate with their histopathological differences.

5 Rhabdomyosarcoma

Rhadomyosarcoma (RMS), the most common soft tissue tumor in childhood, accounts for 10% of all solid tumors in childhood. Chromosome abnormalities have been found in the two major histological forms, the alveolar (aRMS) and embryonal (eRMS) forms.

The most consistent chromosome change in aRMS is a reciprocal translocation t(2;13)(q37;q14). This translocation was first reported by SEIDAL et al. (1982). The tumor was an alveolar form of RMS. We then found a second case and suggested that this translocation was specifically associated with aRMS (TURC-CAREL et al. 1986a). Further publications have brought the number of RMS cases with the t(2;13) up to about 30. These are single cases or some series (DOUGLASS et al. 1987; WANG-WUU et al. 1988; FLETCHER et al. 1991; WHANG-PENG et al. 1992, and other references in it). All these cases are of the alveolar subtype, except two which are of the embryonal subtype. Reciprocal translocations which could be considered variants of the usual t(2;13)(q37;q14) have been described with a breakpoint either at 2q37 (WHANG-PENG et al. 1992) or at 13q14 (DOUGLASS et al. 1987; WHANG-PENG et al. 1992). These three cases are of the alveolar subtype. Of particular interest is the consistent variant translocation t(1;13)(p36;q14) newly described in three aRMS (BIEGEL et al. 1991; DOUGLASS et al. 1991). DOUGLASS et al. suggested that this translocation may characterize a clinical subgroup of aRMS, occurring at an age much younger than the patients with aRMS associated with the t(2;13). Hence, it may be concluded that the consistency of the t(2;13)(q37;q14) or its variant forms is quite remarkable in the alveolar subtype of RMS (29 of 32 published aRMS). Of the three aRMS cases without a t(2;13), there are two cases with a similar tetraploid chromosomal number and double minutes. If in these cases the absence of molecular rearrangements at 2q37 and 13q14 is demonstrated, there would be another defined cytogenetic subentity in aRMS (WANG-WUU et al. 1988). The t(2;13) (and its variant forms) is highly specific for RMS. This specificity is of paramount interest to distinguish RMS (in particular, the poorly differentiated forms of RMS), from other small round cell tumors in children. As for the association of this translocation (and its variant forms) with the aRMS subtype, its frequency is also quite remarkable, although it cannot be excluded that about 10% (three of 32) of these RMS are embryonal forms (DOUGLASS et al. 1987; DAL CIN et al. 1991a). Keeping in mind the need to provide the most reliable markers to differentiate aRMS from eRMS for appropriate clinical management and treatment, it is important that every effort be undertaken to ascertain the histological subtyping of eRMS with t(2;13). In this regard, a molecular differential diagnosis has been proposed (SCRABLE et al. 1989) characterizing the embryonal form as having loss of heterozygosity of loci at the short arm of chromosome 11. In addition, the very recent identification of the molecular rearrangement at the 2q35–37 breakpoint (BARR et al. 1993) could be very valuable for diagnosis, should its specificity to a particular subtype of RMS be demonstrated. We are not aware of published cytogenetic studies of the variant "solid" form of aRMS (ENZINGER and WEISS 1988).

The eRMS form is far from having a clear cytogenetic profile. To date, no completely consistent chromosomal abnormality has been found. There is nonrandom occurrence of trisomy 2 and possibly trisomy 13 as primary or secondary abnormalities (POTLURY and GILBERT 1985; WANG-WUU et al. 1988; WHANG-PENG et al. 1992). Preferential involvement of bands 12q13 (ROBERTS et al. 1992; WANG-WUU et al. 1988) and 8q12–13 (HAYASHI et al. 1988; CALABRESE et al. 1992) has been reported in single translocations. The nonrandom involvement of the short arm of chromosome 3 has also been suggested (TRENT et al. 1985) but not confirmed. As suggested by KOUFOS et al. (1985), it may be that the underlying primary genetic event involved in the pathogenesis of eRMS is the loss of tumor suppressor genes rather than a genetic rearrangement as occurs in aRMS via a chromosomal translocation.

6 Synovial Sarcoma

Synovial sarcoma accounts for approximately 10% of all soft tissue sarcomas. Despite the relatively small number of cases published with chromosomal studies (around 35), the cytogenetics of synovial sarcoma appears, at the present time, to be very solid. A recurrent reciprocal chromosomal translocation t(X;18)(p11;q11) was originally found in four independent cases of the biphasic and the monophasic subtypes of synovial sarcoma (TURC-CAREL et al. 1987). Since then, a number of single cases and several small series (FLETCHER et al. 1991; other references in LIMON et al. 1991) have been reported. The latest and largest series published so far, which includes a review of the literature, gives a comprehensive overview of cytogenetics in synovial sarcoma (LIMON et al. 1991). The consistency of the t(X;18) is quite remarkable (32 cases of the 34 recorded), as is the strength of its association with synovial sarcoma. Only two tumors harbor a translocation t(X;18) without a diagnosis of synovial sarcoma. One was classified as a fibrosarcoma (MANDAHL et al. 1988b). The other involved a recurrence of a tumor initially diagnosed as an MFH outside our institute (TURC-CAREL et al. 1987). Given the difficulties in diagnosing soft tissue tumors, these tumors may well also be synovial sarcomas. Even highly advanced synovial sarcomas have a pseudo- or near diploid chromosome number with few karyotypic aberrations besides the t(X;18). LIMON et al. (1991) found no difference between the karyotype profiles of monophasic versus biphasic subtypes. It can be concluded that the t(X;18)(p11;q11) is an outstanding and reliable diagnostic marker for synovial sarcoma. The translocation can be used in difficult diagnoses of recurrent or metastatic cases as those reported by MOLENAAR et al. (1989), and undifferentiated or poorly differentiated spindle cell sarcomas (FLETCHER et al. 1991; personal unpublished observations).

7 Other Rare Soft Tissue Tumors

7.1 Clear Cell Sarcoma of the Tendons and Aponeuroses/ Malignant Melanoma of the Soft Parts

Two different names for this tumor are in use. This tumor was first named "clear cell sarcoma of the tendons and aponeuroses" by ENZINGER in 1965. It was renamed "malignant melanoma of the soft parts" (ENZINGER and WEISS 1988). The first cytogenetic study of this tumor was not reported until 1990 (BRIDGE et al. 1990b). In one of the two cases, a reciprocal translocation between chromosomes 12 and 22 was found. Since then, in spite of its rarity, about ten cases of this tumor have been investigated and the initial finding confirmed in eight of the ten cases (BRIDGE et al. 1991; PEULVE et al. 1991; STENMAN et al. 1992; REEVES et al. 1992; RODRIGUEZ et al. 1992; TRAVIS and BRIDGE 1992). The translocation t(12;22)(q13;q12-13) is thus another specific chromosome change in soft tissue tumor to be added to the list of potential diagnostic markers. It is potentially useful for distinguishing clear cell sarcoma of the tendons and aponeuroses/malignant melanoma of the soft parts from malignant melanoma.

The t(12;22) translocation may clarify the histogenesis of this tumor. The breakpoint on chromosome 22 is located in the same band as in Ewing's sarcoma. Should it be shown to occur in the very same gene as the Ewing's sarcoma breakpoint on the 22, it would support the neural crest derivation hypothesis suggested by KINDBLOM et al. (1983) on the basis of ultrastuctural and immunohistochemical analyses.

7.2 Extraskeletal Myxoid Chondrosarcoma

Since it was suggested that a reciprocal translocation t(9;22)(q31;q12.2) may characterize the extraskeletal myxoid form of chondrosarcoma (HINRICHS et al. 1985; TURC-CAREL et al. 1988a), only one chromosomal study of this very rare adult soft tissue tumor has, to our knowledge, been reported. This case contained a translocation t(2;13)(q32;p12) but not the t(9;22) (BRIDGE et al. 1989). However, a third case with the t(9;22) that we observed recently (unpublished observations), leads us to consider the t(9;22) as a characteristic chromosome marker that is specific to this very rare form of chondrosarcoma.

7.3 Congenital or Infantile Fibrosarcoma

Four cases of congenital or infantile fibrosarcoma, next to RMS the second most common soft tissue tumor in childhood, have been reported (MANDAHL et al. 1989b; SPELEMAN et al. 1989; ADAM et al. 1991; DAL CIN et al. 1991b). All four cases show a similar karyotypic profile with a combination of exclusively trisomies of the same chromosomes, the most common being trisomies 11 and 20. This profile has no common point with the random structural abnormalities so far observed in adult fibrosarcoma (see references in DAL CIN et al. 1991b), indicating that congenital or infantile fibrosarcoma is a separate entity from adult fibrosarcoma despite their histological simi-larity, a distinction already stated on the basis of their clinical outcome (ENZINGER and WEISS 1988).

7.4 Other Tumors and Tumor-like Lesions of Fibrous (and Other) Tissues

Because of their potential importance in understanding the biology, it is of interest to include in this report the rather scarce data published in the following entities that present with abnormal proliferations of the fibrous (and other) tissue but of uncertain pathogenesis and the true neoplastic or reactive origin of which is still debated (ENZINGER and WEISS 1988).

Within this group, the most studied are the abdominal and extra-abdominal desmoid tumors (aggressive fibromatosis) (27 tumors from 23 patients, three of them with Gardner's syndrome) (KARLSSON et al. 1988; BRIDGE et al. 1992). Normal chromosomes or random nonclonal abnormalities were mostly encountered. However, clonal abnormalities, often multiple and complex, were found in 35% of the cases, suggesting to the authors that desmoid tumors are true neoplasms. Nonrandom interstitial deletions of the long arm of chromosome 5, which include the location of the familial adenomatosis polyposis gene (FAP gene), were observed in a small proportion of patients with and without Gardner's syndrome. Should this be confirmed by molecular analyses, a role may exist for the FAP gene in the biology of desmoid tumors, irrespective of the presence of Gardner's syndrome. The observation of a nonrandom loss of the chromosome Y in desmoid tumors, with similar findings of shared chromosome Y loss in the penile fibromatosis (Peyronie's disease) (GUERNERI et al. 1991) and the palmar fibromatosis (Dupuytren's disease) (SERGOVICH et al. 1983), could be considered indicative of a common origin for these closely related fibromatoses (BRIDGE et al. 1992). Other observations of karyotypes with the following clonal single trisomies have been found in other proliferations of the soft tissues: trisomy 2 in proliferative fasciitis (DEMBINSKI et al. 1992), trisomies 5 and 7 in pigmented villonodular synovitis (RAY et al. 1991). Both the authors of these single case reports stated that the chromosomal finding is suggestive of a neoplastic proliferation rather than a reactive (proliferative fasciitis) or inflamatory process (pigmented villonodular synovitis).

Until recently it was postulated that the observation of a clonal karyotypic abnormality in a particular lesion was synonymous with true neoplastic disease. This generally held opinion must be revised, however, because various clonal chromosomal changes, consisting of trisomies 5, 7, 10 and Y loss, have been reported in non-neoplastic tissues such as kidney, lung, brain (for review see ELVING et al. 1990). Therefore, at the present time, it would be wise to be cautious as to the interpretation of single numerical changes observed in benign and also truly malignant disorders. The question lies in the nature of the cells cytogenetically studied. Are the chromosome abnormalities representative of true neoplastic cells or the intratumoral and surrounding reactive stromal cells or, as recently demonstrated in kidney tumors by DAL CIN et al. (1992a), tumor-infiltrating T4 and T8 lymphocytes. Any and all efforts should be undertaken to clarify this very important question.

8 Summary and Conclusions

Characteristic chromosome abnormalities and karyotype profiles are emerging for the soft tissue tumors. The notable findings are summarized

Table 1. Characteristic chromosome abnormalities and karyotype profiles in soft tissue tumors

Tumor	Chromosome abnormality
Peripheral primitive neuroectodermal tumors	
Extraskeletal Ewing's sarcoma	t(11;22)(q24;q12) FLI-1; EWS[a]
Peripheral neuroepithelioma	t(11;22)(q24;q12) FLI-1; EWS
Askin's tumor	t(11;22)(q24;q12) FLI-1; EWS
Fibrohistiocytic tumors	
Malignant fibrous histiocytoma (myxoid)	Extra ring
Malignant fibrous histiocytoma (pleomorphic)	19p+ marker
Dermatofibrosarcoma protuberans	Extra ring (chromosome 17)
Adipose tissue tumors	
Myxoid liposarcoma	t(12;16)(q13.3;p11.2) CHOP;?
Pleomorphic liposarcoma	Hyperdiploid; complex
Well-differentiated liposarcoma (non-retroperitoneal)/atypical lipoma	Ring(s) or large marker(s) (chromosome 12), MDM2, SAS amplifications, associated with: Simple karyotype
Well-differentiated liposarcoma (retroperitoneal)	Complex karyotype
Lipoma	t(12;var)(q13–15;var)
Rhabdomyosarcoma	
Alveolar rhabdomyosarcoma	t(2;13)(q37;q14) PAX3;?
Alveolar rhabdomyosarcoma (early onset)	t(1;13)(p36;q14)
Synovial sarcoma	t(X;18) (p11;q11)
Other soft tissue tumors	
Clear cell sarcoma of tendons and aponeuroses/malignant melanoma of soft parts	t(12;22)(q13;q12)
Congenital/infantile fibrosarcoma	Trisomies 11, 20
Extraskeletal myxoid chondrosarcoma	t(9;22)(q31;q12.2)

[a] Italics indicate the genes involved in the chromosome changes.

in the Table 1. Within the broad range of solid tumors, it is certainly the soft tissue tumors in which the most spectacular success has occurred with regard to neoplasia-associated chromosome abnormalities. Cytogenetic studies of soft tissue tumors have been encouraged by the early and growing supporting interest of pathologists and clinicians concerned with soft tissue tumors. However, when one considers the variety of types and subtypes of benign and malignant soft tissue tumors, the number that has been so far characterized by a specific chromosome change is still very small. But, as we attempt to demonstrate in this report, these data should be viewed as paradigms for the importance of cytogenetic investigations in solid tumors. Cytogenetic studies of solid tumors are of more than clinical interest. Cytogenetic studies allow molecular investigations of the chromosomal breakpoints. They allow the search to proceed for genes involved in the chromosomal changes, providing a better knowledge of the malignant transformation process. In addition, the fruits of the combined efforts in cytogenetic and molecular technologies, from which has come "molecular cytogenetics," will let us recognize more conveniently, more quickly and, hopefully, less expensively the well-characterized diagnostic chromosome markers in tumor cells. Thus, we may be able to reach the goal of incorporating cytogenetics into standard diagnostic procedures for solid tumors, as has been achieved with hematological malignancies. Molecular cytogenetics including fluorescent in situ hybridization (FISH) technology promises to bring soft tissue tumor cytogenetics into regular diagnostic armamentaria and concurrently speed research into the basis of soft tissue tumors.

Acknowledgement. We thank Pierre Cormier and Prof. Frederick Hecht for their respective helpful clerical assistance and editing of the manuscript. We thank the pathologists of the "Sarcoma Group" of the Fédération Nationale des Centres de Lutte Contre le Cancer" from France for their supportive collaboration.

Addendum to the Proofs. Since the submission of the manuscript, molecular rearrangements resulting in new fusion genes have been found at the breakpoints of most of the consistent and specific translocations described in this manuscript: *ATF1-EWS* at the breakpoints of the t(12;22) in melanoma of the soft part (Zucman J, Delattre O, Desmaze C, Epstein AL, Stenman G, Speleman F, Fletcher CDM, Aurias A, Thomas G (1993). *EWS-ATF1* gene fusion induced by t(12;22) translocation in malignant melanoma of the soft parts. Nature Genet 4: 341–344). *CHOP-FUS* at the breakpoints of the t(12;16) in myxoid liposarcoma (Rabbitts TH, Forster A, Larson R, Nathan P (1993) Fusion of the dominant negative transcription regulator CHOP with a novel gene FUS by translocation t(12;16) in malignant liposarcoma. Nature Gene 4: 175–180). *PAX3-FKHR* at the breakpoints of the t(2;13) in alveolar rhabdomyosarcoma (Galili N, Davis RJ, Fredericks WJ, Mukhopadhyay S, Rauscher III FJ, Emanuel BS, Rovera G, Barr FG (1993) Fusion of a fork head domain gene to *PAX3* in the solid tumor alveolar rhabdomyosarcoma. Nature Genet 5: 230–235). In a subset of Ewing's tumors, a "variant" fusion of *EWS* with *ERG* has been found to be induced by a 21;22 chromosome rearrangement, however not cytogenetically detected (Zucman J, Melot T, Desmaze C, Ghysdael J, Plougastel B, Peter M, Zucker JM, Triche TJ, Sheer D, Turc-Carel C, Ambros O, Combaret V, Lenoir G, Aurias A, Thomas G, Delattre O (1993) EMBO J 12: 4481–4487).

References

Adam LR, Davison EV, Malcolm AJ, Pearson ADJ, Craft AW (1991) Cytogenetic analysis of a congenital fibrosarcoma. Cancer Genet Cytogenet 52: 37–41

Aman P, Ron D, Mandahl N, Fioretos T, Heim S, Arheden K, Willén H, Rydholm A, Mitelman F (1992) Rearrangement of the transcription factor gene CHOP in myxoid liposarcomas with t(12;16)(q13;p11). Genes Chrom Cancer 5: 278–285

Aurias A, Rimbaut C, Buffe D, Dubousset J, Mazabraud A (1983) Chromosomal translocation in Ewing's sarcoma. N Engl J Med 309: 496–497

Barr FG, Galili N, Holick J, Biegel JA, Rovera G, Emanuel BS (1993) Rearrangement of the PAX3 paired box gene in the pediatric solid tumour alveolar rhabdomyosarcoma. Nature Genet 3: 113–117

Becroft DMO, Pearson A, Shaw RL, Zwi LJ (1984) Chromosome translocation in extraskeletal Ewing's tumour. Lancet II: 400

Biegel JA, Meek RS, Parmiter AH, Conard K, Emanuel BS (1991) Chromosomal translocation t(1;13)(p36;q14) in a case of rhabdomyosarcoma. Genes Chrom Cancer 3: 483–484

Bridge JA, Sanger WG, Shaffer B, Neff JR (1987) Cytogenetic findings in malignant fibrous histyocytoma. Cancer Genet Cytogenet 29: 97–102

Bridge JA, Sanger WG, Neff JR (1989) Translocations involving chromosomes 2 and 13 in benign and malignant cartilaginous neoplasms. Cancer Genet Cytogenet 38: 83–88

Bridge JA, Neff JR, Sandberg AA (1990a) Cytogenetic analysis of dermatofibrosarcoma protuberans. Cancer Genet Cytogenet 49: 199–202

Bridge JA, Borek DA, Neff JR, Huntrakon M (1990b) Chromosomal abnormalities in clear cell sarcoma. Implications for histogenesis. Am J Clin Pathol 93: 26–31

Bridge JA, Sreekantaiah C, Neff JR, Sandberg AA (1991) Cytogenetic findings in clear cell sarcoma of tendons and aponeuroses. Cancer Genet Cytogenet 52: 101–106

Bridge JA, Sreekantaiah C, Mourn B, Neff JR, Sandberg AA (1992) Clonal chromosomal abnormalities in desmoid tumors. Cancer 69: 430–436

Calabrese G, Franchi PG, Stuppia L, Rossi C, Bianchi C, Antonucci A, Palka G (1992) Translocation (8;11)(q12–13;q21) in embryonal rhabdomyosarcoma. Cancer Genet Cytogenet 58: 210–211

Cavazzana AO, Miser JS, Jefferson J, Triche TJ (1987) Experimental evidence for a neural origin of Ewing's sarcoma of bone. Am J Pathol 127: 507–518

Christiansen H, Altmannsberger M, Lampert F (1992) Translocation (5;22) in a Askin's tumor. Cancer Genet Cytogenet 62: 203–205

Craig I, Gemmil R, Kucherlapati R (1992) Report of the first international workshop on human chromosome 12 mapping. Cytogenet Cell Genet 61: 244–251

Dal Cin P, Turc-Carel C, Sandberg AA (1988) Consistent involvement of band 12q14 in two different translocations in three lipomas from the same patient. Cancer Genet Cytogenet 31: 237–240

Dal Cin P, Brock P, Aly MS, Casteels-Van Daele M, De Wever I, Van Damme B, Van Den Berghe H (1991a) A variant (2;13) translocation in rhabdomyosarcoma. Cancer Genet Cytogenet 55: 191–195

Dal Cin P, Brock P, Casteels-Van Daele M, De Wever I, Van Damme B, Van Den Berghe H (1991b) Cytogenetic characterization of congenital or infantile fibrosarcoma. Eur J Pediatr 150: 579–581

Dal Cin P, Aly MS, Delabie J, Ceuppens JL, Van Gool S, Van Damme B, Baert L, Van Poppel H, Van Den Berghe H (1992a) Trisomy 7 and trisomy 10 characterize subpopulations of tumor-infiltrarting lymphocytes in kidney tumors and in the surrounding kidney tissue. Proc Natl Acad Sci USA 89: 9744–9748

Dal Cin P, Van Damme B, Hoogmartens M, Van Den Bereghe H (1992b) Chromosome changes in a case of hibernoma. Genes Chrom Cancer 5: 178–180

de Chadarévian JP, Vekemans M, Seemayer TA (1984) Reciprocal translocation in small-cell sarcomas. N Engl J Med 311: 1702–1703

De Jong B, Castedo SMMJ, Oosterhuis JW, Dam A (1988) Trisomy 7 in a case of angiomyolipoma. Cancer Genet Cytogenet 34: 219–222

Debiec-Rychter M, Saryusz-Wolska H, Salagierski M (1992) Cytogenetic analysis of a renal angiomyolipoma. Genes Chrom Cancer 4: 101–103

Dehner LP (1986) Peripheral and central primitive neuroectodermal tumors. A nosologic concept seeking a consensus. Arch Pathol Lab Med 110: 997–1005

Delattre O, Zucman J, Plougastel B, Desmaze C, Melot T, Peter M, Kovar H, Joubert I, De Jong P, Rouleau G, Aurias A, Thomas G (1992) Gene fusion with an ETS DNA-binding domain caused by chromosome translocation in human tumours. Nature 359: 162–165

Dembinski A, Bridge JA, Berger C, Sandberg AA (1992) Trisomy 2 in proliferative fasciitis. Cancer Genet Cytogenet 60: 27–30

Douglass EC, Valentine M, Etcubanas E, Parham D, Webber BL, Houghton PJ, Green AA (1987) A specific chromosomal abnormality in rhabdomyosarcoma. Cytogenet Cell Genet 45:148–155

Douglass EC, Rowe ST, Valentine M, Parham DM, Berkow R, Bowman WP, Maurer HM (1991) Variant translocations of chromosome 13 in alveolar rhabdomyosarcoma. Genes Chrom Cancer 3: 480–482

Elfving P, Cigudosa JC, Lundgren R, Limon J, Mandahl N, Kristoffersson U, Heim S, Mitelman F (1990) Trisomy 7, trisomy 10 and loss of the Y chromosome in short-term cultures of normal kidney tissues. Cytogenet Cell Genet 53: 123–125

Eneroth M, Mandahl N, Heim S, Willén H, Rydolm A, Alberts KA, Mitelman F (1990) Localisation of the chromosomal breakpoints of the t(12;16) in liposarcoma to subbands 12q13.3 and 16p11.2. Cancer Genet Cytogenet 48: 101–107

Enzinger FM, Weiss SW (1988) Soft tissue tumors, 2nd edn. Mosby, St Louis

Enzinger FM, Zhang R (1988) Plexiform fibrohistiocytic tumor presenting in children and young adults. An analysis of 65 cases. Am J Surg Pathol 12: 818–826

Evans HL, Soule EH, Winkelmann RK (1979) Atypical lipoma, atypical intramuscular lipoma, and well differentiated retroperitoneal liposarcoma. A reappraisal of 30 cases formerly classified as well differentiated liposarcoma. Cancer 43: 574–584

Fletcher CDM (1990) Introduction. In: Fletcher CDM, McKee PH (eds) Pathobiology of soft tissue tumors, Churchill Livingstone, Edinburgh, pp 1–7

Fletcher CDM, McKee PH (1990) Progress in malignant soft tissue tumors. In: Fletcher CDM, McKee PH (eds) Pathobiology of soft tissue tumors. Churchill Livingstone, Edinburgh, pp 295–318

Fletcher JA, Kozakewich HP, Hoffer FA, Lage JM, Weidner N, Tepper R, Pinkus GS, Morton CC, Corson JM (1991) Diagnostic relevance of clonal cytogenetic aberrations in malignant soft-tissue tumors. N Engl J Med 324: 436–442

Fletcher JA, Henkle C, Atkins L, Rosenberg AE, Morton CC (1992) Trisomy 5 and trisomy 7 are nonrandom aberrations in pigmented villonodular synovitis. Genes Chrom Cancer 4: 264–266

Gorman AG, Malone M, Pritchard J, Sheer D (1991) Cytogenetic analysis of primitive neuroectodermal tumors. Absence of the t(11;22) in two of three cases and a review of the literature. Cancer Genet Cytogenet 51: 13–22

Guerneri S, Stioui S, Mantovani F, Austoni E, Simoni G (1991) Multiple clonal chromosomes abnormalities in Peyronie's disease. Cancer Genet Cytogenet 52: 181–185

Hayashi K, Inada R, Hanadas R, Yamamoto K (1988) Translocation 2;8 in a congenital rhabdomyosarcoma. Cancer Genet Cytogenet 30: 343–345

Heim S, Mandahl N, Kristoffersson U, Mitelman F, Rööser B, Rydholm A, Willén H (1986) Reciprocal translocation t(3;12)(q27;q13) in lipoma. Cancer Genet Cytogenet 23: 301–304

Heim S, Mandahl N, Rydholm A, Willen H, Mitelman F (1988) Different karyotypic features characterize different clinico-pathologic subgroups of benign lipogenic tumors. Int J Cancer 42: 863–867

Hinrichs SH, Jaramillo MA, Gumerlock PH, Gardner MB, Lewis JP, Freeman AE (1985) Myxoid chondrosarcoma with a translocation involving chromosomes 9 and 22. Cancer Genet Cytogenet 14: 219–226

Huvos AG (1985) The spontaneous transformation of benign into malignant soft tissue tumors (With emphasis on extraskeletal, osseous, lipomatous, and schwannian lesions). Am J Surg Pathol 9(3)[Suppl]: 7–20

Karakousis CP, Dal Cin P, Turc-Carel C, Limon J, Sandberg AA (1987) Chromosomal changes in soft-tissue sarcomas: a new diagnostic parameter. Arch Surg 122: 1257–1260

Karlsson I, Mandahl N, Heim S, Rydholm A, Willén H, Mitelman F (1988) Complex chromosome rearrangements in an extraabdominal desmoid tumor. Cancer Genet Cytogenet 34: 241–245

Kees UR, Rudduck G, Ford J, Spagnolo D, Papadimitriou J, Willoughby MLN, Garson OM (1992) Two malignant peripheral primitive neuroepithelial tumor cell lines established from consecutive samples of one patient. Genes Chrom Cancer 4: 195–204

Kindblom L-G, Lodding P, Angerval A (1983) Clear-cell sarcoma of tendons and aponeurones. An immunohistochemical and electron microscopic analysis indicating neural crest origin. Virchows Arch Pathol Anat 409: 109–128

Koufos A, Hansen MF, Copeland NG, Jenkins NA, Lampkin BC, Cavenee WK (1985) Loss of heterozygoty in three embryonal tumors suggests a common pathogenis mechanism. Nature 316: 330–334

Limon J, Mrozek K, Mandahl N, Nedoszytko B, Verhest A, Rys A, Niezabitowski A, Babinska M, Nosek H, Ochalek T, Kopacz A, Willén H, Rydholm A, Heim S, Mitelman F (1991) Cytogenetics of synovial sarcoma: presentation of ten new cases and review of the literature. Genes Chrom Cancer 3: 338–345

Lipinski M, Braham K, Philip I, Wiels J, Philip T, Goridis C, Lenoir GM, Tursz T (1987) Neuroectodermal-associated antigens on Ewing's sarcoma cell lines. Cancer Res 47: 183–187

Mandahl N, Heim S, Johansson B, Bennet K, Mertens F, Olsson G, Rööser B, Rydholm A, Willén H, Mitelman F (1987) Lipomas have characteristic structural chromosomal rearrangements of 12q13–q14. Int J Cancer 39: 685–688

Mandahl N, Heim S, Arheden K, Rydholm A, Willen H, Mitelman F (1988a) Rings, dicentrics and telomeric association in histiocytomas. Cancer Genet Cytogenet 30: 23–33

Mandahl N, Heim S, Arheden K, Rydholm A, Willén H, Mitelman F (1988b) Multiple karyoytypic rearrangements, including t(X;18)(p11;q11) in a fibrosarcoma. Cancer Genet Cytogenet 30: 323–327

Mandahl N, Heim S, Arheden K, Rydholm A, Willén H, Mitelman F (1988c) Three major cytogenetic subgroups can be identified among chromosomally abnormal solitary lipomas. Hum Genet 79: 203–208

Mandahl N, Heim S, Willén H, Rydholm A, Eneroth M, Nilbert M, Kreicbergs A, Mitelman F (1989a) Characteristic karyotypic anomalies identify subtypes of malignant fibrous histocytoma. Genes Chrom Cancer 1: 9–14

Mandahl N, Heim S, Rydholm A, Willén H, Mitelman F (1989b) Nonrandom numerical chromosome aberrations (+8, +11, +17, +20) in infantile fibrosarcoma. Cancer Genet Cytogenet 40: 137–139

Mandahl N, Heim S, Arheden K, Rydholm A, Willén H, Mitelman F (1989c) Four cytogenetic subgroups can be identified in lipomas. Cancer Genet Cytogenet 41: 230

Mandahl N, Heim S, Willen H, Rydholm A, Mitelman F (1990) Supernumerary ring chromosome as the sole cytogenetic abnormality in a dermatofibrosarcoma protuberans. Cancer Genet Cytogenet 49: 273–275

Molenaar WM, de Jong B, Buist J, Idenburg VJS, Seruca R, Vos AM, Hoekstra HJ (1989) Chromosomal analysis and classification of soft tissue sarcomas. Lab Invest 60: 266–274

Nilbert M, Heim S (1990) Uterine leiomyoma cytogenetics. Genes Chrom Cancer 2: 3–13

Ohjimi Y, Iwasaki H, Kanako Y, Ishiguro M, Ohgami A, Kikuchi M (1992) A case of lipoblastoma with t(3;8)(q12;q11.2). Cancer Genet Cytogenet 62: 103–105

Oliner JD, Kinzler KW, Meltzer PS, George DL, Vogelstein B (1989) Amplification of a gene encoding a p53-associated protein in human sarcomas. Nature 358: 80–83

Örndal C, Mandahl N, Rydholm A, Willén H, Brosjö O, Heim S, Mitelman F (1992) Supernumerary ring chromosomes in five bone and soft tissue tumors of low or borderline malignancy. Cancer Genet Cytogenet 60: 170–175

Pedeutour F, Coindre JM, Nicolo G, Bouchot C, Ayraud N, Turc-Carel (1993) Ring chromosomes in dermatofibrosarcoma protuberans contain chromosome 17 sequences: fluorescent in situ hybridization. Cancer Genet Cytogenet 67: 149

Pedeutour F, Suijkerbuijk RF, Van Gaal J, Van De Klunder W, Coindre JM, Van Haelst A, Collin F, Huffermann K, Turc-Carel (1993) Chromosome 12 origin in rings and giant markers in well-differentiated liposarcoma. Cancer Genet Cytogenet 66: 134–133

Pedeutour F, Suijkerbuijk RF, Forus A, Van Gaal J, Van der Klundert W, Coindre JM, Nicolo G, Collin F, Van Haelst U, Huffermann K, Turc-Carel C (1994) Complex composition and coamplification of SAS and MDM2 in ring and giant rod marker chromosomes in well-differentiated liposarcoma. Genes Chrom Cancer 10: 85–94

Pedeutour F, Coindre JM, Sossi G, Nicolo G, Leroux A, Toma S, Miozzo M, Bouchot C, Hecht F, Turc-Carel C (in press) Supernumerary ring chromosomes containing chromosome

17 sequences. A specific feature of Dermatofibrosarcoma Protuberans. Cancer Genet Cytogenet

Peulvé P, Michot C, Vannier JP, Tron P, Hemet J (1991) Clear cell sarcoma with t(12;22) (q13–14:q12). Genes Chrom Cancer 3: 400–402

Potluri VR, Gilbert F (1985) A cytogenetic study of embryonal rhabdomyosarcoma. Cancer Genet Cytogenet 14: 169–173

Ray RA, Morton CC, Lipinski KK, Corson JM, Fletcher JA (1991) Cytogenetic evidence of clonality in a case of pigmented villonodular synovitis. Cancer 67: 121–125

Reeves BR, Fletcher CDM, Gusterson BA (1992) Translocation t(12;22)(q13;q13) is a nonrandom rearrangement in clear cell sarcoma. Cancer Genet Cytogenet 64: 101–103

Roberts P, Browne CF, Lewis IJ, Bailey CC, Spicer RD, Williams J, Batcup G (1992) 12q13 abnormality in rhabdomyosarcoma. A nonrandom occurence? Cancer Genet Cytogenet 60: 135–140

Rodriguez E, Sreekantaiah C, Reuter VE, Motzer RJ, Chaganti RSK (1992) t(12;22)(q13;q13) and trisomy 8 are nonrandom aberrations in clear-cell sarcoma. Cancer Genet Cytogenet 64: 107–110

Rydholm A, Mandahl N, Heim S, Kreicbergs A, Willén H, Mitelman F (1990) Malignant fibrous histiocytomas with a 19p+ marker chromosome have increased relapse rate. Genes Chrom Cancer 2: 296–299

Sandberg AA (1990) The chromosomes in human cancer and leukemia, 2nd edn. Elsevier, New York

Sandberg AA, Turc-Carel C (1987) The cytogenetics of solid tumors. Relation to diagnosis, classification and pathology. Cancer 59: 387–395

Sandberg AA, Gibas Z, Saren E, Li FP, Limon J, Tebbi CK (1986) Chromosome abnormalities in two benign adipose tumors. Cancer Genet Cytogenet 22: 55–61

Scrable H, Witte D, Shimada H, Seemayer T, Wang-Wuu S, Soukup S, Koufos A, Houghton P, Lampkin B, Cavenee W (1989) Molecular differential pathology of rhabdomyosarcoma. Genes Chrom Cancer 1: 23–35

Seidal T, Mark J, Hagmar B, Angervall L (1982) Alveolar rhabdomyosarcoma: a cytogenetic and correlated cytologic and histological study. Acta Pathol Microbiol Immunol Scand [A] 90: 345–453

Sergovitch FR, Botz JS, McFarlane RM (1983) Nonrandom cytogenetic abnormalities in Dupuytren's disease. N Engl J Med 308: 162–163

Smith S, Fletcher CDM, Smith MA, Gusteron BA (1990) Cytogenetic analysis of a plexiform fibriohistiocytic tumor. Cancer Genet Cytogenet 48: 31–34

Smith SH, Weiss SW, Jankowski SA, Coccia MA, Meltzer PS (1992) SAS amplification in soft tissue sarcoma. Cancer Res 53: 3746–3749

Speleman F, dal Cin P, de Potter K, Laureys G, Roels HJ, Leroy J, van den Berghe H (1989) Cytogenetic investigation of a case of congenital fibrosarcoma. Cancer Genet Cytogenet 39: 21–24

Sreeakantaiah C, Leong SPL, Davis JR, Sandberg AA (1991a) Intratumoral cytogenetic heterogeneity in a benign neoplasm. Cancer 67: 3110–3116

Sreekantaiah C, Leong SPL, Karakousis CP, McGee DL, Rappaport WD, Villar HV, Neal D, Fleming S, Wankel A, Herrington PN et al. (1991b) Cytogenetic profile of 109 lipomas. Cancer Res 51: 422–433

Sreekantaiah C, Karakousis CP, Leong SPL, Sandberg AA (1992) Cytogenetic findings in liposarcoma correlate with histopathologic subtypes. Cancer 69: 2484–2495

Stenman G, Kindblom L-G, Angervall L (1992) Reciprocal translocation t(12;22)(q13;q13) in clear-cell sarcoma of tendons and aponeurones. Genes Chrom Cancer 4: 122–127

Stephenson CF, Berger CS, Leong SPL, Davis JR, Sandberg AA (1992a) Ring chromosome in a dermatofibrosarcoma protuberans. Cancer Genet Cytogenet 58: 52–54

Stephenson CF, Berger CS, Leong SPL, Davis JR, Sandberg AA (1992b) Analysis of a giant marker chromosome in a well-differentiated liposarcoma using cytogenetics and fluorescence in situ hybridization. Cancer Genet Cytogenet 61: 134–138

Travis JA, Bridge JA (1992) Significance of both numerical and structural chromosomal abnormalities in clear cell sarcoma. Cancer Genet Cytogenet 64: 104–106

Trent J, Casper J, Meltzer P, Thompson F, Fogh J (1985) Nonrandom chromosome alterations in rhabdomyosarcoma. Cancer Genet Cytogenet 16: 189–197

Triche TJ, Askin FB (1983) Neuroblastoma and differential diagnosis of small, round, blue-cell tumors. Hum Pathol 14: 569–595

Turc-Carel C (1991) Apport de la cytogénétique au diagnostic du Sarcome d'Ewing et des tumeurs à petites cellules rondes. Bull Cancer (Paris) 78: 77–84

Turc-Carel C, Philip I, Berger MP, Philip T, Lenoir GM (1983) Chromosomal translocation in Ewing's sarcoma. N Engl J Med 309: 497–498

Turc-Carel C, Lizard-Nicol S, Justrabo E, Favrot M, Philip T, Tabone E (1986a) Consistent chromosome translocation in rhabdomyosarcoma. Cancer Genet Cytogenet 19: 361–362

Turc-Carel C, Dal-Cin P, Rao U, Karakousis C, Sandberg AA (1986b) Cytogenetic Studies of Adipose Tissue Tumors. I. A benign lipoma with reciprocal translocation t(3;12)(q28;q14). Cancer Genet Cytogenet 23: 283–289

Turc-Carel C, Limon J, Dal-Cin P, Rao U, Karakousis C, Sandberg AA (1986c) Cytogenetic studies of adipose tissue tumors. II Cancer Genet Cytogenet 23: 291–299

Turc-Carel C, Dal Cin P, Limon J, Rao U, Li FP, Corson JM, Zimmerman R, Parry DM, Cowan JM, Sandberg AA (1987) Involvement of chromosome X in primary cytogenetic change in human neoplasia. Nonrandom translocation in synovial sarcoma. Proc Natl Acad Sci USA 84: 1981–1985

Turc-Carel C, Dal Cin P, Rao U, Karakousis C, Sandberg AA (1988a) Recurrent breakpoints at 9q31 and 22q12.2 in extraskeletal myxoid chondrosarcoma. Cancer Genet Cytogenet 30: 145–150

Turc-Carel C, Aurias A, Mugneret F, Lizard S, Sidaner I, Volk C, Thiery JP, Olschwang S, Philip I, Berger MP, Philip T, Lenoir GM, Mazabraud A (1988b) Chromosomes in Ewing Sarcoma. I. An evaluation of 85 cases and remarkable consistency of the t(11;22)(q24;q12). Cancer Genet Cytogenet 32: 229–238

Turc-Carel C, Dal Cin P, Boghosian L, Leong SPL, Sandberg AA (1988c) Breakpoints in benign lipoma may be at 12q13 or 12q14. Cancer Genet Cytogenet 36: 131–135

Wang-Wuu S, Soukup S, Ballard E, Gotwals B, Lampkin B (1988) Chromosomal analysis of sixteen human rhabdomyosarcomas. Cancer Res 48: 983–987

Whang-Peng J, Triche TJ, Knutsen T, Miser G, Douglass EC, Israel MA (1984) Chromosome translocation in peripheral neuroepithelioma. N Engl J Med 31: 584–585

Whang-Peng J, Knutsen T, Horowitz ME, Triche TJ (1992) Cytogenetic studies in subgroups of rhabdomyosarcoma. Genes Chrom Cancer 5: 299–310

Zucman J, Delattre O, Desmaze C, Plougastel B, Joubert I, Melot T, Peter M, De Jong P, Rouleau G, Aurias A, Thomas G (1992) Cloning and characterization of the Ewing's sarcoma and peripheral neuroepithelioma t(11;22) translocation breakpoints. Genes Chrom Cancer 5: 271–277

DNA Ploidy in Soft Tissue Tumors: An Evaluation of the Prognostic Implications in the Different Tumor Types[*]

W. Mellin, A. Niezabitowski, M. Brockmann, J. Ritter,
P. Wuisman, and V. Krieg

1 Introduction

The prognosis of patients with soft tissue tumors is determined by many factors, among them not only the basic patho-anatomical findings, but also individual influences such as localization, age, overall personal risk factors (operability, etc.), and the chosen therapeutic procedures (Mandard et al. 1989). The patho-anatomical determinants are tumor size, mode and grade of tumor spread at the time of primary diagnosis, histological tumor type or subtype, and histological grading.

Today, tumor spread can be defined with greater accuracy due to the progress in noninvasive imaging methods of investigation, and also with decisive influence on the choice of therapy (Dewhirst et al. 1990). Additional immunohistological characterization has permitted further improvement in detailed tumor classification over these last few years, although the application of such markers is apt to raise new problems of differential

* Supported by Deutsche Forschungsgemeinschaft, Grant Me 895/1-1.

Current Topics in Pathology
Volume 89, Eds. D. Harms/D. Schmidt
© Springer-Verlag Berlin Heidelberg 1995

typing. For instance, the often considerable histomorphological variability of individual sarcomas and of separate sarcoma types (KATENKAMP 1988) is reflected in a corresponding variety of immunophenotypes (BROOKS 1986).

In certain histological types, the grade of malignancy or the prognostic outlook can be predicted by the diagnosis proper (e.g., in the subtypes of rhabdomyosarcoma and liposarcoma, peripheral neuroectodermal tumors); in other sarcomas, mostly of the spindle cell variety, the histological grade of malignancy is more influential on prognosis than the definite histological type, especially in problem cases of typing (COINDRE et al. 1988a; MEISTER 1988; VAN UNNIK et al. 1988; EILBER et al. 1990). With regard to histological grading, there is as yet no generally accepted standard, and reliability depends very much on the subjective diagnostic experience of the pathologist (DONHUIJSEN 1986). The following histological criteria are of relevance in the assessment of malignancy:

1. Grade of cellularity
2. Rate of mitoses
3. Degree of cellular differentiation and pleomorphism
4. Necrosis
5. Quantity of intercellular substance
6. Growth patterns

Among these, parameters 1, 2, and 4 primarily define growth kinetics; 3 and 5 differentiation properties; and 6 the type of histological spread as characterized, for example, by invasiveness, vascular destruction, or the formation of a pseudocapsule.

Some of the different factors are often closely correlated: tumors with immature cells often possess extremely high cellularity with concomitant necrotic trends, and a lower intensity of intercellular substance formation. Proliferation can be assessed distinctively by the use of cell cycle-associated nuclear antigens (Ki-67, PCNA), which may be useful in the choice of radio- or chemotherapy (YU et al. 1991; UEDA et al. 1989).

According to general experience in oncology, cytophotomerically assessed DNA ploidy is another parameter of prognostic relevance, as has been confirmed in some studies of soft tissue sarcomas (KREICBERGS et al. 1987; PERSSON et al. 1988; SCHMIDT et al. 1989; SAPI and BODO 1989; ALVEGARD et al. 1990; LI 1990; ZUBRIKHINA and OL'KHOVSKAJA 1990; STENFERT KROESE et al. 1990; DICTOR et al. 1991; JOVANOVIC et al. 1991). It is still not quite clear how and how much DNA ploidy can be included precisely in the grading of soft tissue sarcomas.

Since the introduction of modern therapeutic concepts (combined surgical and chemotherapy and/or radiotherapy, etc.) in certain tumor types has greatly contributed to improved prognosis, the value and impact of classical patho-anatomical parameters has changed considerably in clinical practice. It appears quite likely that, in some cases, more importance will be attributed to various proliferation markers, DNA ploidy, routine tests for genome aberrations, and other clinical empirical parameters such as intitial response to therapy, etc. as decisive prognostic parameters (GANSLER et al. 1986; KNIGHT 1990; BOURHIS et al. 1991a,b; SHAPIRO et al. 1991; DEWHIRST et al. 1990; DONNER 1991; CARLSEN et al. 1991).

It is intended that the image cytometric DNA analyses on histological slides presented in the following define and explain the degree and prognostic relevance of DNA ploidy in a representative collection of soft tissue tumors ($n = 584$) with various types of differentiation and histogenesis. It is also intended to show practically relevant indications for DNA cytometry in soft tissue sarcomas, and finally to test the methodological validity and practical applicability of DNA image cytometry in paraffin-embedded matrial of soft tissue sarcomas from our archives.

2 Material and Methods

2.1 Classification and Grading of Tumors

Our collection comprised 118 benign and 38 semimalignant (or questionably malignant) soft tissue tumors, and 428 soft tissue sarcomas taken from the soft tissue sarcoma registry of Poland (Cracow University, 220 cases), from the mesothelioma registry (Bochum University, FRG, 53 cases), and from the Gerhard Domagk Institute of Pathology (Münster University, 311 cases). For image cytometrical DNA analysis, formalin-fixed and paraffin-embedded material was at our disposal. The number of cases studied in each sarcoma entity, sex ratio, and mean age are documented in Table 2.

Since the present retrospective study is based on tumor cases from several oncological centers, collected between 1975 and 1991, staging categories for most tumor types were hardly comparable, and so it was only the maximum diameter of every tumor that served as a parameter for tumor expansion. Therapeutic management and clinical course were completely documented in only part of the cases, varying in proportions among the tumor types. Thus, statistically ascertained data about the prognostic relevance of DNA ploidy were possible in only some of the histological types.

2.1.1 Classification

According to general experience in DNA image cytometry (ICM), the behavior and value of DNA ploidy vary considerably from one tumor type to the other, and so careful and exact typing is a prerequisite for the correct evaluation of DNA ploidy. The classification of soft tissue tumors is based on purely histomorphological and conventional histochemical criteria as described in detail by ENZINGER and WEISS (1988) or KATENKAMP and STILLER (1990). Immunohistological differentiation markers were used in addition (MIETTINEN 1990; FISHER 1990), serving mainly to identify intermediate filaments such as cytokeratin, vimentin, desmin, and muscle-specific actin as well as other cellular proteins (S-100, Factor VIII, alpha$_1$-anti trypsin, and alpha$_1$-antichymotrypsin).

Some unexpected expressions of those markers were occasionally observed in several tumor types (BROOKS 1986; BROWN et al. 1987; COINDRE et al. 1988a), and certain immunohistological markers specific for other tumor entities (e.g., malignant lymphomas) may also be expressed in soft tissue sarcomas (MECHTERSHEIMER and MÖLLER 1990); therefore the interpretation of immunohistological findings requires particular caution. Consequently, positive immunohistological labeling was seen as decisive only in those cases that permitted no unequivocal histomorphological differentiation. To ensure the recognition of potentially type-specific data on DNA ploidy, tumors of mixed histological differentiation were not included in the study.

2.1.2 Grading

In our collective, histological grading was based on subjective evaluation of the prognostic cytological criteria mentioned in the introduction (cellularity, mitotic activity, cellular differentiation, and pleomorphism). Restriction to purely cytological criteria was intended to facilitate comparison with the equally cytological parameter of DNA ploidy. Anaplastic tumors of the small and round cell types (e.g., extraskeletal Ewing's sarcoma, peripheral neuroectodermal tumor, alveolar rhabdomyosarcoma, synovioblastic synovial sarcoma) were excluded from the general three-step schedule and listed as grade 4, on account of their minor histological variability and overall high grade of malignancy. As a deviation, sympathicus neuroblastomas were divided in three grades of malignancy according to HUGHES et al. (1974).

All other sarcoma types that are usually manifested in varying degrees of malignancy were classified in three grades. The system was devised to ensure comparability of grading among the different types of sarcoma, and so to verify its general applicability. Admittedly such comparisons carry their own problems: in spindle cell synovial sarcomas, for instance, cytological grading depends, together with proliferation criteria, mainly on the degree of cell maturation. The other spindle cell sarcomas of soft tissue, in contrast, are mainly characterized by the varying degree of cellular atypia (COINDRE et al. 1988a; MANDARD et al. 1989; DONHUIJSEN 1986).

2.2 DNA Image Cytometry

DNA analysis of soft tissue sarcomas as presented here were performed by ICM on Feulgen-stained sections since previous flow cytometric (FCM)

DNA analyses had been found to be rather less useful. The reduced resolution of FCM DNA analysis in paraffin-embedded material (HEDLEY et al. 1983; WERSTO et al. 1991) is particularly marked in spindle cell and fiber-rich sarcomas, the preparation of which is difficult even in fresh material. During the isolation of cells from paraffin-embedded soft tissue sarcomas, nuclei are often damaged with subsequent loss of DNA, thereby hampering even the Feulgen cytometry of smear preparations. Selective damage or destruction may affect especially the larger nuclei which often belong to the tumor cells under investigation.

The specific errors to which DNA measurements of sections are liable, such as nuclear cuts and nuclear overlappings, could be almost completely avoided by optimal sectioning ($10\,\mu$m) and careful focusing of each preparation. For (reliable) calibration we measured 20 local, safely nontumorous, and, if possible, nonproliferating mesenchymal cells which revealed up to 29% higher values than lymphocytes (average 14%); this reflects the well-known error of proportionality in Feulgen cytometry (BÖHM 1968; BIESTER-FELD and BÖCKING 1990), which also affects cytological preparations. The identification of nontumorous mesenchymal cells to be used as reference cells is much more readily possible in sections of soft tissue tumors than in isolated cells. Moreover, the state of preservation and grade of differentiation of the tumor tissues, often very variable in different regions, may be reliably evaluated in sections and accordingly considered in measurements. Despite a usually higher scattering of DNA values, sections would ensure a safer definition of DNA stemline ploidy than the preparations made after cell isolation which are less easily checked for potential errors.

For the DNA analysis of soft tissue tumors performed in this study we chose well-preserved tissue samples which, if possible, represented the highest grade of malignancy found in the individual tumor specimen. If it comprised stronger regional variations of histological malignancy grades, such areas were investigated separately. The 10-μm sections were subjected to hydrolysis in $1\,N$ HCl solution at 37°C for 90 min. Measurements were performed with a microscope photometer (Leitz MPV 3), combined with a DNA cytometry system (Ahrens ACAS) to provide an interactive image analysis. The absorption of matrix immediately surrounding the nuclei (i.e., cytoplasm, as a rule) is taken as reference value for "zero absorption," thereby ensuring due regard to background absorption in each measurement, a factor that may show considerable variation, especially in sections (BIESTERFELD and BÖCKING 1990).

The reference value for DNA diploidy having been established, we proceeded to the measurement of at least 100 tumor cell nuclei in each case. Limited by the number of cells, the resolution of histograms permitted no more than a gross estimate of cell cycle distribution, although tumors with minor proliferation activity are readily distinguished from those with major proliferation activity. The following evaluation of DNA histograms is strictly limited to the assessment of DNA ploidy with principal distinction of single cell and stemline DNA aneuploidy. Single cell aneuploidy defines the proportion of safely aneuploid tumor cells (5c-exceeding rate) in an otherwise peridiploid, unimodal DNA distribution. The relative increase of DNA aneuploid cells also raises the probability of definite malignancy.

Single cell aneuploidy is thus interpreted as an indicator for differentiating benign from malignant tumors, a rather doubtful (problematic) appraisal with regard to soft tissue tumors. Some authors want to use it for DNA grading of malignant tumors, with additional reference to cell cycle distribution in certain algorithms (Böcking and Auffermann 1986). In soft tissue tumors, the presence of appreciable single cell aneuploidies can often be subsumed from routine histology represented in an appropriate grade of nuclear pleomorphism and evidence of giant nuclei in tumor cells.

DNA ploidy in the stricter sense, however, always means DNA stemline ploidy, manifested in a relatively uniform DNA content slightly scattered around a definite modal value (DNA index, DI) which characterizes that tumor stemline. By definition, a DI of 1 describes DNA diploidy. The steps of polyploidy are expressed in DIs 2, 4, 8, 16, etc. DNA contents deviating from these euploid DIs are eventually defined as aneuploidies, always implying chromosomal aneuploidy, too. In contrast, DNA diploidy may include a normal, diploid set of chromosomes, but also numerical and/or structural aberrations (reviewed in Mellin 1990).

With regard to prognostic practice, the most sensible distinction would be to separate tumors with minor stemline deviations from DNA diploidy (= DNA peridiploidy) from those with major deviations (DNA aneuploidy). In our evaluation of histograms, tumors with a DI of 1.0 ± 0.2 were defined as peridiploid, all others (even if polyploid) as DNA aneuploid. These rather pragmatic categories will sufficiently respect certain minor inaccuracies of measurement, especially the errors of Feulgen proportionality, and prevent the identification of false-positive, hyperdiploid stemline aneuploidies. If multiple DNA stemlines were recognized in the DNA histogram, evaluation focused on the stemline with the highest DI (Fig. 1).

3 Results

3.1 Fibrous Tumors and Tumor-like Lesions

3.1.1 Fibroma, Nodular Fasciitis

The analysis comprised ten fibromas and six lesions with nodular fasciitis. Unimodal diploid distribution was ascertained in all these cases (Table 1). Nodular fasciitis differed from fibroma in that the proportion of pro-

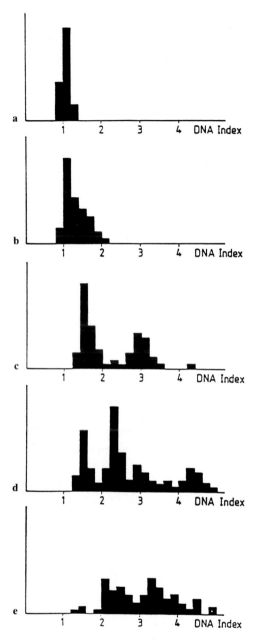

Fig. 1a–e. Typical histograms in ICM: types **a–c** describe unimodal DNA distributions with a rising proportion of proliferating cells (i.e., cells in S and in G_2+M phase). Determination of DNA stemline ploidy is based on the first peak documented in each histogram. Type **d** reflects a bimodal DNA distribution with two DNA aneuploid stemlines ($DI_1 = 1.5$, $DI_2 = 2.3$). Type **e** shows multimodal DNA distribution with poorly delineated DNA stemline peaks ($DI_1 = 2.3$, $DI_2 = 3.3$). In readily measurable preparations, this type may be due to increased scattering of chromosome numbers in the stemlines

Table 1. DNA ploidy in benign, semimalignant, and borderline soft tissue tumors

Histological type	n	DNA stemline aneuploidy (%)	Single cell aneuploidy[a] (%)
Fibroma	10	0.0	0.0
Nodular fasciitis	6	0.0	0.0
Fibromatoses	30	0.0	0.0
Superficial	10	0.0	0.0
Deep	20	0.0	0.0
Dermatofibrohistiocytoma	10	0.0	0.0
Atypical fibroxanthoma	3	66.7	100.0
Dermatofibrosarcoma protuberans	10	10.0	33.3
Lipoma/Angiolipoma	17	0.0	0.0
Leiomyoma	15	0.0	13.3
Hemangioma	20	0.0	0.0
Hemangiopericytoma	5	0.0	0.0
Giant cell tumor of tendon sheath	10	0.0	0.0
Benign schwannoma	10	0.0	30.0
Neurofibroma	10	0.0	20.0

[a] Single cell aneuploidy is only applied in cases without DNA stemline aneuploidy.

liferating cells (S and G_2 phase) was distinctly higher. These results agree in principle with those of EL-JABHOUR et al. (1991).

3.1.2 Fibromatosis

Ten cases of superficial (palmar) fibrosis and 20 cases of deep fibroses (desmoid) were included in the study. Among the latter these were nine abdominal and 11 extraabdominal lesions, chosen at random, but representative of their type with typical distribution of age and sex.

Image cytometry revealed overall diploidy in both superficial and deep fibromatoses, with a variable proportion of S phase cells being evident in DNA histograms. This proportion virtually correlated with the overall cellularity of such lesions, although the proliferative activity was generally distinctly lower than in the sarcoma cases of this study. Since G_2 phase cells and so-called 5c-exceeding events (single cell aneuploidies) were practically nonexistent, no signs of malignancy could be elicited from the DNA histograms (Table 1).

3.1.3 Fibrosarcoma

Currently, "fibrosarcoma" is taken as an exclusive diagnosis acceptable only if the entire tumor consists of fibroblastic cells. Differentiation from fibromatosis, malignant schwannoma, and, in particular, from malignant fibrous histiocytoma (MFH) left only a small number of unequivocal cases in our material. In one case of 12, the tumor was diagnosed as an infantile fibrosarcoma. Of the other 11 cases, six were classified as grade 1, the other five as (less mature) grade 2 tumors. The mean age of patients (predominantly females, 51 years) agrees with general experience (Table 2).

Image cytometry ascertained DNA aneuploidy in only three of these 11 tumors, all classified as grade 2, whereas the infantile fibrosarcoma was peridiploid. None of the cases presented distinguishable single cell aneuploidies. Thus, no conclusions can be drawn about the prognostic relevance of DNA ploidy in fibrosarcoma on account of the small number of evaluable cases in our study.

3.2 Fibrohistiocytic Tumors

3.2.1 Dermatofibrohistiocytoma/Atypical Fibroxanthoma

The ten dermatofibrohistiocytomas subjected to ICM analysis all showed a unimodal peridiploid DNA distribution with only sporadic 5c-exceeding events. Two cases of atypical fibroxanthoma possessed, beside a DNA diploid stemline, another distinct DNA aneuploid stemline plus some additional single cell aneuploidies. Another case revealed considerable single cell aneuploidy in addition to a peridiploid stemline; consequently, tumors of this type fail to reflect any principal differences from MFH (Table 1).

3.2.2 Dermatofibrosarcoma Protuberans

Ten such cases were included, but only one showed a clear hyperdiploid DNA stemline with a DI of 1.4. This dermatofibrosarcoma of the abdominal wall failed, however, to show any clinical difference from the other nine, and neither recurrence nor metastases were observed after the excision of the tumor (Table 1).

3.2.3 Malignant Fibrous Histiocytoma

Under clinical and therapeutic aspects, MFH represents a unique tumor group, but its morphological or rather formal pathogenetic features are suggestive of heterogenous patterns. The fact that MFH may develop from a number of well-defined soft tissue sarcomas in the course of tumor progression is seen as a point in favor of this interpretation (KATENKAMP and STILLER 1990). Accordingly, MFH are separated by morphological patterns into storiform–pleomorphous, myxoid, giant cell, inflammatory, and

Table 2. Clinical and pathological–anatomical data

Histological type	n	Mean age (years)	Sex ratio m/f	Localization				Mean diameter (cm)
				Upper extremities (%)	Lower extremities (%)	Head/neck (%)	Trunk (%)	
Fibrosarcoma	12	51	5/7	–	25.0	25.0	50.0	5.0
MFH	50	59	25/25	14.0	60.0	8.0	18.0	9.2
Liposarcoma	45	52	22/23	8.9	26.7	6.7	57.7	10.3
Lipoma-like/sclerosing/myxoid	23	46	13/10	4.3	34.8	8.7	52.2	10.5
Round cell	7	54	3/4	14.3	28.6	0.0	57.1	42.9
Pleomorphic	15	57	6/9	13.3	13.3	6.7	66.7	9.6
Leiomyosarcoma	60	58	28/32	3.3	25.0	18.3	53.4	10.0
Rhabdomyosarcoma	52	24	23/29	11.5	17.3	34.6	55.8	6.2
Embryonal	29	17	12/17	6.9	13.8	37.9	41.4	6.0
Alveolar	13	16	8/5	23.1	15.3	38.5	23.1	5.0
Pleomorphic	10	58	3/7	10.0	30.0	20.0	40.0	8.6
Angiosarcoma	16	56	8/8	6.3	12.5	37.5	43.7	6.3
Synovial sarcoma	50	30	29/21	14.0	48.0	8.0	30.0	7.5
Spindle cell	26	26	16/10	19.2	57.7	7.7	15.4	6.3
Biphasic	9	31	4/5	11.1	44.4	11.1	33.3	9.8
Synovioblastic	15	36	9/6	6.7	33.3	6.7	53.3	9.9
Diffuse mesothelioma	53	58	49/4	0.0	0.0	0.0	100	–
Epitheloid	29	57	27/2	0.0	0.0	0.0	100	–
Biphasic	20	59	18/2	0.0	0.0	0.0	100	–
Sarcomatous	4	62	4/0	0.0	0.0	0.0	100	–
Malignant schwannoma	46	48	20/26	15.2	34.8	13.1	23.9	13.0
Neuroblastoma	24	3.6	13/11	0.0	0.0	0.0	100	8.4
PNET/Ewing's sarcoma	20	25	11/9	15.0	25.0	15.0	45.0	6.5
Spindle cell sarcomas	168	55	78/90	9.5	38.1	14.3	34.5	10.2
Round cell sarcomas	72	19	41/31	9.7	16.7	12.5	61.1	7.6

angiomatoid subtypes, which also show typical clinical and biological criteria (age, localization, frequency of recurrence, and metastasis).

In our material of 50 MFH, the storiform–pleomorphic subtype was largely predominant (45 cases); two others presented the myxoid, two the inflammatory, and one the giant cell subtype. Histological grading distinguished two tumors of grade 1, nine of grade 2, and 39 of grade 3. The sex distribution was approximately balanced, with a characteristic peak in later adulthood (mean age 59 years). The preferential occurrence at the extremities (74%), with preponderance of the femoral region (60%) was equally typical.

DNA cytometry revealed DNA aneuploid stemlines in 88% (44/50) of cases, and at least some single cell aneuplody in the small number of peridiploid tumors. Compared to the grading categories, the two grade 1 tumors were DNA peridiploid with single cell aneuploidy; both were classified as myxoid MFH. No fundamental differences were found between the grade 2 and grade 3 tumors with regard to rate and degree of DNA stemline aneuploidy. In addition to the aneuploid stemline, a peridiploid stemline was found in 35 of 44 tumors. Like myxoid MFH, the less malignant angiomatoid MFH seem to comprise, according to PETTINATO et al. (1990), a much lower proportion of DNA aneuploid stemlines than all other MFH; this suggests a close correlation between grade of malignancy and DNA stemline ploidy in this tumor category (RADIO et al. 1988; BECKER et al. 1991).

3.3 Lipomatous Tumors

3.3.1 Lipoma, Angiolipoma

From the group of benign lipomatous tumors we recorded and studied five simple lipomas, five spindle cell lipomas, five angiolipomas, and two intramuscular lipomas. All of them were found to be DNA peridiploid in ICM, spindle cell lipomas and angiolipomas bearing a principally higher amount of proliferating cells than the other varieties. No remarkable single cell aneuploidies could be observed in any tumors of the entire group, although pleomorphic and atypical lipomas, however, had not been included.

3.3.2 Liposarcoma

While the different subtypes of lipoma are mainly found in subcutaneous fatty tissue, liposarcomas (LS) arise from immature mesenchymal cells in deeper soft tissue, most frequently affecting the proximal extremities and the trunk, especially the retroperitoneal region (KATENKAMP and STILLER

1990). The 45 liposarcomas analysed in our study showed typical patterns of localization, age, and sex (Table 2).

Histological classification currently distinguishes these tumors (EN-ZINGER and WEISS 1988) as lipoma-like, sclerosing, inflammatory, myxoid, round cell, and pleomorphic subtypes. In 23 cases of mixed differentiation, the tissue variety with the least favorable appearance was appraised for classification. The pattern of LS subtypes corresponds largely to histological grading insofar as lipoma-like and sclerosing LS are recorded as grade 1 malignancies. Among our 21 myxoid LS, six had already attained grade 2, the seven round cell LS were classified as grade 2 or 3, and 15 pleomorphic LS were defined as grade 3, according to schedule. Round cell and pleomorphic LS, metastasizing more frequently and so displaying higher malignancy ($n < 22$) differed from the types with lower malignancy ($n = 23$) also in that they occurred significantly later (mean age of onset 55.2 vs. 46.0 years, $p = 0.01$).

DNA ploidy was found to correlate with subtyping approximately in parallel with histological grading. While lipoma-like and sclerosing LS were DNA peridiploid, six among the 21 myxoid LS were distinctly DNA hyperdiploid (28.6%). Two of 15 peridiploid tumors showed at least a marked single cell aneuploidy. Among round cell LS, three of seven cases were aneuploid (47.9%), while all but two of 15 pleomorphic LS showed distinct aneuploidy of DNA stemlines (86.7%). In these two peridiploid tumors, however, single cell aneuploidy was strongly marked.

Liposarcomas thus showed a considerable correlation between DNA ploidy and histological subtypes. The χ-square test resulted in $p < 0.05$ for lipoma-like, sclerosing, myxoid vs. round cell and pleomorphic LS. Only in myxoid and round cell LS may DNA ploidy offer a criterion with some additional prognostic potential. Correlation of DNA ploidy and cytological grading is equally close, and so the information value of DNA ploidy may not go very much beyond that of histological evaluation in terms of prognosis. The (rather incomplete) clinical course reports are another point in favor. Nevertheless, the results of DNA cytometry may support the validity of histological subtyping with regard to malignancy.

3.4 Smooth Muscle Tumors

3.4.1 Leiomyoma

Ten leiomyomas of the skin, and five such tumors of the deeper soft tissue were studied, but none of them revealed any sign of stemline aneuploidy. Two larger retroperitoneal leiomyomas, partly with regressive changes, showed local evidence of single cell aneuploidy.

3.4.2 Leiomyosarcoma

Leiomyosarcomas (LMS) of soft tissue present, despite considerable histological and cytological uniformity, a rather heterogenous picture with
regard to prognosis, probably due to the impact of their different localizations. We have to distinguish LMS of the retroperitoneal or abdominal
region from those of dermis and subcutis, and also from those of the
vascular wall and deeper peripheral soft tissue (KATENKAMP and STILLER
1990). Retroperitoneal and abdominal LMS are the most frequent, and also
the tumors with the worst prognosis, comprising 36.6% (22/60) of our
material. The entire group is well balanced in its sex distribution and typical
in its age structure with a mean incidence at 58.3 years. Histological grading
revealed a distinct accumulation of grade 2 tumors (Table 3).

The aneuploidy rate of LMS was average with 71.7% (43/60), and with
a slight trend to correlate with tumor diameter. There was also a distinct
increase of aneuploidies in parallel with grading. A comparison of DNA
stemline ploidies between trunkal tumors and those located at the extremities revealed a virtually higher aneuploidy rate in trunkal tumors (81.3%
= 26/32 vs. 64.7% = 11/17), most likely due to the principally larger size of
trunkal tumors, mostly twice that of the limb tumors (12.4 cm vs. 5.7 cm,
$p < 0.01$).

Truly representative survival curves cannot as yet be drawn from the
clinical data at our disposal. Among the 22 patients who have died in the
meantime, six had a peridiploid tumor (6/17 = 35.5%), the remaining 16
had an aneuploid tumor (16/43 = 37.9%), but no clear prognostic significance of DNA ploidy can be deduced from these data. There was, however, a
distinct trend insofar as the death rates increased with the grades: among
grade 1 patients, 3/12 = 25% died; in grade 2, 13/36 = 36.1%; in grade 3,
6/12 = 50%. As mentioned by OLIVER et al. (1991), there was a close
correlation between DNA ploidy and metastatic spread. Metastases occurred in only four of the 17 peridiploid tumors (23.5), but in 22 of the 43
DNA aneuploid tumors (51.2%).

3.5 Rhabdomyosarcoma

Investigations covered a total of 52 rhabdomyosarcomas (RMS); 29 cases
were embryonal RMS, ten pleomorphic RMS, and 13 alveolar RMS. The
group of embryonal RMS comprised 12 male and 17 female patients aged
2–78 years (mean age 17.4 years), that of alveolar RMS consisted of eight
male and five female patients aged 1–34 years (mean age 15.8 years), and
that of pleomorphic RMS three male and seven female patients aged 30–79
years (mean 57.7 years). Seventeen tumors were located in the head and
neck region, ten tumors in the urogenital region, 12 were localized at the

Table 3. Grading, DNA ploidy, and some prognostic data

Histological type	Malignancy grades[a]				DNA stemline aneuploidy (%)	Single cell aneuploidy[b] (%)	Metastases[c] (%)	Died of disease[c] (%)
	1 (n)	2 (n)	3 (n)	4 (n)				
Fibrosarcoma	7	5			25.0	–	33.0	33.0
MFH	2	9	39		88.0	100.0	22.0	22.0
Liposarcoma	17	8	20		48.9	17.4	35.5	42.2
Lipoma-like/ sclerosing| myxoid	17	6			26.1	17.6	26.1	30.4
Round cell		2	5		42.9	0.0	42.9	57.1
Pleomorphic			15		86.7	100.0	46.7	53.3
Leiomyosarcoma	13	31	16		71.7	29.4	43.3	36.7
Rhabdomyosarcoma	8	7	24	13	71.2	3.8	53.8	40.4
Embryonal	8	7	14		55.2	15.4	37.9	41.4
Alveolar				13	84.6	0.0	76.9	46.2
Pleomorphic			10		100.0	0.0	70.0	30.0
Angiosarcoma	1		10		62.5	33.3	37.5	43.8
Synovial sarcoma	3	5	20	7	24.0	0.0	36.0	42.0
Spindle cell	2	20	8		34.6	0.0	38.5	38.5
Biphasic	1	16	4		11.1	0.0	33.3	44.4
Synovioblastic		4		15	13.3	0.0	33.3	46.7
Diffuse mesothelioma	13	24	16		41.5	0.0	0.0	100.0
Epitheloid	13	16			37.9	0.0	0.0	100.0
Biphasic		8	12		45.0	27.3	0.0	100.0
Sarcomatous			4		50.0	50.0	0.0	100.0
Malignant schwannoma	15	23	8		65.2	12.5	21.7	34.8
Neuroblastoma	7	11	6		70.8	0.0	66.7	16.7
PNET/Ewing's sarcoma				20	30.0	0.0	25.0	30.0
Spindle cell sarcomas	37	68	63	72	70.8	29.2	30.4	31.5
Round cell sarcomas					50.0	0.0	50.0	31.9

[a] The definition of grading as applied to the respective tumor type, is given in Sect. 2.1.2.
[b] Single cell aneuploidy is only applied to cases without DNA stemline aneuploidy.
[c] The data on incidence of metastases and on death from the disease are related to all tumors of the respective entity, irrespective of the time of first diagnosis; they are incomplete for several tumor types, and so the whole set gives only a rather vague clue with regard to prognosis.

trunk, and 13 at the extremities. Embryonal RMS were found preferentially in the head and neck and urogenital regions, alveolar RMS predominantly at the extremities, and pleomorphic RMS at the trunk and extremities (Table 2).

In ICM, embryonal RMS showed by far the lowest rate of DNA stemline aneuploidies with 55.2% (16/29). In contrast, lack of aneuploidy is quite exceptional in alveolar and pleomorphic RMS (DNA aneuploidy rates of 84.6% and 100%, respectively). Diploid embryonal RMS occurred mostly in the urogenital region (seven out of ten cases) and, as a rule, in relatively well-differentiated, poorly cellular botryoid RMS. While the RMS of this type had an aneuploidy rate of only 37.3% (in three out of eight cases), the rate was distinctly higher (61.9%, 13/21 cases) in the embryonal RMS of medium or high malignancy. Embryonal RMS differed from the alveolar and pleomorphic types insofar as the grade of DNA aneuploidy was less pronounced. The mean DNA index of aneuploid embryonal RMS was only 1.74, that is, markedly lower ($p < 0.05$) than the mean DI of aneuploid alveolar (1.89) and pleomorphic RMS (2.11). Consequently, RMS show a distinct and close correlation between rate and degree of DNA aneuploidy and the histological grade of malignancy.

Considering the relatively even ratio of peridiploid and aneuploid tumors (rate of aneuploidy: 16/29 = 55.2%), the prognostic aspect of ploidy assessment is of particular interest in embryonal RMS. Clinical follow up for 3 years was available for 18 cases of embryonal RMS. Astonishingly, among the 11 patients with aneuploidies, seven survived this time, whereas only one of seven patients with peridiploidy survived. Possibly the better response of aneuploid tumors to chemotherapy is responsible for this effect (Shapiro et al. 1991); however, three of the seven surviving patients with DNA aneuploidies died after the first 3 years.

3.6 Vascular Tumors

3.6.1 Hemangioma

Ten capillary and ten cavernous hemangiomas of various localizations were investigated. The capillary hemangiomas comprised two juvenile tumors with partly spindle cell components. All hemangiomas showed unimodal DNA diploidy, and there was no evidence of any single cell aneuploidy. A similar bland DNA distribution was observed in an additional case of papillary endothelial hyperplasia (so-called Masson's pseudoangiosarcoma).

3.6.2 Hemangiopericytoma

Five cases of safely diagnosed hemangiopericytoma were studied. Two of them were localized at the femur, the others in the popliteal, cervical, and thyroid region, respectively. There were three male and two female patients aged 28–74 years (mean: 46.2 years). All tumors had been resected locally; three cases had recurrences, and one of them also bone metastases. ICM revealed only one peridiploid DNA distribution with a distinct proportion of cells in S and G_2 phases, and a merely sporadic appearance of hypertetraploid cells. Thus, no criteria of definite malignancy were ascertained (Table 1).

3.6.3 Angiosarcomas

The primary localizations of 16 angiosarcomas investigated in this study were in the thyroid (five), mamma (one), spleen (one), and in the skin or underlying soft tissues (nine). The male/female ratio was 1. The tumor diameters ranged from 1 to 18 cm (mean size: 6.3 cm); most lesions had undergone radical surgery (ten), partly with postoperative radiotherapy.

Histologically, ten of 16 tumors showed high-grade malignancy (grade 3) and a clear stemline aneuploidy with DIs of more than 1.5. In contrast, all other tumors with low or medium-grade malignancy (grades 1–2) manifested DNA peridiploidy. Angiosarcomas thus revealed a particularly close correlation between cytological grading and DNA ploidy. In ten patients with average clinical follow up (3 years), no correlation was found with cytological grade nor with DNA ploidy. Seven of these ten have died in the meantime (Table 3). In contrast to these conventional angiosarcomas, Kaposi's sarcoma nearly always shows DNA peridiploid stemlines (FUKUNAGA and SILVERBERG 1990; DICTOR et al. 1991).

3.7 Synovial Tissue Tumors

3.7.1 Localized Giant Cell Tumor of Tendon Sheath

Ten tumors of this type were studied, always revealing, as expected, diploid DNA distribution with low proliferative activity (Table 1).

3.7.2 Synovial Sarcoma

Among the 50 synovial sarcomas studied, 26 tumors showed almost exclusively spindle cell differentiation, nine clearly biphasic differentiation, and 15 were predominantly or entirely synovioblastic sarcomas (Table 2). The patients, 29 male and 21 female, were aged 8–77 years, with a distinct peak around the age of 30. Twenty-seven tumors were localized at the lower extremity, nine tumors at the upper extremity, and 14 at the trunk or in the head and neck region. Histological differentiation correlated neither with age, nor with sex, nor with localization. Tumor sizes varied between 1 and 20 cm (mean diameter 7.8 cm). Synovioblastic tumors were comparatively larger than the spindle cell variety (mean 9.9 vs. 6.3 cm).

Image cytometry revealed an overall aneuploidy rate of only 24% (12/50). A rather low rate of DNA aneuploidy was also found by EL-NAGGAR et al. (1990). The rate was distinctly higher in spindle cell tumors (34.6% = 9/26) than in biphasic (1/9) and synovioblastic sarcomas (2/15) where aneuploidy is obviously a sporadic event. The grade of DNA aneuploidy was also more marked in spindle cell tumors (average DI 1.62 vs. 1.47). On the whole, DNA aneuploid tumors were only slightly larger than the peridiploid lesions (mean diameters: 8.7 cm vs. 7.5 cm).

Among the 25 patients with 3-year follow up, ten died in this period, and 11 died after the third year, a rate that stresses the known high malignancy of synovial sarcoma. Of eight patients with tumor grades 1 or 2, six survived the first 3 years, but only eight of the 17 patients with grade 3 and 4 tumors, and so we may infer the higher aggressiveness of poorly differentiated tumors. Nevertheless, seven of our eight original collective of grade 1 and 2 patients are now dead, as well as 14 of our original group of 17 grade 3 and 4 cases, and so histological grading seems to have no long-term prognostic significance. Neither was DNA ploidy a truly effective tool: after the first 3 years, about half of the patients were living in the groups with DNA peridiploid (9/18) and with DNA aneuploid tumors (4/7).

3.8 Diffuse Mesothelioma

The diffuse mesotheliomas included in this study were provided by the Mesothelioma Registry of Bochum (Pathologisches Institut, Krankenanstalten Bergmannsheil). The well-documented corpus of 53 pleural mesotheliomas comprised surgical resections in 32 and necropsy material in 21 cases. Dependent on the occupational structure of the case material, only four women were listed. The age distribution was typical. The material showed strictly epitheloid tumors in 29 cases, exclusively spindle cell/sarcomatous differentiation in four cases, and concomitance of both types in the remaining 20 cases.

The overall stemline aneuploidy rate was 41.5% (in 22/53), in approximation to FCM results of such cases (FRIERSON et al. 1987; BURMER et al. 1989; DAZZI et al. 1990; PYRHONEN et al. 1991). In epitheloid tumor sections, the rate was distinctly, though not significantly, lower (32.7% = 11 of 49) than in spindle cell/sarcomatous lesions (45.9% = 11 of 24). This may be interpreted as an indicator of aneuploidy coinciding with advancing dedifferentiation. Since curative management is not possible in most cases of diffuse mesothelioma, DNA ploidy currently does not play any significant role in clinical practice.

In 29 of 53 cases, the density of asbestos bodies within the tissue was more than 1000 per cm^3. These patients were significantly younger than the remaining 24 with lower density values. Aneuploidy rates were virtually higher in patients with a higher asbestos load (52%) than in the cases with lesser values (29%), which suggests an indirect correlation between asbestos load and aneuploidy rates; of course, the observation must be confirmed by further study.

3.9 Tumors of the Peripheral Nerves

3.9.1 Neurofibroma, Benign Schwannoma

Our material on benign tumors of peripheral nerves included ten benign schwannomas and ten neurofibromas. Four of the latter had occurred in the course of Recklinghausen's disease. All were DNA diploid tumors, and the proportion of proliferating cells correlated appreciably with cellularity. Three degenerating benign schwannomas and two partly regressing neurofibromas showed distinct single cell aneuploidies which, however, cannot be taken as signs of malignancy in these cases.

3.9.2 Malignant Schwannoma

The 46 cases of malignant schwannoma (MS) presented, as a rule, as solitary MS unassociated with Recklinghausen's disease; the latter was diagnosed in only six cases. The patients were typically middle aged (mean 47.6 years) with a certain prevalence of females (26/46 = 56.5%). With regard to localization, we found the usual predilection of the extremities near the trunk with, however, an increased occurrence in the head and neck region (6/46). Cytological grading recorded a slight peak in tumors of medium grades (Table 3).

The overall rate of stemline DNA aneuploidy was 65.2%. Four peridiploid tumors showed distinct single cell aneuploidies. The rate of aneuploidies correlated significantly with cytological grading (χ square test: $p = 0.05$). Stemline aneuploidy was found in only one third of grade 1 tumors, but in about 80% of grade 2 and 3 tumors. The only peridiploid tumor of grade 3 had at least a conspicuous single cell aneuploidy reflected by a certain pleomorphism and more or less abundant giant cells visible even in routine histology. In tumors of the trunkal and head and neck region, aneuploidy rates were generally higher than in tumors of the extremities (17/23 vs. 13/23), probably due to the advanced local spread of the former (mean diameters: 13 cm vs. 8.3 cm).

Complete information about clinical 3-year follow up is available in only 12 of our cases, and so we are unable to draw representative Kaplan-Meier curves. Of 16 patients dying over the years, four had peridiploid (4/17 = 23.5%), and the remaining 12 had aneuploid tumors (12/29 = 41.4%), which at least suggests a trend towards the somewhat poorer prognosis of aneuploid tumors. However, the proportion of casualties was no lower among patients with grade 1 tumors (6/15 = 40%) than among patients with grade 2 or 3 tumors (10/31 = 32.3%).

3.10 Neuroblastoma

Included here are only neuroblastomas in the strictest sense, i.e., sympathetic neuroblastomas. In our 24 cases we found a very slight overbalance of the male sex (13/24) and a typical age distribution (under 1–15 years), only four of 24 patients being over 5 years of age. Retroperitoneal or abdominal localization was found in 20 cases. Five tumors were in stage III, 15 in stage IV, and four tumors in stage IVs, all requiring chemotherapy. The tumors measuring up to 15 cm partly showed strong regressive changes. Adopting the classification of HUGHES et al. (1974), we found seven tumors of grade 1, 11 of grade 2, and 6 of grade 3 (Table 3).

Seventeen of our 24 neuroblastomas showed DNA stemline aneuploidy (70.8%) with a distinct accumulation (peak) in the triploid range (13 cases). A further four tumors were tetraploid, and seven were DNA peridiploid. The latter were a bit more frequent among grade 1 tumors than among grades 2 and 3 (3/7 vs. 4/11); similar observations were made by BERGER et al. (1991). The proportion of DNA aneuploidies was higher in the first 2 years than among older patients (9/10 vs. 8/14). The trend correlated with the majority of undifferentiated tumors among the younger patients. No correlation was found between DNA ploidy and tumor stages.

Of seven patients with peridiploid tumors, three have died in the meantime, while of the 17 DNA aneuploid cases 15 are still living. Owing to very different periods of follow up (4–83 months), no reliable data can be derived about the possible prognostic relevance of DNA ploidy. Nevertheless, the apparently favorable course observed in aneuploid tumor cases may help to confirm other studies proposing that DNA aneuploid tumors respond particularly well to chemotherapy (GANSLER et al. 1986; BOURHIS et al. 1991a,b; NAITO et al. 1991).

3.11 Primitive Neuroectodermal Tumor and Extraskeletal Ewing's Sarcoma

Twenty tumors were available in this group, clearly identified as primitive neuroectodermal tumor (PNET) by histomorphological (pseudorosettes) and immunohistological criteria (neuron-specific enolase, NSE, and/or S 100) in 14 cases. The patient group comprised 12 males and eight females aged 8–64 years (mean age 25.4). The six patients with Askin tumor were considerably younger (mean age 20 years). Localizations of the lesions were nine on the trunk, five at the lower extremity, three at the upper extremity, and three in the head and neck region (Table 2).

DNA stemline aneuploidies were found in only six of 20 cases (30%). This rate is not much higher than that assessed for skeletal Ewing's sarcoma (8/38 = 21.1%) investigated by the Bone Tumor Registry of Westphalia in another study (MELLIN et al., in preparation). Distinct single cell aneuploidies were not found. Complete clinical follow up over several years is available in only nine of 20 cases, not permitting any conclusions with regard to the prognostic relevance of DNA ploidy.

3.12 DNA Ploidy and Prognosis in Pleomorphic Sarcomas, Spindle Cell Sarcomas, and in Round Cell Sarcomas

The different types of soft tissue sarcoma partly share some morphological features which may preclude unequivocal classification. Judged by somewhat simplified cytomorphological criteria, soft tissue sarcomas may be differentiated into spindle cell, small and round cell, and pleomorphic tumors.

The pleomorphic sarcomas (e.g., pleomorphic LS, RMS, MFH, or dedifferentiated LMS, MS) must be appraised in principle as highly malignant lesions, as reflected in a high rate of DNA stemline aneuploidy (63/70 = 90.0%). Since the few peridiploid cases show at least pronounced single cell aneuploidies, DNA cytometry fails to provide additional information of clinical relevance in these types.

Conditions in soft tissue sarcomas of spindle cell morphology are quite different on account of the wide spectrum, from low to high malignancy, reflected in the varied grading.

In this respect, fibrosarcomas belong mainly to the lesions of lower or intermediate malignancy, while MFH are predominantly of higher malignancy; LMS and MS, however, show a relatively even distribution among all grades. In fact, grading in these tumors depends mainly on criteria of cell proliferation and the amount of cellular atypia, which may suggest that considering them as a group is appropriate. In contrast, spindle cell synovial sarcomas display only different grades of cell maturation, and they were therefore excluded from prognostic evaluation in common with other spindle cell sarcomas.

Among our collective of 168 spindle cell sarcomas we distinguished 60 LMS, 46 MS, 50 MFH, and 12 fibrosarcomas. By cytological grading they were classified as 37 tumors of grade 1, 68 of grade 2, and 63 of grade 3.

Grading results were largely independent of tumor size (maximum average diameters 9.6 cm in grade 1, 9.9 cm in grade 2, 10.1 cm in grade 3 tumors).

DNA stemline aneuploidies were identified in 120 tumors (71.7%). The mean size of aneuploid tumors was barely greater than that of peridiploid tumors (9.9 cm vs. 9.2 cm), so we failed to define any significant correlation between tumor size and DNA ploidy. Ploidy rates did increase in parallel with the grade of malignancy (Fig. 2): the rate of aneuploidies was significantly lower in grade 1 than in grades 2 and 3, the latter showing only a certain trend of gradual difference. In 14 of 48 cases with DNA peridiploid stemlines we noted some single cell aneuploidies, and seven of these 14 were identified as grade 3 tumors.

Sufficiently complete clinical data of 3-year follow up were available in only 74 cases. The clinical course of DNA aneuploid tumors was distinctly worse than in DNA peridiploid lesions (Fig. 3). Among the patients with peridiploid tumors, mortality was higher in those with evidence of single cell aneuploidy (5/8 vs. 7/19), most likely due to the higher proportion of grade 3 tumors. Cytological grading, however, yielded a better stratification than the assessment of DNA ploidy, although the low number of cases failed to give statistical significance (Fig. 4). All in all, our results suggest that DNA stemline ploidy will not offer much additional prognostic data for spindle cell sarcomas beyond the results obtained by cytological grading. Some relevance, however, may be gathered in grade 1 tumors of this kind since the presence of DNA aneuploidies would predict a less favorable course.

If the above group of spindle cell type (soft tissue) sarcomas ($n = 168$) is compared with spindle cell synovial sarcomas ($n = 26$), the most striking feature is the significantly lower rate of aneuploidies in the latter ($9/26 = 34.6\%$ vs. $120/168 = 71.7\%$; $p < 0.0005$). In 16 synovial spindle cell sarcomas with documented clinical follow up during the first 3 years,

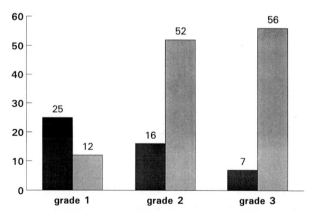

Fig. 2. Grades of malignancy and DNA stemline ploidy in spindle cell sarcomas. *Dark columns*, DNA peridiploid; *light columns*, DNA aneudiploid

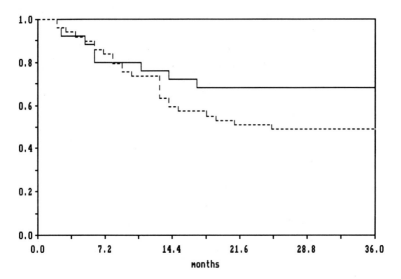

Fig. 3. Kaplan-Meier curves of DNA peridiploid (*solid line*; n = 25) and DNA aneuploid (*broken line*; n = 49) spindle cell sarcomas. Not significant

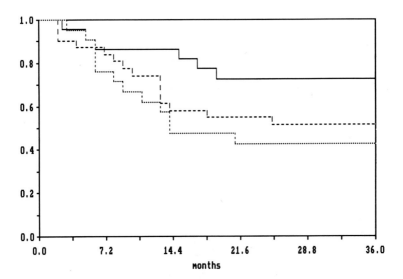

Fig. 4. Kaplan-Meier curves of spindle cell sarcomas in malignancy grades 1 (*solid line*; n = 22), 2 (*broken line*; n = 31) and 3 (*dotted line*; n = 21). Not significant

no prognostic differences could be observed between DNA peridiploid and DNA aneuploid tumors, and this would also be a distinctive difference from the remaining larger group of spindle cell (soft tissue) sarcomas.

The group of small and round cell (soft tissue) sarcomas comprised 72 cases, i.e., 24 neuroblastomas, 20 PNETs or extraskeletal Ewing's sarcomas, 15 synovioblastic synovial sarcomas, and 13 alveolar RMS. Aneuploidy rates varied rather strongly among these types. With the exception of two cases, alevolar RMS were DNA aneuploid (84.6%) with a typical peak in the tetraploid region (8/11). Still above 50% was the aneuploidy rate among sympathetic neuroblastomas (17/24 = 70.8%), with a typical peak of aneuploid indexes in the triploid region (13/17). The six aneuploid cases of PNET/Ewing's sarcoma (30%), too, showed DIs in the triploid region, while the two synvioblastic synovial sarcomas (2/15 = 13.3%) had DIs of 1.3 and 1.7, respectively.

The only currently evaluable prognostic data were collected in neuroblastomas, as already mentioned. In alveolar RMS, in synovioblastic synovial sarcomas, and in PNET/Ewing's sarcoma there is no convincing material suggesting a prognostic relevance of DNA ploidy assessment, since even peridiploid lesions are eventually to be classified as anaplastic tumors. Whether DNA aneuploid tumors will actually respond better to chemotherapy, as has been shown in neuroblastoma and in childhood RMS (GANSLER et al. 1986; BOURHIS et al. 1991a,b; NAITO et al. 1991; SHAPIRO et al. 1991), must be carefully ascertained in the other types of round cell sarcomas.

While sympathetic neuroblastomas are readily diagnosed, in general, by way of characteristic clinical and morphological findings, the differential diagnostic distinction of all other round cell sarcomas is much more difficult. Transitional forms between synovioblastic synovial sarcoma, for instance, and extraskeletal Ewing's sarcoma are often fleeting, and even immunohistological markers are usually unhelpful in this field. Since aneuploidy rates are comparatively low in both skeletal and extraskeletal Ewing's sarcomas as well as in synovioblastic synovial sarcomas, ploidy assessment cannot assist differential diagnosis either. If, however, cytometry reveals peritetraploid round cell sarcomas, alveolar RMS will be the first diagnosis to be considered (MOLENAAR et al. 1988; SHAPIRO et al. 1991).

4 Conclusions

That no DNA stemline aneuploidy was found among the 118 clearly benign soft tissue tumors investigated in this study, may emphasize the high specificity of this marker for malignancy, but also means the absence of false positivity in the evaluation of histological slides subjected to DNA ICM on the basis of our definition of DNA stemline aneuploidy (DI over 1.2). This is particularly important when the method is applied to diagnostic practice. Single cell aneuploidy, in contrast, was by no means uncommon in benign tumors (especially in leiomyoma, benign schwannoma, neurofibroma), and so cannot be taken as a criterium for evaluating the biological behavior of soft tissue tumors.

All our 20 cases of aggressive fibromatosis were peridiploid (even without single cell aneuploidies), whereas DNA stemline aneuploidy was found in one of the ten dermatofibrosarcomas. DNA stemline aneuploidy was also present in two of three atypical fibroxanthomas studied, which must be interpreted as of at least a doubtful biological nature. Nevertheless, a third of these cases showed stronger single cell aneuploidy. None of our five hemangiopericytomas showed DNA stemline aneuploidy, although one of them was identified as a malignant tumor with positive evidence of metastases.

In the group of sarcomas proper, the round cell/anaplastic types predominant in childhood and young adults have to be distinguished from the types predominating the adult and older groups. Among round cell sarcomas, synovioblastic synovial sarcomas, Ewing's sarcomas, and PNETs are characterized by a rather minor aneuploidy rate (maximum 30%), in contrast to their high actual malignancy, with a typical absence of single cell aneuploidies. In contrast, alveolar RMS are characterized by a very high aneuploidy rate (11/13 = 84.6%) with typically tetraploid DIs, which may even serve as a differential diagnostic criterium. Neuroblastomas are predominantly aneuploid with typical DIs in the triploid range.

The spindle cell group of soft tissue sarcomas (fibrosarcoma, MS, LMS, MFH) are characterized by a close correlation between cytological grading of malignancy, and DNA stemline aneuploidy plus single cell aneuploidy. In fact, the expression of DNA ploidy may influence, more or less consciously, the performance of grading which additionally reflects the cytological criteria of proliferation. This may be one important reason why cytological grading secures a better stratification than the assessment of DNA stemline ploidy. As far as we can judge today, DNA cytometry will be of practical (prognostic) value only in grade 1 tumors where the evidence of DNA aneuploidy predicts a less favorable outcome.

Spindle cell synovial sarcomas occupy an extra position among the whole group of spindle cell sarcomas due to their rather low aneuploidy rate (9/26 = 34.6%). The particular character also results from the occasional occurrence of immature, synovioblastic areas, and from the average onset at a distinctly younger age. Beyond this, DNA ploidy appears prognostically rather meaningless in synovial sarcomas of generally high malignancy.

Pleomorphic sarcomas are principally seen as highly malignant tumors with almost exclusive DNA aneuploidy, and so DNA cytmetry may be superfluous as an additional method. LS show a particularly close correlation of DNA ploidy with histological subtyping and grading, and here, too, DNA cytometry will not offer much additional information. Angiosarcomas also show the close correlation between DNA ploidy and grading, but the actual prognostic relevance of ploidy is hard to ascertain. In diffuse mesotheliomas we see an appropriate balance of DNA peridiploid and aneuploid tumors but, on account of their overall poor prognosis, this information is of merely academic interest at present.

In contrast, embryonal RMS with DNA stemline aneuploidy will show a more favorable clinical course than those with DNA peridiploidy, most likely due to a better response of aneuploid tumors to chemotherapy. A comparable behavior has been observed in sympathetic neuroblastoma. Similar favorable results from new modes of therapy may eventually induce a change in the prognostic relevance of DNA stemline ploidy, also in some other types of soft tissue sarcomas.

References

Alvegard TA, Berg NO, Baldetrop B, Fernö M, Kilander D, Ranstam J, Rydholm A, Akerman M (1990) Cellular DNA content and prognosis of high-grade soft tissue sarcoma: the Scandinavian Sarcoma Group experience. J Clin Oncol 8: 538–547

Becker RL, Venzon D, Lack EE, Mikel UV, Weiss SW, O'Leary TJ (1991) Cytometry and morphometry of malignant fibrous histiocytoma of the extremities. Prediction of metastasis and mortality. Am J Surg Pathol 15: 957–964

Berger K, Harms D, Denk H, Beck JD (1991) Impulse cytophotometric determination of the DNA content of paraffin-fixed neuroblastoma. Monatsschr Kinderheilkd 139: 216–219

Biesterfeld S, Böcking A (1990) Methodological requirements for precise measurements using DNA single cell cytometry. Verh Dtsch Ges Pathol 74: 199–202

Böcking A, Auffermann W (1986) Algorithm for DNA-cytophotometric diagnosis and grading of malignancy. Anal Quant Cytol 8: 363–369

Böhm N (1968) Einfluß der Fixierung und der Säurekonzentration auf die Feulgen-Hydrolyse bei 28°C. Histochemie 14: 201–211

Bourhis J, De-Vathaire F, Wilson GD, Hartmann O,, Terrier-Lacombe MJ, Boccon-Gibod L, McNally NJ, Lemerle J, Riou G, Benard J (1991a) Combined analysis of DNA ploidy index and N-myc genomic content in neuroblastoma. Cancer Res 51: 33–36

Bourhis J, Dominici C, McDowell H, Raschella G, Wilson G, Castello MA, Plouvier E, Lemerle J, Riou G, Benard J, et al. (1991b) N-myc genomic content and DNA ploidy in stage IVs neuroblastoma. J Clin Oncol 9: 1371–1375

Brooks JJ (1986) The significance of double phenotypic patterns and markers in human sarcomas: a new model of mesenchymal differentiation. Am J Pathol 125: 113–123

Brown DC, Theaker JM, Banks PM, Gatter KC, Mason DY (1987) Cytokeratin expression in smooth muscle tumours. Histopathology 11: 477–486

Burmer GC, Rabinovitch PS, Kulander BG, Rusch V, McNutt MA (1989) Flow cytometric analysis of malignant pleural mesotheliomas. Hum Pathol 20: 777–783

Carlsen NL, Mortensen BT, Andersson PK, Larsen JK, Nielson OH, Tommerup N (1991) Chromosome abnormalities, cellular DNA content, oncogene amplification and growth pattern in agar culture of human neuroblastomas. Anticancer Res 11: 353–358

Coindre JM, Bui NB, Bonichon F, de Mascarel I, Trojani M (1988a) Histopathologic grading in spindle cell soft tissue sarcomas. Cancer 61: 2305–2309

Coindre JM, de Mascarel A, Trojani M, de Mascarel I, Pages A (1988b) Immunohistochemical study of rhabdomyosarcoma. Unexpected staining with S-100 protein and cytokeratin. J Pathol 155: 127–132

Dazzi H, Thatcher N, Hasleton PS, Chatterjee AJ, Lawson AM (1990) DNA analysis by flow cytometry in malignant pleural mesothelioma: relationship to histology and survival. J Pathol 162: 51–55

Dewhirst MW, Sostman HD, Leopold KA et al. (1990) Soft tissue sarcomas: MR imaging and MR spectroscopy for prognosis and therapy monitoring. Radiology 174: 847–853

Dictor M, Ferno M, Baldetorp B (1991) Flow cytometric DNA content in Kaposi's sarcoma by histologic stage. Comparison with angiosarcoma. Anal Quant Cytol Histol 13: 201–208

Donhuijsen K (1986) Reproducibility and significance in grading of malignancy. Hum Pathol 17: 1122–1125

Donner LR (1991) Cytogenetics and molecular biology of small round-cell tumors and related neoplasms. Current status. Cancer Genet Cytogenet 54: 1–10

Eilber FR, Huth JF, Mirra J, Rosen G (1990) Progress in the recognition and treatment of soft tissue sarcomas. Cancer 65: 660–666

El-Jabhour JN, Wilson GD, Bennett MH, Burke MM, Davey AT, Eames K (1991) Flow cytometric study of nodular fasciitis, proliferative fasciitis, and proliferative myositis. Hum Pathol 22: 1146–1149

El-Naggar AK, Ayala AG, Abdul-Karim FW, McLemore D, HTL (ASCP), Ballance WW, Garnsey L, Ro JY, Batsakis JG (1990) Synovial sarcoma. A DNA flow cytometric study. Cancer 65: 2295–2300

Enzinger F, Weiss S (1988) Soft tissue tumors. Mosby, St Louis

Fisher C (1990) The value of electron microscopy and immunohistochemistry in the diagnosis of soft tissue sarcomas: a study of 200 cases. Histopathology 16: 441–454

Frierson HF, Mills SE, Legier JF (1987) Flow cytometric analysis of ploidy in immunohisto-chemically confirmed examples of malignant epithelial mesothelioma. Am J Clin Pathol 90: 240–243

Fukunaga M, Silverberg SG (1990) Kaposi's sarcoma in patients with acquired immune deficiency syndrome. A flow cytometric DNA analysis of 26 lesions in 26 patients. Cancer 66: 758–764

Gansler T, Chatten J, Varello M, Bunin GR, Atkinson B (1986) Flow cytometric DNA analysis of neuroblastoma. Correlation with histology and clinical outcome. Cancer 58: 2453–2455

Hedley DW, Friedlander ML, Taylor IW, Rugg CA, Musgrove EA (1983) Method for analysis of cellular DNA content of paraffin-embedded pathological material using flow cytometry. J Histochem Cytochem 31: 1333–1335

Hughes M, Marsden HB, Palmer HK (1974) Histologic patterns of neuroblastoma related to prognosis and clinical staging. Cancer 34: 1706–1712

Jovanovic R, Hacker GW, Falkmer UG, Falkmer S, Mendel L, Graf AH, Hoog A, Kanjuh V, Silfversward C, Grimelius L (1991) Paragangliomas: neuroendocrine features and cytometric DNA distribution patterns. A clinico-pathological study of 22 cases. Virchows Arch [A] 419: 455–461

Katenkamp D (1988) Cellular heterogeneity. Explanation for changing of tumor phenotype and biologic behaviour in soft tissue sarcomas. Pathol Res Pract 183: 698–705

Katenkamp D, Stiller D (1990) Weichgewebstumoren. Pathologie, histologische Diagnose und Differentialdiagnose. Barth, Leibzig

Knight JC (1990) The molecular genetics of soft tissue sarcomas. Br J Cancer 26: 511–513

Kreicbergs A, Tribukait B, Willems J, Bauer HCF (1987) DNA flow analysis of soft tissue tumors. Cancer 59: 128–133

Li S (1990) Flow cytometric analysis of DNA from 98 cases of soft tissue tumors and its clinical significance. Chung Hua Wai Ko Tsa Chih 28: 281–284

Mandard AM, Petiot JF, Marnay J, Mandard JC, Chasle J, de Ranieri E, Dupin P, Herlin P, de Ranieri J, Tanguy A, Boulier N, Abbatucci S (1989) Prognostic factors in soft tissue sarcomas. Cancer 63: 1437–1451

Mechtersheimer G, Möller P (1990) Expression of Ki-1 antigen (CD 30) in mesenchymal tumors. Cancer 66: 1732–1737

Meister P (1988) Weichgewebssarkome, Klassifizierung und/oder Graduierung? Zentralbl Allg Pathol Pathol Anat 134: 355–362

Mellin W (1990) Cytophotometry in tumor pathology. A critical review of methods and applications, and some results of DNA analysis. Pathol Res Pract 186: 37–62

Mellin W, Roessner A, Edel G, Ritter J, Wuisman P, Jürgens H (1995) DNA ploidy in round cell sarcomas (in preparation)

Miettinen M (1990) Immunohistochemistry of soft tissue tumors. Possibilities and limitations in surgical pathology. Pathol Annu 25: 1–36

Molenaar WM, Dam-Meiring A, Kamps WA, Cornelisse CJ (1988) DNA aneuploidy in rhabdomyosarcomas as compared with other sarcomas of childhood and adolescence. Hum Pathol 19: 573–579

Naito M, Iwafuchi M, Ohsawa Y, Uchiyama M, Hirota M, Matsuda Y, Inuma Y (1991) Flow cytometric DNA analysis of neuroblastoma: prognostic significance of DNA ploidy in unfavorable group. J Pediatr Surg 26: 834–837

Oliver GF, Reiman HM, Gonchoroff NJ, Muller SA, Umbert IJ (1991) Cutaneous and subcutaneous leiomyosarcoma: a clinicopathological review of 14 cases with reference to antidesmin staining and nuclear DNA patterns studied by flow cytometry. Br J Dermatol 124: 252–257

Persson S, Willems JS, Kindblom LG, Angervall L (1988) Alveolar soft part sarcoma. An immunohistochemical, cytologic and electron-microscopic study and a quantitative DNA analysis. Virchows Arch [A] 412: 499–513

Pettinato G, Manivel JC, De-Rosa G, Petrella G, Jaszcz W (1990) Angiomatoid malignant fibrous histiocytoma: cytologic, immunohistochemical, ultrastructural, and flow cytometric study of 20 cases. Mod Pathol 3: 479–487

Pyrhonen S, Laasonen A, Tammilehto L, Rautonen J, Anttila S, Mattson K, Holsti LR (1991) Diploid predominance and prognostic significance of S-phase cells in malignant mesothelioma. Eur J Cancer 27: 1978–2000

Radio SJ, Wooldridge TN, Linder J (1988) Flow cytometric DNA analysis of malignant fibrous histiocytoma and related fibrohistiocytic tumors. Hum Pathol 19: 74–77

Sapi Z, Bodo M (1989) DNA cytometry of soft tissue tumors with TV image-analysis system. Pathol Res Pract 185: 363–367

Schmidt D, Leuschner I, Harms D, Sprenger E, Schäfer HJ (1989) Malignant rhabdoid tumor. A morphological and flow cytometric study. Pathol Res Pract 184: 202–210

Shapiro DN, Parham DM, Douglass EC, Ashmun R, Webber BL, Newton WA Jr, Hancock ML, Maurer HM, Look AT (1991) Relationship of tumor-cell ploidy to histologic subtype and treatment outcome in children and adolescents with unresectable rhabdomyosarcoma. J Clin Oncol 9: 159–166

Stenfert Kroese MC, Rutgers DH, Wils IS et al. (1990) The relevance of the DNA index and proliferation rate in the grading of benign and malignant soft tissue tumors. Cancer 65: 1782–1788

Ueda T, Aozasa K, Tsujimoto M, Ohsawa M, Uchida A, Aoki Y, Ono K, Matsumoto K (1989) Prognostic significance of Ki-67 reactivity in soft tissue sarcomas. Cancer 63: 1607–1611

van Unnik JAM, Coindre JM, Contesso G, Albus-Lutter CE, Schiodt T, Garcia Miralles T, Sylvester R, Thomas D, Bramwell V (1988) Grading of soft tissue sarcomas: experience of the EORTC Soft Tissue and Bone Sarcoma Group. In: Ryan JR, Baker LO (eds) Recent concepts in sarcoma treatment. Kluwer, Utrecht, pp 7–13

Wersto RP, Liblit RL, Koss LG (1991) Flow cytometric DNA analysis of human solid tumors: a review of the interpretation of DNA histgrams. Hum Pathol 22: 1085–1098

Yu CC-W, Hall PA, Fletcher CDM, Camplejohn RS, Waseem NH, Lane DP, Levison DA (1991) Haemangiopericytomas: the prognostic value of immunohistochemical staining with a monoclonal antibody to proliferating cell nuclear antigen (PCNA). Histopathology 19: 29–33

Zubrikhina GN, Ol'khovskaja IG (1990) Flow cytometry in the evaluation of the prognosis and course of malignant soft-tissue tumors. Arkh Patol 52: 29–33

Heterogeneity in Malignant Soft Tissue Tumors

D. Katenkamp and H. Kosmehl

1 Heterogeneity – A General Phenomenon in Tumors

Heterogeneity exists in all tumors and should thus be acknowledged as a fundamental and inherent characteristic of soft tissue tumors as well. As all pathologists know from their diagnostic work, particularly malignant soft tissue tumors may show marked heterogeneity at the morphological and/or functional level (Fidler 1978; Heppner 1984; Katenkamp 1988; Rubin 1990). The term heterogeneity as applied here can be defined as a diversity of cellular and structural features and functional determinants. This is not identical with the term "heterogeneity" used by biologists who define it with clonality only, i.e., in a heterogeneous tumor there must occur at least two different cell clones. In contrast, we use a more comprehensive definition and include all phenomena of both interclonal differences and intra-clonal variabilites (compare Heppner 1984; Heppner and Miller 1989).

In contrast to carcinomas, where the question of clonal origin is still open, all or at least the overwhelming majority of malignant soft tissue tumors seem to be of monoclonal derivation (cf. Iannacone et al. 1987; Heim et al. 1988). This concept does not conflict with the tenet of tumor heterogeneity. Experimentally it can easily be shown that in vitro single cell clones develop and diversify to different cell subpopulations distinguishable due to their cellular features and behavioral properties (Okabe et al. 1983; Gerharz et al. 1990a,b).

Current Topics in Pathology
Volume 89, Eds. D. Harms/D. Schmidt
© Springer-Verlag Berlin Heidelberg 1995

The development of heterogeneity in general may be explained by genetic alterations due to random somatic mutations. These appear as point mutations, chromosomal aberrations and translocations, gene deletions, amplifications, and neo-insertions resulting from postgenetic changes at the posttranscriptional or posttranslational level and from influences of the microenvironment comprising all external factors having a modifying effect on tumor cells (cellular interactions, influences of hormones, enzymes, growth and other factors, effects of the extracellular matrix, etc. – NICOLSON 1987). In the development of heterogeneity the latter epigenetic mechanisms causing nonmutational DNA modifications (see also HORIO et al. 1991) probably play a larger role in cellular diversification than genotypic instability.

Taking into consideration the many factors and mechanisms which produce heterogeneity one recognizes the surprising stability tumors possess which forms the basis for interpretation, classification, and prognostication of neoplasms, and for identifying general tendencies in clinical oncology. According to HEPPNER (1989) tumors have an inclination to form cell societies which achieve a balance, similar to that in an ecosystem, ensuring a relatively constant phenotype over a certain time period if no additional selection pressure operates (e.g., radio- and/or chemotherapy).

Although it is generally known how heterogeneity develops during tumor progression (for review see NICOLSON 1987; PITOT 1989; BOYLAN et al. 1990), there are only speculations about causes and the realization factors of a regularly appearing heterogeneity as seen in biphasic tumors (synovial sarcoma, mesothelioma, etc.) or in cellularly mixed neoplasms like Triton tumors (cf. HALL and LEVISON 1989). And lastly, nothing is known about what we call evolutionary heterogeneity of cells. We cannot explain why differently committed cells with defined morphological features may transform to a common phenotype (e.g., granular or rhabdoid cells – see Sect. 5).

What can be heterogeneous? Heterogeneity is possible for all parameters important in the morphological diagnosis: cellular and structural features, histochemical and immunohistochemical findings, cytogenetic characteristics as well as oncogene expression and the pertinent oncogene products. Tumors are heterogeneous in terms of growth kinetics, DNA content of cells, the ability to invade host tissue and produce metastases as well as the response to immunological and nonimmunological defence mechanisms of the host and to therapy measures. In the following we want to address the phenomenon of heterogeneity in malignant soft tissue tumors with emphasis on those aspects relevant to diagnosis.

2 Heterogeneity and Light-Microscopic Diagnosis

It must first be defined in what form heterogeneity may appear in routinely stained hematoxylin and eosin sections. In principle, this phenomenon may manifest by different cytological features within the same tumor or occur as the presence of various structures side by side. Usually the two possible forms of heterogeneity expression occur in combination, structural variability is generally linked with different cytological features and exceptions are rare.

As generally known, cells of malignant neoplasms are phenotypically different. However, if the cells originate from one lineage but are at different stages of maturity, this cannot be called heterogeneity in the proper sense. At the cellular level this term should be reserved for tumors containing different cell types such as malignant Schwann cell tumors with rhabdomyoblastic cells (malignant Triton tumors – DAIMARU et al. 1984; DUCATMAN and SCHEITHAUER 1984; BROOKS et al. 1985; ENJOJI and HASHIMOTO 1990; WONG et al. 1991).

In some tumors heterogeneity is consistently present and thus represents a morphological criterion for diagnosis (biphasic synovial sarcoma, malignant mesenchymoma and ectomesenchymoma, gangliorhabdomyosarcoma, malignant glandular schwannoma, etc. – WOODRUFF 1976; TAKAHARA et al. 1979; COZZUTTO et al. 1982; URI et al. 1984; KODET et al. 1986; KAWAMOTO et al. 1987; BROOKS 1988; NEWMAN and FLETCHER 1987). Other neoplasms display heterogeneity to a greater or lesser degree. Especially malignant schwannomas tend to show different structures which may considerably hamper a correct diagnosis, particulary if only a small tissue sample is available from a large tumor (Fig. 1) (ENZINGER and WEISS 1988; KATENKAMP and STILLER 1990).

The cells of some structurally heterogeneous tumors obviously exhibit the same basic differentiation. This holds true for some endothelial tumors. Spindle cell hemangioendotheliomas are composed of cells with endothelial differentiation but show areas resembling cavernous hemangiomas and Kaposi's sarcomas side by side (WEISS and ENZINGER 1986; FLETCHER et al. 1991a). Recently, vascular tumors have been documented in the literature which, beside structures of spindle cell hemangioendothelioma, demonstrate foci like epithelioid hemangioendothelioma (ZOLTIE and ROBERTS 1989). A further pertinent example is the recently reported congenital infiltrating giant cell angioblastoma (GONZALES-CRUSSI et al. 1991). But even seemingly heterogeneous tumors at the light-microscopic level (e.g., synovial sarcomas, glandular schwannomas) have more common differentiation immunohistochemically than found in hematoxylin and eosin sections (FERRY and DICKERSIN 1988; DARDICK et al. 1991). Heterogeneity may be recognized by the simultaneous occurrence of undifferentiated regions and well-differentiated structures. A group of such tumors is nowadays termed "dedifferentiated" sarcomas (ENJOJI and HASHIMOTO 1990). First reported in chondrosarcomas, the phenomenon of "dedifferentiation" can be observed in liposarcomas, malignant schwannomas, rhabdomyosarcomas, leiomyosarcomas, extraskeletal osteosarcomas, and extraskeletal chondrosarcomas (ENJOJI and HASHIMOTO 1990) and is said to be generated by the abrupt emergence of a new, undifferentiated cell clone responsible for the resulting

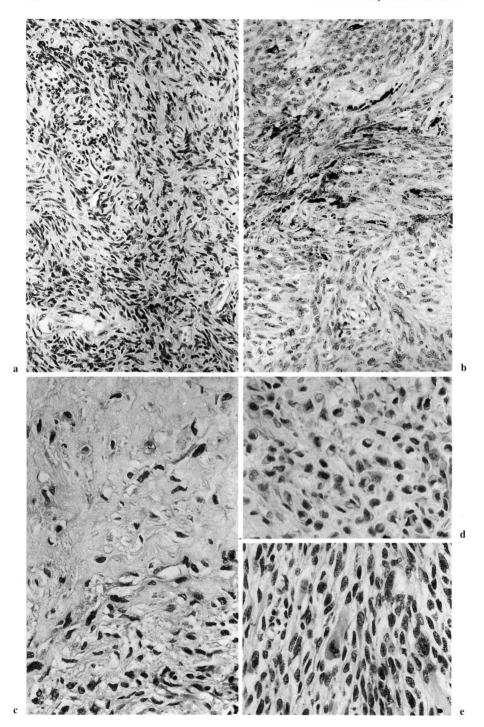

double phenotypic pattern (BROOKS 1986). "Dedifferentiation" implies a certain pathway of evolution, namely a reverse transformation, which certainly does not apply to all of these tumors. The designation "soft tissue sarcomas with additional anaplastic components" seems to be more neutral and thus more appropriate (HASHIMOTO et al. 1990). Dermatofibrosarcoma protuberans is another example of tumors possibly expressing a structurally heterogeneous feature, as documented by reports on occurrence of fibrosarcomatous or malignant fibrous histiocytoma (MFH) areas (DOWD and LAIDLER 1988; WROTNOWSKI et al. 1988; DING et al. 1989) or regions with the picture of giant cell fibroblastoma (cf. ALGUACIL-GARCIA 1991; SHMOOKLER et al. 1989). Although belonging to this group from their description, the heterogeneously structured mesenchymal chondrosarcomas with undifferentiated and chondroid regions should not be included because the anaplastic mesenchymal component represents per definition a feature of this entity (BERTONI et al. 1983; NAKASHIMA et al. 1986; CHETTY 1990).

Finally, metaplasia in soft tissue sarcomas should be addressed. Osseous and chondroid metaplasia are the most frequent types. The occurrence of metaplasia can be a diagnostic aid as it is expressed more frequently in some tumors (e.g., malignant schwannomas, leiomyosarcomas, liposarcomas, and certain MFH variants – BHAGAVAN and DORFMAN 1982; DUCATMAN and SCHEITHAUER 1984, 1986; FLETCHER 1990) than in others. Moreover, the development of metaplastic structures may occur in non-neoplastic cells of sarcomatous tissue as well as in sarcoma cells themselves.

3 Heterogeneity at the Electron-Microscopic Level

Electron-microscopic examination of malignant soft tissue tumors reveals somewhat varying cellular phenotypes mostly due to different levels of maturity. Fibroblast- and histiocyte-like cells are difficult to define electron-microscopically because otherwise committed cells may transform to them. In this chapter the term "heterogeneity" will be restricted to cell mixtures composed of cells obviously belonging to different differentiation lineages.

←

Fig. 1a–e. Heterogeneous cellular appearance, growth pattern, and matrix formation in a malignant peripheral nerve sheath tumor (MPNST). Characteristic features of MPNST: sweeping fascicles of spindle cells with elongated nuclei and whorl-like formations in the periphery (**a**); focal melanin synthesis in tumor cells of another area (**b**); in addition to cell-rich tumor areas, region with formations of a prominent extracellular chondroid-like hyaline matrix (**c**); tumor area with polygonal signet cell-like cells (**d**); heterologous cellular elements in MPNST representing rhabdomyoblasts (**e**). **a,b** H&E, ×180; **c–e** H&E, ×300

Heterogeneity viewed at the light-microscopic level is reflected by a corresponding ultrastructural cytology. However, electron-microscopic examination reveals additional details extending the spectrum of heterogeneous findings to include many not discovered in hematoxylin and eosin sections. MFH serve as a good example of this. Cytologically, MFH is well defined consisting of fibroblast- and histiocyte-like cells together with undifferentiated cells and frequent giant cells (JABI et al. 1987; LAGACÉ 1987). Electron-microscopically, unexpected and perplexing findings were obtained: epithelial cells with tonofilaments were seen in a storiform–pleomorphic MFH and in cultured MFH cells (HIROSE et al. 1989; ROHOLL et al. 1991a), while muscle cells with striated muscular differentiation (Z-lines) or smooth muscle features (myofilaments and attachment points) could be viewed in an angiomatoid MFH (LEU and MAKEK 1982; see also LAGACÉ 1987).

Observations of this kind stimulated discussions on the cellular origin of MFHs and seemed to bear out the theory of development from undifferentiated mesenchymal stem cells (FU et al. 1975; ALGUACIL-GARCIA et al. 1978; FUKADA et al. 1988). Similarly, other malignant soft tissue tumors with an ultrastructurally heterogeneous cellular composition were interpreted as being derivatives of undifferentiated mesenchymal progenitor cells, e.g., experimental soft tissue sarcomas (KATENKAMP and STILLER 1975), malignant mesenchymomas (KLIMA et al. 1975), human botryoid sarcomas (KATENKAMP et al. 1979), and postirradiation sarcomas (SEO et al. 1985; for review see KATENKAMP and RAIKHLIN 1985).

In addition to aiding in the confirmation of heterogeneity, electron microscopy may also contribute to the interpretation of cells in these tumors. In glandular malignant schwannomas particular emphasis was placed on explaining the nature of glandular structures within sarcomatous tissue. From reported ultrastructural findings we can infer that these sarcomas are not identical in their glandular components which were said to be of intestinal (URI et al. 1984), ependymal (DE SCHRYVER and SANTA GRUZ 1984), or schwannian type (FERRY and DICKERSIN 1988), or we must concede that several ultrastructural details are ambiguous, thus preventing the confident classification of cell differentiation, requiring additional histochemical and/or immunohistochemical findings for interpretation.

The diagnostic value of electron-microscopic techniques is often impaired by the availability of only small tissue samples. The pathologist may be misled by such samples, falling victim to sampling error. Nevertheless, electron microscopy, as is true of other adjunct methods of morphology, is an important tool for defining tumors cytologically. Thus, this method must also be considered when developing new tumor concepts (e.g., the monophasic "fibrous" synovial sarcomas redefined as spindle cell carcinomas of soft tissue – DARDICK et al. 1991).

4 Heterogeneous Findings in Diagnostic Immunohistochemistry with Regard to Cellular Differentiation Markers

Immunohistochemistry is currently one of the major ancillary methods used by pathologists to more precisely classify tumors possessing features considered ambiguous in the light-microscopic examination (DE LELLIS and DAYAL 1987). The advent of this technique raised many hopes for a tool to easily determine cellular differentiation. But with time immunohistochemistry proved to be more complicated in the interpretation of results than originally thought. Pathologists came to recognize that considerable heterogeneity could result from (a) immunohistochemical markers which were less specific than initially assumed and hence marking epitopes in different cellular lineages; and (b) from unexpected or aberrant marker expressions (MIETTINEN 1990). No completely reliable diagnostic antibody is available at present, thus requiring the use of a panel of antibodies as well as cautious interpretation of conventional histological findings and clinical data (KATENKAMP 1986; DARBYSHIRE et al. 1987; GRAY et al. 1989; FISHER 1990).

The diagnostic value of individual antibodies has been determined in large series of normal tissues and tumors. Despite the use of respective "diagnostic" antibodies in nearly all malignant soft tissue tumors, an uneven immunohistochemical pattern is observed as not all tumor cells react with the so-called diagnostic antibody (ROHOLL et al. 1985). This may be caused by methodical error (e.g., inadequate fixation reduces the antigenicity) or by the presence of less differentiated or undifferentiated tumor cells, in any case hindering the diagnostic interpretation. Tumors composed of cells with and without certain antigenic sites can be shown to be immunohistochemically heterogeneous just as tumors that demonstrate different differentiation markers side by side. In the following, we discuss some heterogeneous reaction patterns of antibodies to certain noncytoskeletal and cytoskeletal proteins. To serve as an example of the former group reaction patterns of S100 protein antibodies shall be presented.

In cases of malignant schwannomas a heterogeneous binding of S100 protein antibodies is the usual finding, apart from the 30%–60% of tumors lacking S100 protein positivity at all (DAIMARU et al. 1985; WICK et al. 1987; SWANSON et al. 1987; CHRISTENSEN et al. 1988; GRAY et al. 1989; FLETCHER 1990, 1992; JOHNSON et al. 1991). Beside the fact that tumorous Schwann cells could have lost this marker, another possibility must be taken into consideration. In neural tumors, antibodies to S100 protein are said to mark only cells with schwannian differentiation. The only partial immunostaining may therefore be explained by a nonhomogeneous cellularity of these tumors consisting not only of cells with schwannian characteristics but also of cells with peri- and endoneurial fibroblastic features as shown by electron microscopy (HIROSE et al. 1988). For purposes of nomenclature it seems justified to consider this fact and accordingly replace the designation "malignant schwannoma" by the more comprehensive term "malignant peripheral nerve sheath tumor (MPNST)" (cf. GIANGASPERO et al. 1989; FLETCHER 1990; FISHER et al. 1992).

S100 protein antibodies are known to react not only with Schwann cells and their derivatives but also with cells of lipoblastic and chondroblastic differentiation as well as immunoaccessory cells or cells of malignant melanomas (HASHIMOTO et al. 1984; OTTO et al. 1987; SCHMITT and BACCHI 1989). In individual cases an unexpected positive marking of cells in soft tissue tumors outside this spectrum of cellular differentiation is possible representing a further expression of immunohistochemical heterogeneity. There are reports of cells reacting with antibodies to S100 protein in tumors like MFH (COCCHIA et al. 1983; OHMORI et al. 1986; DONHUIJSEN et al. 1988), synovial sarcomas (FISHER and SCHOFIELD 1991; DICKERSIN 1991), leiomyosarcomas (SWANSON et al. 1987; WICK et al. 1988; JOHNSON et al. 1988; GIANGASPERO et al. 1989), epithelioid sarcomas (CHASE and ENZINGER 1985; SCHMIDT and HARMS 1987; WICK et al. 1988), and rhabdomyosarcomas (MIERAU et al. 1985; COINDRE et al. 1988; SCHMIDT et al. 1989a, 1990a). Such observations need not be associated with an aberrant schwannian, lipoblastic, or chondroblastic differentiation in otherwise defined soft tissue tumors. Unexpected positivity of antibodies to S100 protein might also merely indicate the existence of an unspecific epitope recognizable by these antibodies. This may also be valid for other unexpected antibody reactions (FISHER 1990).

Vimentin is the principal intermediate filament of malignant soft tissue tumors (Fig. 2) (cf. ALTMANNSBERGER and OSBORN 1987). The atypical occurrence of cytoskeletal filaments, demonstrable using antibodies to cytokeratin, desmin, neurofilament, glial fibrillary acidic protein, and actins was of particular importance for some modifications in understanding the biology of these tumors. Some years ago it was postulated that intermediate filaments in tumors correspond to the alleged tissue of origin, resulting in the assumption that cytokeratins are specific of epithelial, desmin, and certain actin isoforms of muscular, neurofilaments of neuroblastic and glial fibrillary acidic protein (outside of the central nervous system) of some nerve sheath tumors. Special attention has been directed to cytokeratin occurrence in soft tissue tumors. After recognizing cytokeratins as regularly coexpressed intermediate filaments in synovial sarcomas, epithelioid sarcomas, and mesotheliomas, their demonstration in cells of other soft tissue tumors was perplexing. First detected in leiomyosarcomas (BROWN et al. 1987; NORTON et al. 1987; RAMAEKERS et al. 1988; MIETTINEN 1988a, 1989, 1990; FISHER 1990; TAUCHI et al. 1990), they are now known to occur in cells of some MFH (ENZINGER

Fig. 2a–d. Immunohistochemical heterogeneity of MFH. Expression of vimentin (a) as the characteristic intermediate filament in all tumor cells, cytokeratin (b), desmin (c), and S100 protein (d) in single cells of MFH. PAP technique, ×300

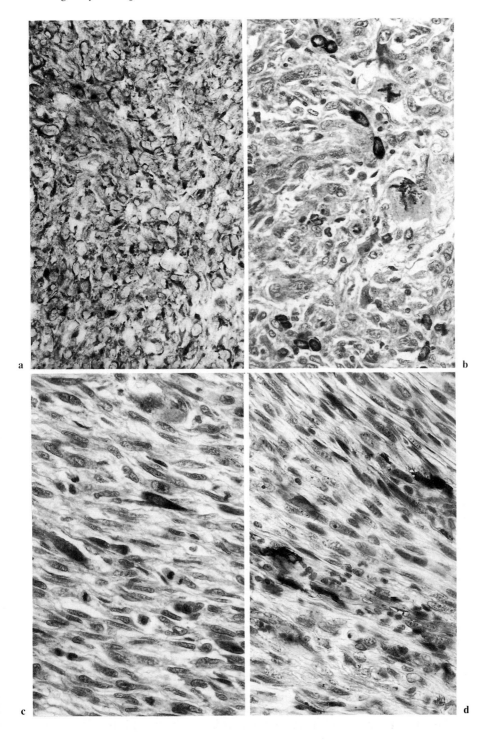

and WEISS 1988; WEISS et al. 1988; HIROSE et al. 1989; MIETTINEN and SOINI 1989), malignant schwannomas including Triton tumors (GRAY et al. 1989; SCHMIDT et al. 1990b; MIETTINEN 1989, 1991), malignant peripheral neuro-ectodermal tumors (SCHMIDT et al. 1991), rhabdomyosarcomas (ENZINGER and WEISS 1988; COINDRE et al. 1988; SCHMIDT et al. 1989a, 1990; CARTER et al. 1990; PARHAM et al. 1991), liposarcomas (ENZINGER and WEISS 1988), malignant hemangiopericytomas, fibrosarcomas (MEIS and ENZINGER 1991) as well as of some rhabdoid (ENJOJI and HASHIMOTO 1990) and angiomatous tumors (ENJOJI and HASHIMOTO 1990; EUSEBI et al. 1990; VAN HAELST et al. 1990; FLETCHER et al. 1991b). The controversy stemming from the search for explanations for this phenomenon is not yet over. Interpretations include, for instance, the assumption of technical artifacts owing to methodical error (SWANSON 1991), as well as the opinion that simple cytokeratins should not be surprising in soft tissue tumors because nontumorous mesenchymal cells are able to at least transiently form cytokeratins as well (MIETTINEN and KOVATICH 1991). The latter view applies to embryonal and adult smooth muscle cells (BROWN et al. 1987; GOWN et al. 1988; JOHN and FRANKE 1989), to embryonal fibroblasts and embryonal mesenchyme in general (KULESH and OSHIMA 1988; MIETTINEN 1990), and also to striated muscle cells (KOSMEHL et al. 1990a). We consider cytokeratin expression in some malig-nant soft tissue tumors to be a re-emergence of early embryonal charac-teristics, comparable to retrodifferentiation (URIEL 1979). Furthermore, if not verified by biochemical or immunoblot techniques, the staining with cytokeratin antibodies does not necessarily indicate the existence of the respective intermediate filaments, but, as already mentioned above for S100 antibodies, rather may merely indicate a suitable cellular epitope for this reaction. The latter statement also holds true for other immunohistochemical heterogeneity: the unexpected reaction of some tumor cells with neurofila-ment antibodies in rhabdomyosarcomas (MIETTINEN and RAPOLA 1989; MIETTINEN 1990; PARHAM et al. 1991), MFH (HIROSE et al. 1989), and epithelioid sarcomas (GERHARZ et al. 1990a,b), or with desmin antibodies in fibrosarcomas (MIETTINEN et al. 1982; WICK et al. 1988), MFH (MIETTINEN 1988b; LEADER et al. 1987; DONHUIJSEN et al. 1988; WICK et al. 1988; HASHIMOTO et al. 1990; DONNER and DE LANEROLLE 1990; ROHOLL et al. 1990a; FLETCHER 1991), ordinary malignant schwannomas (WICK et al. 1988; JOHNSON et al. 1991), liposarcomas (LEADER et al. 1987; MIETTINEN 1988b; ROHOLL et al. 1990a), and epithelioid sarcomas (SCHMIDT and HARMS 1987). The widespread occurrence of myofibroblasts has also been cited as an explanation for desmin expression because these cells may exhibit desmin filaments under pathological conditions (SKALLI et al. 1988; HASEGAWA et al. 1990). The heterogeneity of cytoskeletal filaments in malignant soft tissue tumors is also related to actin filaments and their isoforms (SKALLI et al. 1988; SCHÜRCH et al. 1987; ROHOLL et al. 1990a). Relevant pertinent immu-nohistochemical investigations have demonstrated that the boundary between rhabdomyosarcomas and leiomyosarcomas is somewhat indistinct and overlapping between both entities does occur (for references, see KATENKAMP and KOSMEHL 1993).

Immunohistochemical heterogeneity is not a rare phenomenon, knowledge of which should provide for a prudent interpretation of immunohistochemical findings (MIETTINEN 1989). But occasionally such an interpretation will be impossible, as in the case of polyphenotypic tumors of childhood and adolescence (SWANSON et al. 1988) or in the case of rhabdoid-like tumor with the coincidental expression of five classes of intermediate filaments (NAKAZATO et al. 1991).

5 Immunohistochemical Heterogeneity and the Concept of Histogenetic Classification

As emphasized earlier, one has to be aware of a minor or major degree of immunohistochemical heterogeneity in nearly all tumors posing a serious challenge to exact classification in some cases. For some years the position has been held that a "histogenetic" classification with defining the cellular genesis of tumors should be replaced by a classification based on the actual differentiation without histogenetic aspects (GOULD 1986; LANGBEIN et al. 1988; MEISTER 1991) as German pathologists already called for in the first half of this century (HUECK 1939). Comments on heterogeneous immunohistochemical findings in rhabdoid cells and MFH may exemplify the need to omit histogenetic aspects in soft tissue tumor classification.

First, rhabdoid cells were described as cellular constituents of kidney tumors in infancy and early childhood. These tumors were called rhabdoid tumors and were believed to be a nephroblastoma variant (BECKWITH and PALMER 1978; PALMER and SUTOW 1983). More recently, tumors indistinguishable from renal rhabdoid tumors by light microscopy were described in different organs and soft tissue (TSUNEYOSHI et al. 1987; SCHMIDT et al. 1989b; TSOKOS et al. 1989). Light microscopy revealed large cells with vesicular nuclei, prominent single nucleoli and abundant cytoplasm with an inclusion-like hyaline globular structure, and electron microscopy disclosed hyaline globules consisting of tangled filaments. With both methods relatively homogeneous findings were obtained. However, immunohistochemical examinations often showed heterogeneous patterns, only few authors could find only vimentin as the sole marker of rhabdoid cells (BIGGS et al. 1987; DERVAN et al. 1987; HARRIS et al. 1987; MATIAS et al. 1990). The most common example of heterogeneity in intermediate filaments was the co-expression of vimentin and cytokeratin (BALATON et al. 1987; SCHMIDT et al. 1989b; TSOKOS et al. 1989; ORDONEZ et al. 1990; KODET et al. 1991a). However, numerous additional other markers are possible comprising EMA, desmin, myoglobin, actin, S100 protein. Leu-7, NSE, GFAP, CEA, and A1ACT (EKFORS et al. 1985; KENT et al. 1987; PARHAM et al. 1987;

TSUNEYOSHI et al. 1987; JAKATE et al. 1988; TSOKOS et al. 1989; ORDONEZ et al. 1990). From this astonishing marker heterogeneity the question arose whether or not rhabdoid cells represent a unique cell type at all. Currently, most authors believe that the term "rhabdoid" cell stands only for a defined cellular phenotype regardless of the original cellular lineage which it is derived from (BITTESINI et al. 1992). The occurrence of rhabdoid cells is said to be indicative of a particular aggressiveness and corresponding high malignancy (PERRONE et al. 1989; WEEKS et al. 1989). The purely descriptive significance of the term "rhabdoid" has been confirmed by observations of rhabdoid cells in different tumors as epithelioid sarcomas, synovial sarcomas, extraskeletal myxoid chondrosarcomas, malignant mesotheliomas, and (with reservation) in rhabdomyosarcomas (TSUNEYOSHI et al. 1987; ORDONEZ et al. 1990; KODET et al. 1991b; MIRRA et al. 1992). A cellular phenotype with comparable immunohistochemical diversity is reputed to be the granular cell, which is the main cellular element in granular cell tumors (including the congenital gingival variant) but may also be found in myomas, nerve sheath tumors, in dermatofibrosarcoma protuberans, MFH, and in angiosarcomas (MCWILLIAM and HARRIS 1985; TANIMURA et al. 1985; ABENOZA and SIBLEY 1987; RAJU and O'REILLY 1987; BULEY et al. 1988; BANERJEE et al. 1990; FUJITA and OKABE 1990). The occurrence of rhabdoid and granular cells in different tumors contributes to their cellular heterogeneity at the light-microscopic level and stresses the questionable value of drawing histogenetic conclusions from phenotypic cellular features (ULRICH et al. 1987; BITTESINI et al. 1992).

The heterogeneity of MFH has already been referred to. Using light and electron microscopy it is easily recognized, potentially posing problems in the diagnostic interpretation. The cellular heterogeneity of MFHs is explained as the result of the derivation from undifferentiated mesenchymal precursor cells capable of developing into fibroblast- and histiocyte-like cells (for review see MEISTER 1988). Apart from angiomatoid MFH, nowadays assumed to be a separate tumor type (PETTINATO et al. 1990; SMITH et al. 1991), other MFH variants were found with an allegedly true histio-monocytic cellular component, requiring that this concept be somewhat modified (STRAUCHEN and DIMITRIU-BONA 1986; SOINI and MIETTINEN 1991). Other authors, however, were unable to confirm these observations (IWASAKI et al. 1992). Regardless of this heterogeneity, conventional MFHs were declared to be a true entity (cf. MEISTER 1988). This may in fact be true. However, it must be acknowledged that tumors with the MFH phenotype may also be disguised non-MFH soft tissue sarcomas whose origin is found in the dedifferentiation processes during tumor progression (BROOKS 1986; DEHNER 1988; KATENKAMP 1988; KOSMEHL et al. 1990b). This fact has challenged the idea of the existence of MFH as being an independent entity (DONHUIJSEN et al. 1987; MIETTINEN and SOINI 1989; FLETCHER 1992). Related to this, the demonstration of some cytokeratin-positive cells in MFHs (see above) need not be interpreted as aberrant intermediate filament synthesis, but might be indicative of a tumor located at the end of the tumor progression pathway of synovial sarcoma, epithelioid sarcoma, or chordoma (BELZA and URICH 1986; FLETCHER 1989). Likewise, S100 protein-positive cells could point to a development from malignant nerve sheath tumors or melanomas (cf. HERRERA et al. 1982; BROOKS 1986; FLETCHER 1990) and expression of desmin in some tumor cells could indicate a derivation from rhabdo- or leiomyosarcomas (ROHOLL et al. 1988a, 1990a). Accordingly, the marker diversity in MFHs may have at least two roots: (a) it could represent the heterogeneity of a true MFH; or (b) it could indicate another sarcoma mimicking MFH morphology (secondary MFH). Transplantation studies in fact revealed a masked schwannian or muscular differentiation in some MFHs (ROHOLL et al. 1988b). Likewise, the possible heterogeneity of extracellular matrix in MFHs could speak in favor of different "histogenetic" origins. In principle, MFHs belong to the group of non-basement membrane-forming sarcomas (MIETTINEN et al. 1983; BEHAM et al. 1986). However, a focal laminin and collagen IV immunostaining in MFH and the expression of mRNA for laminin in cells of some MFH have been reported (SOINI and AUTIO-HARMAINEN 1991). The occurrence of such unusual extracellular matrix components could indicate a non-fibrohistiocytic differentiation, at least in some tumor regions. MFH exemplifies the situation in soft tissue tumors: most if not all are derivatives of uncharacteristic mesenchymal precursor cells (KATENKAMP and RAIKHLIN 1985) and, as stated above, attempts at histogenetic classification should be omitted in favor of demonstrating the lineage differentiation of tumor cells.

To substantiate the impossibility of a histogenetic classification, small cell tumors in young patients with striking heterogeneous differentiation are mentioned. These include Ewing's sarcomas (MOLL et al. 1987) as well as polyphenotypic tumors in childhood (SWANSON et al. 1988; WICK et al. 1988) and intraabdominal desmoplastic small cell tumors with divergent differentiation (GERALD and ROSAI 1989; GONZALEZ-CRUSSI et al. 1990; GAFFNEY 1991; SCHRÖDER and TESSMANN 1991; LAYFIELD and LENARSKY 1991).

6 Heterogeneity of DNA Content, Genes, Gene Products, Growth Factors and Their Receptors

More or less autonomous growth is considered a basic attribute of malignant tumors. Much effort has been made to elucidate the complex mechanisms involved in stimulating or inhibiting the proliferation processes and thus determining the biological behavior of tumors. Accordingly, this subject of basic research is of utmost importance for establishing a prognosis in tumors. Pathologists have recently focused their attention on cytogenetic alterations, DNA content, and gene expression as well as on growth factors and their receptors. However, findings on these objects are complicated by heterogeneity. Some pertinent aspects will be discussed briefly.

It is widely accepted that karyotypic anomalies may emerge during soft tissue tumor development, usually appearing early and possibly being useful in diagnostic considerations (KNIGHT 1990; COOPER and STRATTON 1991). This applies to some chromosomal translocations, suggesting a relationship between chromosomal breakpoints and morphological phenotype (MOLENAAR et al. 1989a). Chromosomal rearrangements are well known (KNIGHT 1990; Turc-Carel et al., this volume). However, chromosomal anomalies of a given type are never found in all cells of a soft tissue tumor. Moreover, different chromosomal aberrations are possible in the same tumor. Cytogenetic findings are therefore in line with clonal heterogeneity in clinically manifested soft tissue sarcomas (STENMAN et al. 1990; BRIDGE et al. 1990, 1991). Against this background the functional heterogeneity of genetic material cannot be surprising (cf. COOPER and STRATTON 1991).

Karyotypic anomalies evolving during tumor progression may be reflected in changes of the DNA profile (MOLENAAR et al. 1988). Again, there may be a striking diversity of findings for cell ploidy within one tumor. Despite initially optimistic reports, reliable discriminations between benign and malignant soft tissue tumors based on the measurement of DNA content can fail (XIANG et al. 1987) and, additionally, highly malignant tumors (e.g., rhabdoid tumors) may exhibit only minimal karyotypic changes (MOLENAAR et al. 1989b; DOUGLASS et al. 1990). Nevertheless, this method has a practical value: the nondiploid DNA pattern is more common in high-grade than in low-grade sarcomas and there is a statistically significant relationship between aneuploidy and an unfavorable clinical outcome (RADIO et al. 1988). This statement holds true in spite of the known variations in ploidy. However, if results of different series are to be compared, the definition of heterogeneity must include the number of nuclei permissible at peaks beyond the diploid peak without having to speak of an aneuploid tumor.

To confirm the hypothesis of an autocrine stimulation of soft tissue tumor proliferation, numerous growth factors and corresponding receptors have been examined during recent years (Fig. 3a,b) (PEROSIO and BROOKS 1989; ROHOLL et al. 1991b). It could be shown that the expression of growth factors and their receptors is related to the biological potential of malignancy (PEROSIO and BROOKS 1989). The growth factor distribution and receptor pattern was frequently nonuniform not only in sarcomas but also in benign proliferations like fibromatoses (ROHOLL et al. 1991b; own observations). In some sarcomas the heterogeneity of growth factors and growth factor receptors could be recognized in correlation with structural heterogeneity (e.g., in biphasic synovial sarcomas), but in most malignant soft tissue

Fig. 3a–d. Heterogeneous expression of growth factor and growth factors receptors in human rhabdomyosarcoma cells. Demonstration of EGF (**a**), EGF receptor (**b**), bFGF receptor (**c**), and PDGF receptor (**d**) in several cells and cell groups. **a–d** cryosection, APAAP technique, ×300

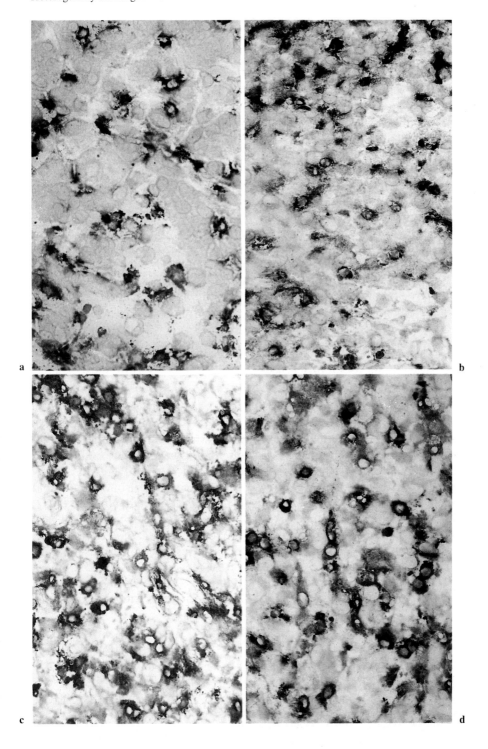

tumors the distribution seemed independent of phenotypic patterns (ROHOLL et al. 1991b). This heterogeneity should be considered in common with the heterogeneity of the functional state of the genetic material, especially since it is known that some oncogene and suppressor gene products are involved in regulation of growth factor and growth factor receptor expression (Fig. 3c,d) (HUANG et al. 1984; LEITH and DEXTER 1986). The heterogeneity of oncogene and suppressor gene expression in soft tissue sarcomas concerns not only quantitative alterations (DIAS et al. 1990; PORTER et al. 1992) but also qualitative abnormalities such as mutations (STRATTON et al. 1990).

Another new class of transmembranous protein receptors, the receptor family of the integrin type (for review see ALBELDA and BUCK 1990), seems to promise new insights into the dynamic heterogeneity of soft tissue sarcomas. In most, if not all, soft tissue sarcomas the development of a defined cellular phenotype is closely associated with the formation of specialized cell–cell and cell–matrix contacts (BEN-ZEÉV 1985; LANGBEIN et al. 1990). The integrin-type receptors are involved in cellular adhesion and in forming cell–matrix contacts. Again, it can be assumed that investigations on cellular phenotype, extracellular matrix formation, and integrin status aid in understanding phenotypic and functional heterogeneity in sarcoma cells (Fig. 4).

7 Heterogeneity and Some Implications for Clinical Pathology

Problems caused by heterogeneity in the histological diagnosis have already been discussed. Another fact deserving mention is the possible change of the histological phenotype due to tumor progression (MATTHEWS and GAZDAR 1985). This phenomenon made possible by heterogeneity may be the cause of different diagnoses if the primary tumor and recurrent growth are examined by two pathologists who have insufficient clinical information and exchange. From our own experiments (KATENKAMP and NEUPERT 1982; KATENKAMP 1988; KOSMEHL et al. 1990b) and numerous clinicopathological observations we conclude that a transformation of at least the common soft tissue sarcomas in MFH-like tumors is possible (cf. Sect. 5; see also SNOVER et al. 1982; BROOKS 1986; McGREGOR et al. 1987; O'DOWD and LAIDLER 1988; ENJOJI and HASHIMOTO 1990; FLETCHER 1992). Even some carcinomas, cystosarcoma phyllodes, lymphomas, and melanomas are able to mimic

Fig. 4a–d. Heterogeneous distribution of extracellular matrix and matrix receptors of integrin type in MFH. Diffuse extracellular fibronectin network (a); focal accumulation of an extracellular laminin matrix (*upper part*, b); demonstration of the fibronectin receptor subunit (α5-chain) in most cells (c) and of laminin receptor subunit (α6-chain) only in some spindle cells (d). Cryosections, APAAP technique; a,b,d ×180, c ×150

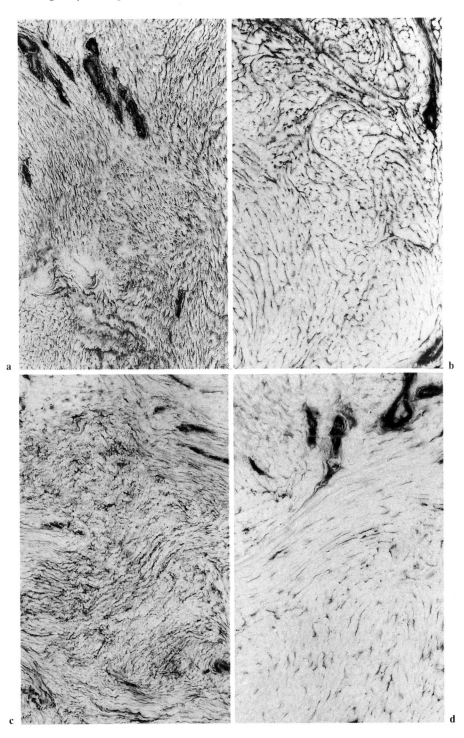

MFHs (BLOM et al. 1983; Ro et al. 1987; LODDING et al. 1990; MENTZEL et al. 1991; FLETCHER 1992).

In addition, increasing differentiation may be seen in the course of tumor disease (e.g., in rhabdomyosarcomas or liposarcomas; see MOLENAAR et al. 1984; BUI et al. 1984). Especially poorly differentiated rhabdomyosarcomas may reveal distinct myogenic differentiation after radiation or chemotherapy (LOLLINI et al. 1989; TAKIZAWA et al. 1989). Differing potentials of individual cell subpopulations to differentiate may explain such phenomena indicative of another aspect of tumor cell heterogeneity.

The question arises whether or not the phenotypic shift is merely an academic problem without associated clinical equivalents and consequences. Strictly speaking, clinically important questions are addressed; the different behavior possible in true and secondary MFHs with regard to clinical aggressiveness, route of metastatic dissemination, and therapeutic responsiveness. Up to now there seems to be some need for clarity relevant to this, warranting further clinicopathological research. However, the diagnostic examination should be aimed at making a diagnosis in order to avoid devaluating the term "MFH" from that of an entity to a wastebasket for unclassifiable sarcomas (Fig. 5) (FLETCHER 1987; DONHUIJSEN et al. 1987). Other soft tissue phenotypes which could be produced due to progression of an otherwise defined sarcoma are features of fibrosarcoma or completely undifferen-

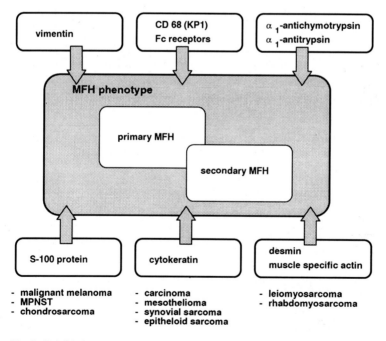

Fig. 5. Possible heterogeneous expression of marker proteins in neoplasia with MFH phenotype indicating relations to other tumor entities

tiated anaplastic sarcoma. In some cases recognition of the original differentiation is first possible after culturing the tumor cells and adding differentiation inducers to the culture medium, or after transplanting tumor tissue to nude mice. Success in detecting diagnostically decisive differentiations by these procedures is well documented (FRESHEY 1985; GARVIN et al. 1986; GABBERT and GERHARZ 1988; GABBERT et al. 1988; LLOMBART-BOSCH et al. 1988). Especially in tumors of childhood and adolescence clear differentiation along one cell line is often lacking and virtually no histotypic markers can be demonstrated or the tumors display complex patterns of multiple lineage differentiation with coexpression of neural, mesenchymal, and epithelial traits (MOLL et al. 1987). To distinguish these neoplasms from similar tumors or dedifferentiated neoplasms for purposes of a diagnosis, consideration of the clinical pattern is indispensable. The immunohistochemical analysis of neural cell adhesion molecules may facilitate diagnostic decisions (GARIN-CHESA et al. 1991). Furthermore, cytogenetic techniques and methods of molecular pathology can be employed in revealing cellular differentiations unrecognizable in conventionally stained sections, the result being the ability to classify the tumor as an entity with a definable cellular lineage. In situ hybridization or Northern blotting may be used to test for typical chromosomal anomalies (see the Ch. 5 by Turc-Carel et al., this volume) or certain DNA or RNA expressions (e.g., Myo D1 expression in rhabdomyosarcomas – SCRABLE et al. 1989; DIAS et al. 1990).

Another problem of practical importance in soft tissue tumor pathology is the difficulty of malignancy grading. Apart from the fact that different grading procedures are used and that no agreement has been reached as to the most suitable method and to guidelines of application (for references see the chapter by Meister, this volume; KATENKAMP and HÜNERBEIN 1992), an exact grading may be decisively hampered by tumor heterogeneity. This situation requires that many tissue specimens be taken to ensure examination of tissue areas representative for the whole neoplasm. Conflicting results of studies correlating tumor malignancy and therapy results may be explained by this last point.

Heterogeneity in malignant soft tissue tumors involves, as shown above, many different aspects and manifests itself at all levels of examination. Thus, diagnostic interpretation of tumors must always take this phenomenon into account.

The maxim never to rely on only a single finding may be taken as a golden rule. Heterogeneity may show varying appearances and generate unexpected, perplexing, and seemingly contradictory immunohistochemical findings. However, if findings of conventional histological examination, data of ancillary methods such as histochemistry, immunohistochemistry, and electron microscopy, and, if necessary, cell culture, transplantation, and molecular characterization are considered and, while also considering clinical observations, an exact diagnosis will nearly always be possible in spite of tumor heterogeneity.

142   D. Katenkamp and H. Kosmehl

References

Abenoza P, Sibley RK (1987) Granular cell myoma and schwannoma: fine structural and immunohistochemical study. Ultrastruct Pathol 11: 19–28

Albelda SM, Buck CA (1990) Integrins and other cell adhesion molecules. FASEB J 4: 2868–2888

Alguacil-Garcia A (1991) Giant cell fibroblastoma recurring as dermatofibrosarcoma protuberans. Amer J Surg Pathol 15: 798–801

Alguacil-Garcia A, Unni KK, Goellner JR (1978) Malignant fibrous histiocytoma – an ultrastructural study of six cases. Amer J Clin Pathol 69: 121–129

Altmannsberger M, Osborn M (1987) Mesenchymal tumor markers: intermediate filaments. In: Seifert G (ed) Morphological tumor markers. Current Topics in Pathology 77, Springer, Berlin Heidelberg New York, pp 155–178

Balaton AJ, Vaury P, Videgrain M (1987) Paravertebral malignant rhabdoid tumor in an adult – a case report with immunocytochemical study. Pathol Res Pract 182: 713–716

Banerjee SS, Harris M, Eyden BP, Hamid NA (1990) Granular cell variant of dermatofibrosarcoma protuberans. Histopathology 17: 375–378

Beckwith JB, Palmer NF (1978) Histopathology and prognosis of Wilms' tumor – results from the first National Wilms' tumor study. Cancer 41: 1937–1948

Beham A, Wirnsberger G, Schmid C (1986) Immunhistochemische Untersuchungen zur Differentialdiagnose des malignen fibrösen Histiozytoms. Wien Klin Wschr 98: 617–622

Belza MG, Urich H (1986) Chordoma and malignant fibrous histiocytoma: evidence for transformation. Cancer 58: 1082–1087

Ben-Zeév A (1985) Cell–cell interactions and cell configuration related control of vimentin and cytokeratin expression in epithelial cells and fibroblasts. Ann NY Acad Sci 455: 597–613

Bertoni F, Picci P, Bacchini P, Capanna R, Innao V, Bacci G, Campanacci M (1983) Mesenchymal chondrosarcoma of bone and soft tissue. Cancer 52: 533–541

Bhagavan BS, Dorfman HD (1982) The signifigance of bone and cartilage formation in malignant fibrous histiocytoma of soft tissue. Cancer 49: 480–488

Biggs PJ, Caren PD, Powers JM, Garvin AJ (1987) Malignant rhabdoid tumor of the central nervous system. Human Pathol 18: 332–337

Bissell M, Hall HG, Parry G (1982) How does extracellular matrix direct gene expression? J Theor Biol 99: 31–68

Bittesini L, Tos APD, Fletcher CDM (1992) Metastatic malignant melanoma showing a rhabdoid phenotype – further evidence of a non-specific histological pattern. Histopathology 20: 167–170

Blom PG, Stenwig AE, Sobel HS, Johannessen JV (1983) Metastasizing malignant melanoma mimicking a malignant fibrous histiocytoma. Ultrastruct Pathol 5: 307–313

Boylan JF, Jackson J, Steiner MR, Shih TY, Duigou GJ, Roszman T, Fisher PB, Zimmer SG (1990) Role of the HA-ras (Ras^H) oncogene in mediating progression of the tumor cell phenotype (review). Anticancer Res 10: 717–724

Bridge JA, Sanger WG, Neft JR, Hess MM (1990) Cytogenetic findings in a primary malignant fibrous histiocytoma of bone and the lung metastasis. Pathology 22: 16–19

Bridge JA, Sreekantaiah C, Neft JR, Sandberg AA (1991) Cytogenetic findings in clear cell sarcomà of tendons and aponeuroses; malignant melanoma of soft parts. Cancer Genet Cytogenet 52: 101–106

Brooks JJ (1986) The significance of double phenotypic patterns and markers in human sarcomas: a new model of mesenchymal differentiation. Am J Pathol 125: 113–123

Brooks JJ (1988) Malignant schwannomas with divergent differentiation including the "Triton" tumor. In: Williams CJ, Krikorian JG, Greene MR, Raghavan D (eds) Textbook of uncommon cancer. John Wiley, New York, pp 653–668

Brooks JJ, Freeman M, Enterline HT (1985) Malignant "Triton" tumors: natural history and immunohistochemistry of nine new cases with literature review. Cancer 55: 2543–2549

Brown DC, Theaker JM, Banks PM, Gatter KC, Mason DY (1987) Cytokeratin expression in smooth muscle and smooth muscle tumours. Histopathology 11: 477–486

Bui NB, Coindre JM, Maree D, Trojani M (1984) Liposarcoma: patterns of tumor differentiation following induction chemotherapy. Oncology 41: 170–173

Buley ID, Gatter KC, Kelly PMA, Heryet A, Millard PR (1988) Granular cell tumors revisited – an immunohistochemical and ultrastructural study. Histopathology 12: 263–274

Carter RL, Jameson CF, Philip ER, Pinkerton CR (1990) Comparative phenotypes in rhabdomyosarcomas and developing skeletal muscle. Histopathology 17: 301–309

Chase DR, Enzinger FM (1985) Epithelioid sarcoma – diagnosis, prognostic indicators and
treatment. Am J Surg Pathol 9: 241–263

Chetty R (1990) Extraskeletal mesenchymal chondrosarcoma of the mediastinum. Histopathology 17: 261–263

Christensen WN, Strong EW, Bains MS, Woodruff JM (1988) Neuroendocrine differentiation
in the glandular peripheral nerve sheath tumor: pathologic distinction from the biphasic
synovial sarcomas with glands. Am J Surg Pathol 12: 417–426

Cocchia D, Lauriola L, Stolfi VM, Tallini G, Michetti F (1983) S-100 antigen labels neoplastic
cells in liposarcoma and cartilaginous tumours. Virchows Arch A 402: 139–145

Coindre JM, de Mascarel A, Trojani M, de Mascarell I, Pages A (1988) Immunohistochemical
study of rhabdomyosarcoma – unexpected staining with S100 protein and cytokeratin. J
Pathol 155: 127–132

Cooper CS, Stratton MR (1991) Soft tissue tumors – the genetic basis of development.
Carcinogenesis 12: 155–165

Cozzutto C, Comelli A, Bandelloni R (1982) Ectomesenchymoma – report of two cases.
Virchows Arch A 398: 185–195

Daimaru Y, Hashimoto H, Enjoji M (1984) Malignant "Triton" tumors: a clinicopathologic
and immunohistochemical study of nine cases. Human Pathol 15: 768–778

Daimaru Y, Hashimoto H, Enjoji M (1985) Malignant peripheral nerve-sheath tumors (malignant schwannomas). Am J Surg Pathol 9: 434–444

Darbyshire PJ, Bourne SP, Allan PM, Berry J, Oakhill A, Kemshead JT, Coakham HB (1987)
The use of a panel of monoclonal antibodies in pediatric oncology. Cancer 59: 726–730

Dardick I, Ramjohn S, Thomas MJ, Jeans D, Hammar SP (1991) Synovial sarcoma – interrela-
tionship of the biphasic and monophasic subtypes. Pathol Res Pract 187: 871–885

Dehner LP (1988) Malignant fibrous histiocytoma: nonspecific morphologic pattern, specific
pathologic entity, or both? Arch Pathol Lab Med.112: 236–237

De Lellis RA, Dayal Y (1987) The role of immunohistochemistry in the diagnosis of poorly
differentiated malignant neoplasms. Sem Oncol 14: 173–192

Dervan PA, Cahalane SF, Kneafsey P, Mynes A, McAllister K (1987) Malignant rhabdoid
tumour of soft tissue – an ultrastructural and immunohistological study of a pelvic tumor.
Histopathology 11: 183–190

De Schryver K, Santa Gruz DJ (1984) So-called glandular schwannoma: ependymal differentiation in a case. Ultrastruct Pathol 6: 167–175

Dias P, Kumar P, Marsden HB, Gattamaneni HR, Heighway J, Kumar S (1990) N-myc gene is
amplified in alveolar rhabdomyosarcomas (RMS) but not in embryonal RMS. Int J Cancer
45: 593–596

Dias P, Parham DM, Shapiro DN, Webber BL, Houghton PJ (1990) Myogenic regulatory
protein (MyoD1) expression in childhood solid tumors – diagnostic utility in rhabdomyosarcoma. Am J Pathol 137: 1283–1291

Dickersin GR (1991) Synovial sarcoma: a review and update, with emphasis on the ultrastructural characterization of the nonglandular component. Ultrastruct Pathol 15: 379–402

Ding J, Hashimoto H, Enjoji M (1989) Dermatofibrosarcoma protuberans with fibrosarcomatous areas: a clinicopathologic study of nine cases and a comparison with allied tumors.
Cancer 64: 721–729

Donhuijsen K, Schmidt U, Metz K, Leder LD (1987) Malignant fibrous histiocytoma (MFH):
hotchpotch or entity? Blut 55: 365

Donhuijsen K, Metz K, Leder LD (1988) Desmin and S-100-protein positive malignant fibrous
histiocytomas: practical and theoretical implications. Pathologe 9: 261–267

Donner LR, de Lanerolle P (1990) Expression of myogenic markers in mesenchymal tumors.
Lab Invest 62: 27A

Douglass EC, Valentine M, Rowe ST, Parham DM, Williams JA, Sanders JM, Houghton PJ
(1990) Malignant rhabdoid tumor: a highly malignant childhood tumor with minimal karyotypic changes. Genes, Chromosomes & Cancer 2: 210–216

Dowd JO, Laidler P (1988) Progression of dermatofibrosarcoma protuberans to malignant
fibrous histiocytoma: report of a case with implications for tumor histogenesis. Human Pathol
19: 368–370

Ducatman BS, Scheithauer BW (1984) Malignant peripheral nerve sheath tumors with divergent
differentiation. Cancer 54: 1049–1057

Ducatman BS, Scheithauer BW (1986) Malignant peripheral nerve sheath tumors: a clinico-
pathologic study of 120 cases. Cancer 57: 2006–2021
Ekfors TO, Aho HJ, Kekomäki M (1985) Malignant rhabdoid tumor of the prostatic region –
immunohistochemical and ultrastructural evidence for epithelial origin. Virchows Arch A
406: 381–388
Enjoji M, Hashimoto H (1990) Pathology of soft tissue sarcomas – selected current issues. Acta
Pathol Jpn 40: 863–870
Enzinger FM, Weiss SW (1988) Soft Tissue Tumors. Mosby, St Louis
Eusebi V, Carcangiu ML, Dina R, Rosai J (1990) Keratin-positive epithelioid angiosarcoma of
thyroid: a report of four cases. Am J Surg Pathol 14: 737–747
Ferry JA, Dickersin GR (1988) Pseudoglandular schwannoma. Am J Clin Pathol 89: 546–552
Fidler IJ (1978) Tumor heterogeneity and the biology of cancer invasion and metastasis. Cancer
Res 38: 2651–2660
Fisher C (1990) The value of electronmicroscopy and immunohistochemistry in the diagnosis of
soft tissue sarcomas: a study of 200 cases. Histopathology 16: 441–454
Fisher C, Schofield JB (1991) S-100 protein positive synovial sarcoma. Histopathology 19:
375–377
Fisher C, Carter RL, Ramachandra S, Thomas DM (1992) Peripheral nerve sheath differentia-
tion in malignant soft tissue tumours: an ultrastructural and immunohistochemical study.
Histopathology 20: 115–125
Fletcher CDM (1987) Commentary: malignant fibrous histiocytoma. Histopathology 11: 433–437
Fletcher CDM (1989) Postirradiation malignant fibrous histiocytoma expressing cytokeratin: a
question of diagnostic criteria. Am J Surg Pathol 13: 428–432
Fletcher CDM (1990) Peripheral nerve sheath tumors: a clinicopathologic update. Pathol Annu
25: 53–74
Fletcher CDM (1991) Angiomatoid malignant fibrous histiocytoma – an immunohistochemical
study indicative of myoid differentiation. Human Pathol 22: 563–568
Fletcher CDM (1992) Pleomorphic malignant fibrous histiocytoma – fact or fiction? – A critical
reappraisal based on 159 tumors diagnosed as pleomorphic sarcoma. Am J Surg Pathol 16:
213–228
Fletcher CDM, Beham A, Schmid C (1991a) Spindle cell haemangioendothelioma – a clinicopathological and immunohistochemical study indicative of a non-neoplastic lesion. Histopathology 18: 291–301
Fletcher CDM, Beham A, Bekir S, Clarke AMT, Marley NJE (1991b) Epithelioid angiosarcoma
of deep soft tissue – a distinctive tumor readily mistaken for an epithelial neoplasm. Am J
Surg Pathol 15: 915–924
Freshey RI (1985) Induction of differentiation in neoplastic cells. Anticancer Res 5: 111–130
Fu YS, Gabbiani G, Kaye GI, Lattes R (1975) Malignant soft tissue tumors of probable
histiocytic origin (malignant fibrous histiocytomas): general considerations and electron
microscopic and tissue culture studies. Cancer 35: 176–198
Fujita TH, Okabe SH (1990) Immunohistochemical study of congenital gingival granular cell
tumor (congenital epulis). J Oral Pathol Med 19: 492–496
Fukada T, Tsuneyoshi M, Enjoji M (1988) Malignant fibrous histiocytoma of soft parts: an
ultrastructural quantitative study. Ultrastruct Pathol 12: 117–129
Gabbert H, Gerharz CD (1988) Differenzierungsinduktion in malignen Tumoren. Verh Dtsch
Ges Path 72: 115–127
Gabbert H, Gerharz CD, Engers R, Müller-Klieser W, Moll R (1988) Terminally differentiated
postmitotic tumor cells in a rat rhabdomyosarcoma cell line. Virchows Arch B 55: 255–261
Gaffney EF (1991) Intra-abdominal neuroectodermal tumor of childhood with divergent dif-
ferentiation. Histopathology 19: 390
Garin-Chesa P, Fellinger EJ, Huvos AG, Beresford HR, Melamed MR, Triche TJ, Rettig EJ
(1991) Immunohistochemical analysis of neural cell adhesion molecules – differential expres-
sion in small round cell tumors of childhood and adolescence. Am J Pathol 139: 275–286
Garvin AJ, Stanley WS, Bennett DD, Sullivan JL, Sens DA (1986) The in vitro growth,
heterotransplantation, and differentiation of a human rhabdomyosarcoma cell line. Am J
Pathol 125: 208–217
Gerald WL, Rosai J (1989) Desmoplastic small cell tumor with divergent differentiation.
Pediatr Pathol 9: 177–183

Gerharz CD, Moll R, Ramp U, Mellin W, Gabbert HE (1990a) Multidirectional differentiation in a newly established human epithelioid sarcoma cell line (GRU-1)N with co-expression of vimentin, cytokeratin and neurofilament proteins. Int J Cancer 45: 143–152

Gerharz CD, Moll R, Meister P, Knuth A, Gabbert HE (1990b) Cytoskeletal heterogeneity of an epithelioid sarcoma with expression of vimentin, cytokeratins and neurofilaments. Am J Surg Pathol 14: 274–283

Giangaspero F, Fratamico FCM, Ceccarelli C (1989) Malignant peripheral nerve sheath tumors and spindle cell sarcomas: an immunohistochemical analysis of multiple markers. Appl Pathol 7: 134–144

Gonzalez-Crussi F, Crawford SE, Sun CCJ (1990) Intra-abdominal desmoplastic small-cell tumors with divergent differentiation: observation on three cases of childhood. Am J Surg Pathol 14: 633–642

Gonzalez-Crussi F, Chou P, Crawford SE (1991) Congenital, infiltrating giant-cell angioblastoma – a new entity. Am J Surg Pathol 15: 175–183

Gould VE (1986) Histogenesis and differentiation: a re-evaluation of these concepts as criteria for the classification of tumors. Human Pathol 17: 212–215

Gown AM, Boyd HC, Chang Y, Ferguson M, Reichler B, Tippens D (1988) Smooth muscle cells can express cytokeratins of "simple" epithelium. Am J Pathol 132: 223–232

Gray MH, Rosenberg AE, Dickersin GR, Bhan AK (1989) Glial fibrillary acidic protein and keratin expression by benign and malignant nerve sheath tumors. Human Pathol 20: 1089–1096

Hall PA, Levison DA (1989) Biphasic tumours: clues to possible histogenesis in developmental processes. J Pathol 159: 1–2

Harris H, Eyden BP, Joglekar VM (1987) Rhabdoid tumour of the bladder: a histological, ultrastructural and immunohistochemical study. Histopathology 11: 1083–1096

Hasegawa T, Hirose T, Kudo E, Abe JI, Hizawa K (1990) Cytoskeletal characteristics of myofibroblasts in benign neoplastic and reactive fibroblastic lesions. Virchows Arch A 416: 375–382

Hashimoto T, Daimaru Y, Enjoji M (1984) S-100 protein distribution in liposarcoma – an immunoperoxidase study with special reference to the distinction of liposarcoma from myxoid malignant fibrous histiocytoma. Virchows Arch A 405: 1–10

Hashimoto T, Daimaru Y, Tsuneyoshi M, Enjoji M (1990) Soft tissue sarcoma with additional anaplastic components: a clinicopathologic and immunohistochemical study of 27 cases. Cancer 66: 1578–1589

Heim S, Mandahl N, Mitelman F (1988) Genetic convergence and divergence in tumor progression. Cancer Res 48: 5911–5916

Heppner GH (1984) Tumor heterogeneity. Cancer Res 44: 2259–2265

Heppner GH (1989) Tumor cell societies. J Natl Cancer Inst 81: 648–649

Heppner GH, Miller BE (1989) Therapeutic implications of tumor heterogeneity. Sem Oncol 16: 91–106

Herrera G, Reiman BEF, Salinas JA (1982) Malignant schwannomas presenting as malignant fibrous histiocytomas. Ultrastruct Pathol 3: 253–261

Hirose T, Sano T, Hizawa K (1988) Heterogeneity of malignant schwannomas. Ultrastruct Pathol 12: 107–116

Hirose T, Kudo E, Hasegawa T, ABE JI, Hizawa K (1989) Expression of intermediate filaments in malignant fibrous histiocytomas. Human Pathol 20: 871–877

Horio K, Yoshikura H, Kawabata M, Odawara T, Sudo K, Fujitani Y, Lee GH, Iwamoto A (1991) Epigenetic control of tumor cell morphology. Japan J Cancer Res 82: 676–685

Huang JS, Huang SS, Deuel TF (1984) Transforming protein of simian sarcoma virus stimulates autocrine growth of SSV-transformed cells through PDGF cell-surface receptors. Cell 39: 79–83

Hueck W (1939) Über das Mesenchym. III. Mesenchymale Tumoren. Beitr Path Anat 103: 308–349

Iannacone PM, Weinberg WC, Deamant FD (1987) On the clonal origin of tumors – a review of experimental models. Int J Cancer 39: 778–784

Iwasaki H, Isayama T, Ohjimi Y, Nickuchi M, Yoh S, Shinohara N, Yoshitake K, Eshiguro M, Kamada N, Enjoji M (1992) Malignant fibrous histiocytoma – a tumor of facultative histiocytes showing mesenchymal differentiation in cultured cell lines. Cancer 69: 437–447

Jabi M, Jeans D, Dardick I (1987) Ultrastructural heterogeneity in malignant fibrous histiocytoma of soft tissue. Ultrastruct Pathol 11: 583–592

Jakate SM, Marsden HB, Ingram L (1988) Primary rhabdoid tumor of the brain. Virchows
Arch A 412: 393–397

John L, Franke WW (1989) High frequency of cytokeratin-producing smooth muscle cells in
human atherosclerotic plaques. Differentiation 40: 55–62

Johnson MD, Glick AD, David BW (1988) Immunohistochemical evaluation of Leu 7, myelin
basic protein, S 100 protein, glial fibrillary acidic protein, and LN3 immunoreactivity in nerve
sheath tumors and sarcomas. Arch Pathol Lab Med 112: 151–160

Johnson TL, Lee MW, Meis JM, Zarbo RJ, Crissman (1991) Immunohistochemical characterization of malignant peripheral nerve sheath tumors. Surg Pathol 4: 121–135

Katenkamp D (1986) Electron microscopy and immunohistochemistry in soft tissue sarcoma
diagnosis – problems and limitations. 14th Int Cancer Congr, Budapest, August 21–27,
Abstracts, vol 3, p 9

Katenkamp D (1988) Cellular heterogeneity – explanation for changes of tumor phenotype and
biologic behaviour in soft tissue sarcomas. Path Res Pract 183: 698–702

Katenkamp D, Hünerbein R (1992) Untersuchunger zur prognostischen Bedeutung von
Entzündungszellen in malignen Weichgewebstumoren des Menschen. Zugleich ein Beitrag
zur Malignitätsgraduierung. Zentralbl Pathol 138: 21–25

Katenkamp D, Kosmehl H (1993) Letter to the case (leiomyomatous rhabdomyosarcoma).
Pathol Res Pract 189: 107–108

Katenkamp D, Neupert G (1982) Experimental tumors with features of malignant fibrous
histiocytomas. Exp Pathol 22: 11–27

Katenkamp D, Raikhlin NT (1985) Stem cell concept and heterogeneity of soft tissue tumors –
a challenge for diagnostics and therapy. Exp Pathol 28: 3–11

Katenkamp D, Stiller D (1975) Structural patterns and histological behaviour of experimental
sarcomas. II. Ultrastructural cytology. Exp Pathol 11: 190–206

Katenkamp D, Stiller D (1990) Weichgewebstumoren. Pathologie, histologische Diagnose und
Differentialdiagnose. Barth, Leipzig

Katenkamp D, Stiller D, Kütter K, Möller HJ (1979) Untersuchungen zur submikroskopischen
Zytologie botryoider (Rhabdomyo-) Sarkome des Nasen-Rachens. Zbl Allg Pathol 123:
508–519

Kawamoto EH, Weidner N, Agostini RM, Jaffe R (1987) Malignant ectomesenchymoma of
soft tissue: report of two cases and review of the literature. Cancer 59: 1791–1802

Kent AL, Mahoney DH, Gresik MV, Steuber CP, Fernbach DJ (1987) Malignant rhabdoid
tumor of the extremity. Cancer 60: 1056–1059

Klima M, Smith M, Spjut HJ, Root EN (1975) Malignant mesenchymoma – case report with
electron microscopic study. Cancer 36: 1086–1094

Knight JC (1990) The molecular genetics of soft tissue sarcomas. Br J Cancer 26: 511–513

Kodet R, Kasthuri N, Marsden HB, Coad AG, Raafat F (1986) Gangliorhabdomyosarcomas: a
histopathological and immunohistochemical study of three cases. Histopathology 10: 181–193

Kodet R, Newton WA, Sachs N, Hamoudi AB, Raney RB, Asmar L, Gehan EA (1991a)
Rhabdoid tumors of soft tissues – a clinicopathologic study of 26 cases enrolled in the
intergroup rhabdomyosarcoma study. Human Pathol 22: 674–684

Kodet R, Newton WA, Hamoudi AB, Asmar L (1991b) Rhabdomyosarcomas with intermediate-
filaments inclusions and features of rhabdoid tumors – light microscopic and immunohistochemical study. Am J Surg Pathol 15: 257–267

Kosmehl H, Langbein L, Katenkamp D (1990a) Transient cytokeratin expression in skeletal
muscle during murine embryogenesis. Anat Anz 171: 39–44

Kosmehl H, Langbein L, Katenkamp D (1990b) Experimental rhabdomyosarcoma with regions
like malignant fibrious histiocytoma (MFH) – a true double phenotypic pattern? J Pathol 160:
135–140

Kulesh DA, Oshima RG (1988) Cloning of human keratin 18 gene and its expression in
nonepithelial mouse cells. Mol Cell Biol 8: 1540–1550

Lagacé R (1987) The ultrastructural spectrum of malignant fibrous histiocytoma. Ultrastruct
Pathol 11: 153–159

Langbein L, Kosmehl H, Katenkamp D (1988) Intermediate filament typing in tumour diagnostics – an aid in histogenetic classification? Acta Morph Hung 36: 215–225

Langbein L, Kosmehl H, Katenkamp D, Neupert G, Stiller KJ (1990) Experimentally induced rhabdomyosarcomas – correlation between cellular contacts, matrix formation and cellular differentiation. Differentiation 44: 185–196

Layfield LJ, Lenarsky C (1991) Desmoplastic small cell tumors of the peritoneum coexpressing mesenchymal and epithelial markers. Am J Clin Pathol 96: 536–543

Leader M, Collins M, Patel J, Henry K (1987) Desmin: its value as a marker of muscle derived tumours using a commercial antibody. Virchows Arch A 411: 345–349

Leith JT, Dexter DL (1986) Mammalian tumor cell heterogeneity. CRC Press, Bocan Raton

Leu HJ, Makek M (1982) Angiomatoid malignant fibrous histiocytoma – case report and electron microscopic findings. Virchows Arch A 395: 99–107

Llombart-Bosch A, Carda C, Boix J, Pellin A, Peydro-Olaya A (1988) Value of nude mice xenografts in the expression of cell heterogeneity of human sarcomas of bone and soft tissue. Path Res Pract 183: 683–692

Lodding P, Kindblom LG, Angervall L, Stenman G (1990) Cellular schwannoma – a clinicopathologic study of 29 cases. Virchows Arch A 416: 237–248

Lollini PL, Degiovanni D, Delre B, Landuzzi L, Nicoletti G, Prodi G, Scotlandi K, Nanni (1989) Myogenic differentiation of human rhabdomyosarcoma cells induced in vitro by antineoplastic drugs. Cancer Res 49: 3631–3636

Matias C, Nunes JFM, Vicente LF, Almeida MO (1990) Primary malignant rhabdoid tumor of the vulva. Histopathology 17: 576–578

Matthews MJ, Gazdar AF (1985) Changing histology in malignant tumors: diagnostic and therapeutic significance. Eur J Cancer Clin Oncol 21: 549–552

McGregor DH, Dixon AY, Moral L, Kanabe S (1987) Liposarcoma of pleural cavity with recurrence as malignant fibrous histiocytoma. Ann Clin Lab Sci 17: 83–92

McWilliam LJ, Harris M (1985) Granular cell angiosarcoma of the skin: histology, electron microscopy and immunohistochemistry of a newly recognized tumour. Histopathology 9: 1205–1216

Meis JM, Enzinger FM (1991) Inflammatory fibrosarcoma of the mesentery and retroperitoneum – a tumor loosely simulating inflammatory pseudotumor. Am J Surg Pathol 15: 1146–1156

Meister P (1988) Malignant fibrous histiocytoma – history, histology, histogenesis. Path Res Pract 183: 1–7

Meister P (1991) Weichgewebstumoren: Definition, Klassifizierung und Graduierung. 27. Symposium der Int. Akademie für Pathologie, Deutsche Abtlg. e.V., Bonn, Februar 1991

Mentzel T, Kosmehl H, Katenkamp D (1991) Metastasizing phyllodes tumour with malignant fibrous histiocytoma-like areas. Histopathology 19: 557–560

Mierau GW, Berry FJ, Orsini EN (1985) Small round cell neoplasms: can electron microscopy and immunohistochemical studies accurately classify them? Ultrastruct Pathol 9: 99–111

Miettinen M (1988a) Immunoreactivity for cytokeratin and epithelial membrane antigen in leiomyosarcomas. Arch Pathol Lab Med 112: 637–640

Miettinen M (1988b) Antibody specific to muscle actins in the diagnosis and classification of soft tissue tumors. Am J Pathol 130: 205–215

Miettinen M (1989) Intermediate filament proteins in soft tissue sarcomas: new findings suggest a complex pattern of expression. In: Osborn M, Weber K (eds) Cytoskeletal proteins in tumor diagnosis. Cold Spring Harbor Lab, New York, pp 63–68

Miettinen M (1990) Immunohistochemistry of solid tumours. Brief review of selected problems. APMIS 98: 191–199

Miettinen M (1991) Keratin subsets in spindle cell sarcomas – keratins are widespread but synovial sarcomas contain a distinctive keratin polypeptide pattern and desmoplakins. Am J Pathol 138: 505–513

Miettinen M, Kovatich A (1991) Keratins in soft tissue sarcomas – common phenomenon or technical artifact? Am J Clin Pathol 96: 673–674

Miettinen M, Rapola J (1989) Immunohistochemical spectrum of rhabdomyosarcoma and rhabdomyosarcoma-like tumors – expression of cytokeratin and 68-kD neurofilament protein. Am J Surg Pathol 13: 120–132

Miettinen M, Soini Y (1989) Malignant fibrous histiocytoma – heterogeneous patterns of intermediate filament proteins by immunohistochemistry. Arch Pathol Lab Med 113: 1363–1366

Miettinen M, Lehto VP, Badley RA, Virtanen I (1982) Expression of intermediate filaments in soft-tissue sarcomas. Int J Cancer 30: 541–546

Miettinen M, Foidart JM, Ekblom P (1983) Immunohistochemical demonstration of laminin, the major glycoprotein of basement membranes, as aid in the diagnosis of soft tissue tumors. Am J Clin Pathol 73: 306–311

Mirra JM, Kessler S, Bhuta S, Eckardt J (1992) The fibroma-like variant of epithelioid sarcoma – a fibrohistiocytic/myoid cell lesion often confused with benign and malignant spindle cell tumors. Cancer 69: 1382–1395

Molenaar WM, Oosterhuis JW, Kamps WA (1984) Cytologic "differentiation" in childhood rhabdomyosarcomas following polychemotherapy. Human Pathol 15: 973–979

Molenaar WM, Dam-Meiring A, Kamps WA, Cornelisse CJ (1988) DNA-aneuploidy in rhabdomyosarcomas as compared with other sarcomas of childhood and adolescence. Human Pathol 19: 573–579

Molenaar WM, deJong B, Buist J, Idenburg VJS, Seruca R, Vos AM, Hoekstra HJ (1989a) Chromosomal analysis and the classification of soft tissue sarcomas. Lab Invest 60: 266–274

Molenaar WM, deJong B, Dam-Meiring A, Postma A, Hoekstra HJ (1989b) Epithelioid sarcoma or malignant rhabdoid tumor of soft tissue? Epithelioid immunophenotype and rhabdoid karyotype. Human Pathol 20: 347–351

Moll R, Lee I, Gould VE, Berndt R, Roessner A, Franke WW (1987) Immunohistochemical analysis of Ewing's tumors – pattern of expression of intermediate filaments and desmosomal proteins indicate cell type heterogeneity and pluripotential differentiation. Amer J Pathol 127: 288–304

Nakashima Y, Unni KK, Shives TC, Swee RG, Dahlin DC (1986) Mesenchymal chondrosarcoma of bone and soft tissue: a review of 111 cases. Cancer 57: 2444–2453

Nakazato Y, Hirato J, Nakanishi Y, Tamaki O, Yazaki C (1991) Immunohistochemical localization of five classes of intermediate filaments in a benign pelvic soft tissue tumor of rhabdoid appearance. Acta Pathol Jpn 41: 65–72

Newman PL, Fletcher CDM (1987) Malignant mesenchymoma – clinicopathologic analysis of a series with evidence of low-grade behaviour. Am J Surg Pathol 15: 607–614

Nicolson GL (1987) Tumor cell instability, diversification, and progression to the metastatic phenotype: from oncogene to oncofetal expression. Cancer Res 47: 1473–1487

Norton AJ, Thomas JA, Isaacson PG (1987) Cytokeratin-specific monoclonal antibodies are reactive with tumours of smooth muscle derivation – an immunohistochemical and biochemical study using antibodies to intermediate filament cytoskeletal proteins. Histopathology 11: 487–499

O'Dowd J, Laidler P (1988) Progression of dermatofibrosarcoma protuberans to malignant fibrous histiocytoma: report of a case with implications for tumor histogenesis. Human Pathol 19: 368–370

Ohmori T, Arita N, Sano A, Watanabe Y (1986) Malignant fibrous histiocytoma showing cytoplasmic hyaline globules and stromal osteoids – a case report with light and electron microscopic, histochemical and immunohistochemical study. Acta Pathol Jpn 36: 1931–1941

Okabe T, Suzuki A, Hirono M, Tamaoki N, Oshimura M, Takaku F (1983) Establishment of different clonal strains from a human sarcoma of the stomach: tumorigenic heterogeneity in athymic nude mice. Cancer Res 43: 5456–5461

Ordonez NG, Mahfouz SM, MacKay B (1990) Synovial sarcoma – an immunohistochemical and ultrastructural study. Human Path 21: 733–749

Otto HF, Berndt R, Schwechheimer K, Möller P (1987) Mesenchymal tumor markers: special proteins and enzymes. Current Topics Pathol 77: 197–205

Palman G, Bowenpope DF, Brooks JJ (1992) Plastelet-derived growth factor receptor (beta-subunit) immunoreactivity in soft tissue tumors. Lab Invest 66: 108–115

Palmer NF, Sutow W (1983) Clinical aspects of the rhabdoid tumor of the kidney: a report of the National Wilm's Tumor Study Group. Med Pediatr Oncol 11: 242–245

Parham DM, Jenkins JJ, Holt H, Callihan TR (1987) Phenotypic diversity in pediatric rhabdoid tumors: a morphologic and immunohistochemical study. Lab Invest 56: 58A

Parham DM, Webber B, Holt H, Williams WK, Maurer H (1991) Immunohistochemical study of childhood rhabdomyosarcomas and related neoplasms – results of an intergroup Rhabdomyosarcoma Study project. Cancer 67: 3072–3080

Perosio PM, Brooks JJ (1989) Expression of growth factor receptors in soft tissue tumors – implications for the autocrine hypothesis. Lab Invest 60: 245–253

Perrone T, Swanson PE, Twiggs L, Ulbright TM, Dehner LP (1989) Malignant rhabdoid tumor of the vulva: is distinction from epithelioid sarcoma possible? A pathologic and immunohistochemical study. Am J Surg Pathol 13: 848–858

Pettinato G, Manivel JC, De Rosa G, Petrella G, Jaszcz W (1990) Angiomatoid malignant fibrous histiocytoma: cytologic, immunohistochemical, ultrastructural and flow cytometric study of 20 cases. Mod Pathol 3: 479–487

Pitot HC (1989) Progression: the terminal stage in carcinogenesis. Jpn Cancer Res 80: 599–607

Porter PL, Gown AM, Kramp SG, Coltrera MD (1992) Widespread p53 overexpression in human malignant tumors. Am J Pathol 140: 145–153

Radio SE, Woolridge TN, Lindner J (1988) Flow cytometric DNA analysis of malignant fibrous histiocytoma and related fibrohistiocytic tumors. Human Pathol 19: 74–77

Raju GC, O'Reilly AP (1987) Immunohistochemical study of granular cell tumour. Pathology 19: 402–406

Ramaekers FC, Pruszczynski M, Smedts F (1988) Cytokeratins in smooth muscle cell and smooth muscle tumours. Histopathology 12: 558–561

Ro JY, Ayala AG, Sella A, Samuels ML, Swanson DA (1987) Sarcomatoid renal cell carcinoma: a clinicopathologic study of 42 cases. Cancer 59: 516–526

Roholl PJM, deJong ASH, Albus-Lutter CE, Ramaekers FCS (1985) Application of markers in the diagnosis of soft tissue tumours. Histopathology 9: 1019–1035

Roholl PJM, deJong ASH, Albus-Lutter CE, van Unnik JAM (1988a) Leiomyosarcomas: the three cases with desmin positive tumour cells, lacking ultrastructural features of smooth muscle cells. Histol Histopathol 3: 389–394

Roholl PJM, Rutgers DH, Ramaekers FCS, De Weger RA, Elbers JRJ, van Unnik JAM (1988b) Characterization of human soft tissue sarcomas in nude mice: evidence for histogenetic properties of malignant fibrous histiocytomas. Am J Pathol 131: 559–568

Roholl PJM, Elbers JRJ, Prinsen I, van Unnik JAM (1990a) Distribution of actin isoforms in sarcomas – an immunohistochemical study. Human Pathol 21: 1269–1274

Roholl PJM, Skottner A, Prinsen I, Lips CJM, Den Otten W, van Unnik JAM (1990b) Expression of insulin-like growth factor 1 in sarcomas. Histopathology 16: 455–460

Roholl PJM, Weima SM, Prinsen I, Ramaekers LPHM, Hsu SM, van Unnik JAM (1991a) Two cell lines with epithelial cell-like characteristics established from malignant fibrous histiocytomas. Cancer 68: 1963–1972

Roholl PJM, Weima SM, Prinsen I, De Weger RA, Den Otten W, van Unnik JAM (1991b) Expression of growth factors and their receptors in human sarcomas. Immunohistochemical detection of platelet-derived growth factor, epidermal growth factor and their receptors. Cancer J 4: 83–88

Rubin H (1990) The signifigance of biological heterogeneity. Cancer Metastasis Rev 9: 1–20

Schmidt D, Harms D (1987) Epithelioid sarcoma in children and adolescents – an immuno-histochemical study. Virchows Arch A 410: 423–431

Schmidt D, Steen A, Voss C (1989a) Immunohistochemical study of rhabdomyosarcoma: unexpected staining with S-100 protein and cytokeratin. J Pathol 157: 83

Schmidt D, Leuschner I, Harms D, Sprenger E, Schäfer HJ (1989b) Malignant rhabdoid tumor – a morphological and flow cytometric study. Path Res Pract 184: 202–210

Schmidt D, Leuschner I, Moeller R, Harms D (1990a) Immunohistochemische Befunde bei Rhabdomyosarkomen. Pathologe 11: 283–289

Schmidt D, Harms D, Leuschner I (1990b) Cytokeratin expression in malignant Triton tumor. Path Res Pract 186: 507–511

Schmidt D, Herrmann C, Jürgens H, Harms D (1991) Malignant peripheral neuroectodermal tumor and its necessary distinction from Ewing's sarcoma – a report from the Kiel Pediatric Tumor Registry. Cancer 68: 2251–2259

Schmitt FC, Bacchi CE (1989) S-100 protein: is it useful as tumour marker in diagnostic immunohistochemistry? Histopathology 15: 281–288

Schröder S, Tessmann D (1991) Maligner desmoplastischer kleinzelliger Tumor des Peritoneums mit divergenter Differenzierung. Pathologe 12: 334–340

Schürch W, Skalli O, Seemayer TA, Gabbiani G (1987) Intermediate filament proteins and actin isoforms as markers for soft tissue tumor differentiation and origin. I. Smooth muscle tumors. Am J Pathol 128: 91–103

Schürch W, Skalli O, Lagacé R, Seemayer TA, Gabbiani G (1990) Intermediate filament proteins and actin isoforms as markers for soft tissue tumor differentiation and origin. 3. Hemangiopericytomas and glomus tumors. Am J Pathol 136: 771–786

Scrable H, Witte D, Shimada H, Seemayer TA, Wang-Wuu S, Soukup S, Koufos A, Houghton P, Lampkin B, Cavenee W (1989) Molecular differentiation pathology of rhabdomyosarcoma. Genes Chromosomes Cancer 1: 23–35

Seo IS, Warner TFCS, Warren JS, Bennett JE (1985) Cutaneous postirradiation sarcoma – ultrastructural evidence of pluripotential mesenchymal cell derivation. Cancer 56: 761–767

Shmookler BM, Enzinger FM, Weiss SW (1989) Giant cell fibroblastoma: a juvenile form of dermatofibrosarcoma protuberans. Cancer 64: 2154–2161

Skalli O, Gabbiani G, Babai F, Seemayer TA, Pizzolato G, Schürch W (1988) Intermediate filament proteins and actin isoforms as markers for soft tissue tumor differentiation and origin: II. Rhabdomyosarcoma. Am J Pathol 130: 515–531

Smith MEF, Costa MJ, Weiss SW (1991) Evaluation of CD68 and other histiocytic antigens in angiomatoid malignant fibrous histiocytoma. Am J Surg Pathol 15: 757–763

Snover DC, Sumner HW, Dehner LP (1982) Variability of histologic pattern in recurrent soft tissue sarcomas originally diagnosed as liposarcoma. Cancer 49: 1005–1015

Soini Y, Autio-Harmainen H (1991) Tumor cells of malignant fibrous histiocytomas express mRNA for laminin. Am J Pathol 139: 1061–1067

Soini Y, Miettinen M (1991) Immunohistochemistry of markers of histiomonocytic cells in malignant fibrous histiocytomas – a monoclonal antibody study. Path Res Pract 186: 759–767

Stenman G, Kindblom LG, Willems J, Angervall L (1990) A cell culture, chromosomal and quantitative DNA analysis of a metastatic epithelioid sarcoma: deletion 1p. a possible primary chromosomal abnormality in epithelioid sarcoma. Cancer 65: 2006–2013

Stratton MR, Moss S, Warren W, Patterson H, Clark J, Fisher C, Fletcher CDM, Ball A, Thomas M, Gusterson BA, Cooper CS (1990) Mutation of p53 gene in human soft tissue sarcomas: association with abnormalities of the RB1 gene. Oncogene 5: 1297–1301

Strauchen JA, Dimitriu-Bona A (1986) Malignant fibrous histiocytoma – expression of monocyte/macrophage differentiation antigens detected with monoclonal antibodies. Am J Pathol 124: 303–309

Swanson PE (1991) Heffalumps, jagulars, and cheshire cats – a commentary on cytokeratins and soft tissue sarcomas. Am J Clin Pathol 95(Suppl I): S2–S7

Swanson PE, Manivel JC, Wick MR (1987) Immunoreactivity for Leu-7 in neurofibrosarcoma and other spindle cell sarcomas of soft tissue. Am J Pathol 126: 546–560

Swanson PE, Dehner LP, Wick MR (1988) Polyphenotypic small cell tumors of childhood. Lab Invest 68: 9P

Takahara O, Nakayama I, Yokoyama S, Moriuchi A, Muta H, Uchida Y (1979) Malignant neurofibroma with glandular differentiation (glandular schwannoma). Acta Pathol Jpn 40: 597–606

Takizawa T, Matsui T, Maeda Y, Okabe S, Mochizuki M, Tanaka A, Kawaguchi K, Fukayama M, Funata N, Koike M, Mastuda T (1989) X-radiation-induced differentiaton of xenotransplanted human undifferentiated rhabdomyosarcoma. Lab Invest 69: 22–29

Tanimura A, Nagayama K, Nakamura Y, Tanaka S, Tanaka T (1985) Malignant fibrous histiocytoma with granular cells, mimicking a granular cell tumor – light, electron microscopic and immunohistochemical observations of a case. Acta Pathol Jpn 35: 1555–1560

Tauchi K, Tsutsumi Y, Yoshimura S, Watanabe K (1990) Immunohistochemical and immunoblotting detection of cytokeratin in smooth muscle tumours. Acta Pathol Jpn 40: 574–580

Tsokos M, Kouraklis G, Chandra RS, Bhagavan BS, Triche TJ (1989) Malignant rhabdoid tumor of the kidney and soft tissues – evidence for a diverse morphological and immunocytochemical phenotype. Arch Pathol Lab Med 113: 115–120

Tsuneyoshi M, Daimaru Y, Hashimoto H, Enjoji M (1987) The existence of rhabdoid cells in specified soft tissue sarcomas. Virchows Arch A 411: 509–514

Ulrich J, Heitz PU, Fischer T, Obrist E, Gullotta F (1987) Granular cell tumors: evidence for heterogeneous tumor cell differentiation – an immunohistochemical study. Virchows Arch B 53: 52–57

Uri AK, Witzleben CL, Raney RB (1984) Electron microscopy of glandular schwannoma. Cancer 53: 493–497

Uriel J (1979) Retrodifferentiation and fetal patterns of gene expression in cancer. Adv Canc Res 29: 127–174

van Haelst UGJM, Pruszcznski M, Cate LN, Mravunac M (1990) Ultrastructural and immunohistochemical study of epithelioid hemangioendothelioma of bone: coexpression of epithelial and endothelial markers. Ultrastruct Pathol 14: 141–149

Weeks DA, Beckwith JB, Mierau CW (1989) Rhabdoid tumor – an entity or a phenotype? Arch Pathol Lab Med 113: 113–114

Weiss SW, Enzinger FM (1986) Spindle cell hemangioendothelioma: a low-grade angiosarcoma resembling a cavernous hemangioma and Kaposi's sarcoma. Am J Surg Pathol 10: 521–530

Weiss SW, Bratthauer GL, Morris PA (1988) Postirradiation malignant fibrous histiocytoma expressing cytokeratin – implications for the immunodiagnosis of sarcomas. Am J Surg Pathol 12: 554–558

Wick MR, Swanson PE, Scheithauer BW, Manivel JC (1987) Malignant peripheral nerve sheath tumor: an immunohistochemical study of 62 cases. Am J Clin Pathol 87: 425–433

Wich MR, Manivel JC, Swanson PE (1988) Contributions of immunohistochemical analysis to the diagnosis of soft tissue tumors: a review. Progr Surg Pathol 8: 197–249

Wong SY, Teh M, Tan YO, Best PV (1991) Malignant glandular Triton tumors. Cancer 67: 1076–1081

Woodruff JM (1976) Peripheral nerve tumors showing glandular differentiation (glandular schwannomas). Cancer 37: 2399–2413

Wrotnowski U, Cooper PH, Shmookler BM (1988) Fibrosarcomatous change in dermatofibrosarcoma protuberans. Am J Surg Pathol 12: 287–293

Xiang JH, Spanier SS, Bensen NA, Braylan RC (1987) Flow cytometric analysis of DNA in bone and soft tissue tumors using nuclear suspensions. Cancer 59: 1951–1958

Zoltie N, Roberts PF (1989) Spindle cell haemangioendothelioma in association with epithelioid haemangioendothelioma. Histopathology 15: 544–546

Grading of Soft Tissue Sarcomas: Proposal for a Reproducible, Albeit Limited Scheme

P. Meister

In order to treat malignant tumors of mesenchymal origin one must first learn to recognize them. (Stout 1964)

1 Grading: General Remarks

1.1 Grading in the TNM Classification

After determination of the histological type a grading has to be carried out according to accepted criteria including cellularity, pleomorphism, mitotic activity and necrosis. The presence of intercellular substances, collagenous or mucoid, ought to be considered as favorable factor judging the degree of differentiation.

This statement is taken from the TNM classification of malignant tumors by the International Union Against Cancer (UICC; comparable to the AJCC) (Hermanek et al. 1987). Histopathological grading is defined as: Gx – grade of differentiation cannot be determined; G1 – well differentiated; G2 – moderately differentiated; G3/4 – poorly differentiated/ undifferentiated. Obviously differentiation as a parameter for grading is

Current Topics in Pathology
Volume 89, Eds. D. Harms/D. Schmidt
© Springer-Verlag Berlin Heidelberg 1995

also being applied without having specifically been mentioned among the "accepted criteria" cited above.

Also, according to this TNM classification, grading is the basis for staging, as stages I, II, and III, respectively, are determined by the grades G1, G2, or G3/4. Tumor size (T1 – below, T2 – above 5 cm maximal diameter) only influences subdivision of stages into Ia or Ib, etc. Only stage IV is defined by the presence of metastasis irrespective of grading: IVa – lymphogenic spread, IVb – hematogenous spread.

In summary it has to be critically emphasized that not only is precise information lacking on how to evaluate accepted criteria of grading, such as pleomorphism and mitoses, but there is also an additional (independent?) parameter introduced, namely differentiation without any further definition. Finally, staging which is supposed to be paramount for prognostic and therapeutic evaluation, is based on these vague grading parameters. The fact that staging according to the TNM classification only rests on weak histo-morphological foundations of grading, which is supposedly inferior to staging has obviously been ignored! This fact becomes especially evident in apparently exact, scientific therapeutic studies with a histomorphological background which can actually be traced back to "criteria" which could not even be called arbitrary.

1.2 Grading in the WHO Classification of Soft Tissue Tumors

The second edition of the WHO classification of soft tissue tumors (WEISS 1993) could be called "arbitrary," recommending not one, but several proposed grading schemes which will be discussed in the following. The decision to declare one system as the best has been postponed, as advantages and disadvantages are being discussed for several proposals. As a compromise, it has been recommended that the individual grading scheme applied should at least be used consistently. In the first edition of the WHO classification (ENZINGER 1967), it was only mentioned that, for instance, the diagnosis liposarcoma is quite meaningless for prognosis and adequate therapy without reference to its histological subtype as "notable differences in the clinical course exist not only between neoplasms of different histological type, but also between morphological different subvarieties of certain soft tissue tumors." It is further stated that the term differentiation is used to indicate maturity, or resemblance of neoplastic cells to the cells of corresponding normal adult tissue. Thus, "in most instances the degree of differentiation is a reliable indicator of the future clinical behaviour. But sometimes differentiation is misleading" (!). The different weighting of the "degree of differentiation" for different tumor types as well as of the individual "accepted criteria for grading" ought to be especially emphasized. Moreover, grading criteria as well as the biological behavior of given tumor types may also depend on other factors influencing prognosis such as local-ization (the region involved and the depth!) and the age and possibly also the sex of the patient (HAJDU 1979; ENZINGER and WEISS 1988). Last but not least, especially for soft tissue tumors, intratumoral variations which may concern criteria of grading as well as typing have to be pointed out (KATENKAMP and STILLER 1990; MEISTER 1992). Therefore it is mandatory to examine several sections from various portions of a given tumor, which should include all areas with varying optic appearance or consistency (FIDDER 1987; MEISTER 1988).

1.3 Grading Problems Related to Heterogeneity of Soft Tissue Tumors

Regional morphological differences, synchronous or metachronous, demand standardized procedures regarding the minimal requirements for the quantity of tissue to be examined and the criteria for final tumor characterization (RABES and MEISTER 1979; MEISTER 1988; QUINN and WRIGHT 1990). The latter can be based either solely on the presence of certain morphological features, or on their predominance, and not so much on their absence. As exact guidelines are lacking, soft tissue sarcomas are chiefly classified ac-cording to the highest grade of malignancy, even if only focally present, and according to the tumor type exhibiting the best defined criteria (SCHMIDT et al. 1986; MEISTER 1988). Changing histological features with the course of time, also during radio- or chemotherapy, deserve special consideration (WEISS et al. 1988; KATENKAMP 1988; KATENKAMP and STILLER 1990). This is of utmost importance with tumors undergoing adjuvant or even neoadjuvant therapy, where an evaluation of the response is required. Heterogeneity, including immunohistochemical, fine-structural, and even cytogenetic criteria demands exact definitions in relation to unexpected, "aberrant" findings (MIETTINEN et al. 1982; BROOK 1982; ERLANDSON 1984; ALTMANNSBERGER et al. 1986; BROOKS 1986, 1989; BROWN et al. 1987; COINDRE et al. 1988a; KATENKAMP 1988; IWASAKI et al. 1987).

1.4 Grading: Requirements, Outlooks

In conclusion: a reproducible, simple and effective system of grading has to be implemented to fulfill all the requirements for exact tumor characteriza-tion as required, for instance, in the TNM classification (HERMANEK et al. 1987). Empirically this grading system has to be related to the specific tumor type, as interdependency between grading and typing may play an albeit varying role for prognosis (ENZINGER and WEISS 1988; MEISTER 1988).

Additionally more sophisticated methods such as immunohistochemical evaluation of proliferative markers and DNA analysis (flow cytophometry) deserve further consideration, especially to broaden the general understanding of biological behavior in soft tissue tumors, as well as to solve certain specific problems such as prognosis for individual tumors (DONHUIJSEN 1986; MEISTER 1988).

2 Overview of Various Grading Systems

2.1 Historical Development of Grading

In 1933 BRODERS (BRODERS et al. 1939) proposed a grading system for carcinomas, especially adenocarcinomas of the colon, based on maturity, or resemblance to corresponding normal tissue. For the colon carcinoma, uniformity of cell size and shape, and formation of glandular structures expressed high differentiation or low-grade malignancy. High-grade malignancy, in contrast, would show loss of differentiation with marked cellular pleomorphism and loss of glandular pattern with solid growth, occasionally also loss of epithelial cohesion and sarcoma-like features. Later, in 1939, BRODERS et al. adapted this grading scheme to mesenchymal tumors, for instance fibrosarcoma (Table 1). In analogy fibrosarcomas were graded according to cellular uniformity and differentiation, that is distinct collagen formation and fasciculation as low-grade malignant (O = G1), or with marked cellular pleomorphism, loss of collagen production, and fascicular orientation as high-grade malignant (= G3/4) (Figs. 1, 2). Applying this concept to studies of prognosis in fibrosarcomas, which previously showed a wide range of varying survival rates, good separation between low-grade G1 tumors and high-grade malignant grade 3/4 tumors became evident. However, problems arose for "intermediate" G2 cases. In one study these cases were closer to low-, in another to high-grade malignancies in their prognosis. The intermediate G2 group is by "compromise" the largest. More precise grading schemes are required to assign G2 cases as often as possible either to the low or the high malignancy group, with correspondingly differing therapy (MACKENZIE 1964; CASTRO et al. 1973; PRITCHARD et al. 1974; RUSSELL et al. 1977; SCOTT et al. 1989).

Table 1. Grading according to BRODERS et al. (1939)

1. Cellularity
2. Pleomorphism/anaplasia
3. Mitoses (number and atypia)
4. Degree of necrosis
(5. Growth pattern: expansive vs. invasive)

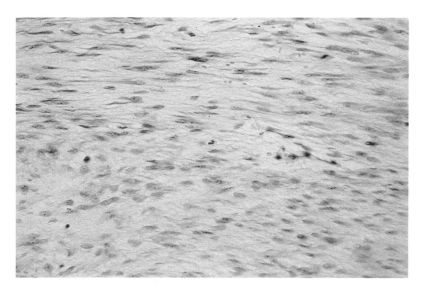

Fig. 1. Fibrosarcoma G1: distinct fasciculation with intercellular collagen. Neither remarkable cellular atypia nor mitotic activity. Histologic features compatible with low-grade malignancy. H&E

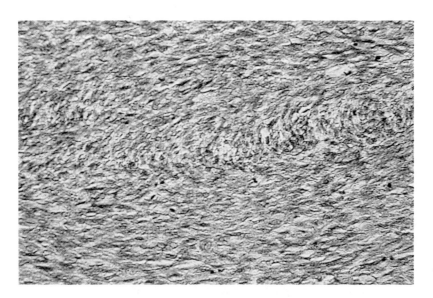

Fig. 2. Fibrosarcoma G3: fascicles still recognizable, however, no collagenous intercellular substance. High cellularity of immature cells with only moderate atypia, but high mitotic activity as signs of high-grade malignancy. H&E

2.2 Grading and Subtypes

Criteria such as differentiation and also atypia, and later mitotic activity and necrosis had already been generally introduced into tumor pathology, especially for soft tissue sarcomas (HERMANEK et al. 1987). However, with some soft tissue sarcomas, for instance, liposarcomas, myxoid, round cell and pleomorphic types were not only distinguished by morphology but also by prognosis (ENZINGER and WINSLOW 1962; EVANS 1979; EVANS et al. 1979; ENZINGER and WEISS 1988). Myxoid liposarcoma obviously presents with immaturity and hardly any recognizable lipoblasts as a "bad sign." On the other hand, there is a lack of cellular pleomorphism, low mitotic activity and low cellularity, and abundant (mucoid) ground substance as "good signs," an impression marred by necrosis as a bad sign again (Fig. 3). With the related round cell-type immaturity, high cellularity and mitotic activity are signs of high-grade malignancy, although cellular pleomorphism is missing. Only pleomorphic liposarcoma fulfills all criteria of high-grade malignancy showing marked atypia, anaplasia with giant cells, mitoses, necrosis, cellularity, and quite often, but not always, a lack of lipoblastic differentiation (Fig. 4). Problematic, again, is the grading of highly differentiated lipoma-like liposarcoma. Some of these cases may be underdiagnosed as lipoma and recur. Others, even in the presence of pleomorphism, way behave benignly, if located superficially! Reclassification of these tumors as "pleomorphic lipoma" has been proposed (EVANS et al. 1979) (Figs. 5, 6).

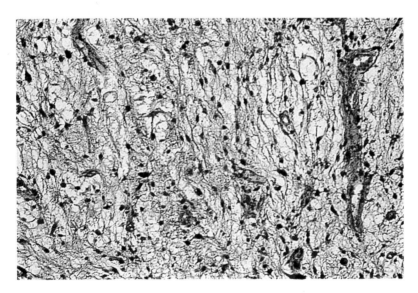

Fig. 3. Myxoid liposarcoma/G1, immature with hardly recognizable lipoblasts. Otherwise features compatible with low-grade malignancy as low cellularity, lack of atypia and mitoses. H&E

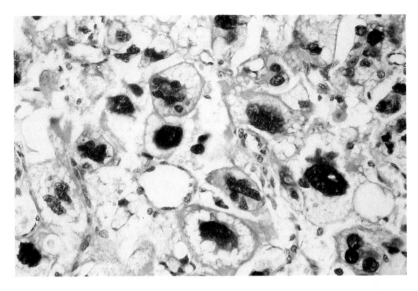

Fig. 4. Pleomorphic liposarcoma/G3 exhibiting marked cellular atypia with bizarre giant cells and questionable mitosis, compatible with high-grade malignancy – albeit clearly recognizable lipoblastic differentiation. H&E

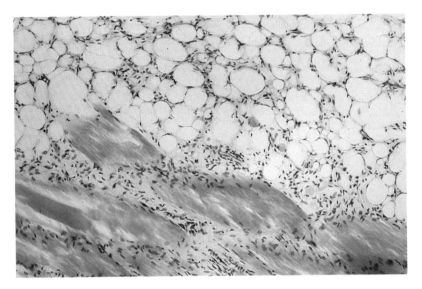

Fig. 5. Well-differentiated lipoma-like liposarcoma/G1, chiefly mature fat cells, with only a few small foci of immature cells, without recognizable mitotic activity, leading to the false diagnosis of lipoma. Accepted histologic features of malignancy are only suggested. The tumor periphery is remarkable with higher cellularity and infiltration of muscle cells. H&E

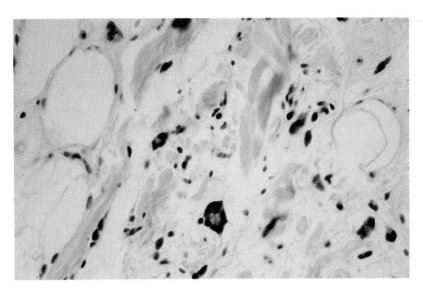

Fig. 6. Pleomorphic lipoma with superficial localization. Alarming cellular atypia, occasional floret-cell type giant cells and fibrosis as in sclerosing type of wel-differentiated liposarcoma but benign lesion. Discrepancy between "bad looks" and good behavior. H&E

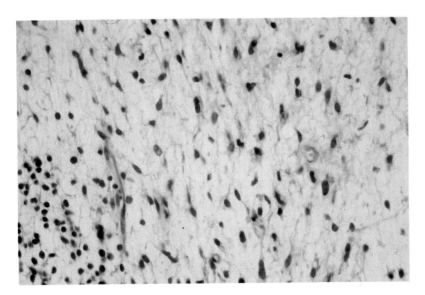

Fig. 7. Embryonal rhabdomyosarcoma/G3, hypocellular chiefly myxoid sarcoma similar to botryoid type. Muscular differentiation could only be demonstrated by expression of muscle-characteristic intermediate filament – desmin. Example of high-grade malignancy in absence of marked cellular atypia, high cellularity, necrosis or high mitotic activity! H&E

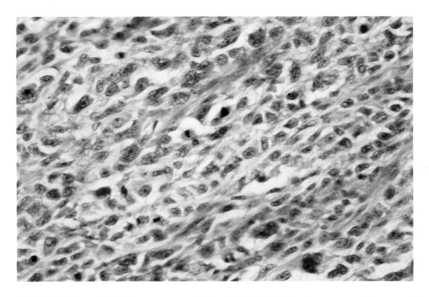

Fig. 8. Embryonal rhabdomyosarcoma/G3 with histologic features generally compatible with high-grade malignancy as cellular atypia, high cellularity, and distinct mitotic activity. However, in contrast to distinct histomorphologic differences to Fig. 7, no significant differences as to prognosis, if localization of tumor and age of patient are comparable. H&E

The example of liposarcoma subtypes emphasizes the relativity of single grading criteria, especially if interpreted out of context with other morphological and clinical parameters (ENZINGER and WEISS 1988; MEISTER 1988). To stress individual misleading grading parameters even further, embryonal rhabdomyosarcomas may be cited as an example of immaturity, lack of cellular atypism and pleomorphism, and low cellularity on the one hand, but in contrast to the similar myxoid liposarcomas they do not display low- but high-grade malignancy (Fig. 7). However, prognosis and response to therapy may be similar to that in their highly cellular counterparts, with all the "accepted" attributes of high-grade malignancy (Fig. 8). This experience supports the concept that for some tumors, like rhabdomyosarcomas, prognosis is ruled by the tumor type (SULSER 1979; COSTA et al. 1984; SCHMIDT et al. 1986; HAWKINS et al. 1987; ENZINGER and WEISS 1988).

For leiomyosarcoma, a spindle cell tumor extending over the entire range from low- to high-grade malignancy, several controversial studies are known, stressing on the one hand the significance of grading by atypia, mitosis, and necrosis, but, on the other hand, pointing out differences in weighing of these criteria dependent on the localization of these tumors, that is, soft tissue, uterus or gastrointestinal tract, etc. (SILVERBERG 1976; APPLEMAN 1986; COSTA et al. 1982; PERRONE and DEHNER 1988).

2.3 Development of Reproducible Grading Schemes

With due consideration to the differences regarding types, subtypes, localization, and also age (ENZINGER and WEISS 1988), the search for a simple,
reproducible grading system continued. In 1982 (COSTA et al.), following a
study of 161 soft tissue sarcomas, a grading system was tested which was
based on empirical interdependencies between tumor (sub)type and prognosis:
myxoid liposarcomas were automatically classified as low-grade, rhabdomyosarcomas as high-grade malignant (Table 2). However, in addition,
"accepted" criteria for grading such as differentiation, atypia, mitosis and
necrosis were applied for a large group of sarcoma types which extended
over the entire range from G1 to G3/4 as fibro- and leiomyosarcoma, and
malignant fibrous histiocytoma, graded between G2 and G3. At last necrosis
was found to be statistically most significant, graded either as absent or
maximally 15%, or as moderate to marked (over 15%).

In 1983 (MYHRE-JENSEN et al.) an intriguing grading scheme was proposed and tested with clinicopathologic correlation in a collective of 261
surgically treated cases. To enhance reproducibility, grading was based on a
score consisting of (a) the number of mitoses/ten high power fields of
$2.5 \, mm^2$; and in addition (b) a mean score of $1-3$ based on a semiquanita-
tive evaluation of cellularity, anaplasia, and necrosis. Whereas (a) is clearly
reproducible with three groups defined by (1) less than one mitosis; (2) one
to five mitoses; (3) more than five mitoses, score (b) is subject to personal
interpretation. As an example, G3 tumors could be characterized either by
(a) moderate mitotic activity (score 2) and maximal values for (b) (score 3),
or by a maximal number of mitoses over five (score 3) and any values for the
(b) score $(1-3)$.

In 1986 the French Federation of Cancer Centers (COINDRE et al. 1988)
(Table 3) tested reproducibility in the grading of 25 soft tissue sarcomas
independently by 15 pathologists. Surprisingly, the agreement as to grading
turned out to be higher (75%) than that concerning typing (61%)! A grading
score was based on a mixture of: (a) differentiation: score (1) sarcoma
closely resembling mature adult tissue, score (2) sarcoma with certain typing
and (3) with doubtful typing, or undifferentiated, as well as embryonal
tumors; (b) number of mitoses: score (1) 0–9, (2) 10–19, (3) over 20

Table 2. Grading according to COSTA et al. (1984)

1. Mitotic activity: "low or high" (6–10 HPF)
2. Necrosis: absent, minimal, moderate, massive
3. Cellularity: low, intermediate, high
4. Pleomorphism: absent, minimal, moderate, marked

The single best parameter for prediction of recurrence and
survival according to this study is *necrosis*!

Table 3. Grading according to COINDRE et al. (1986)

1. Differentiation: 1, resembling normal tissue
                     2, certain typing
                     3, uncertain typing, undifferentiated or
                       embryonal
2. Mitotic activity: 1, 0–9/10 HPF
                    2, 10–19/10 HPF
                    3, over 20/10 HPF
3. Necrosis: 0, absent
              1, up to 50%
              2, over 50%

G1 sarcomas, scores 2, 3; G2, scores 4, 5; G3, scores 6–8.

mitoses/ten high power fields measuring $0.1734 \, mm^2$; (c) tumor necrosis was scored 0 if absent, 1 with under and 2 with over 50%. Thus G1 was defined by a total score of 2–3, G2 4–5, and G3 6–8. This system appears to be quite logical. It is also advantageous that undifferentiated sarcomas can be evaluated. In practice, particularly differentiation proved to be very much subjective, especially regarding the distinction between scores (1) and (2). Myxoid liposarcoma, for instance, would be contradictory, presenting doubtful typing (score 3) and necrosis (score 1). Thus this tumor could be graded as G2 even with low mitotic activity, which is usually not correct as its prognosis is actually compatible with G1.

2.4 EORTC Experience of Grading

In 1987 the European Organization for Cancer Research (EORTC) (VAN UNNIK et al. 1987), which included coworkers of the above-mentioned French study group, undertook a study to abolish subjective grading parameters and to make everything simpler, but based on mathematical results. The material comprised 169 patients of a trial therapeutic study, with a variety of sarcoma types, some of them admittedly underrepresented, for instance, rhabdomyosarcoma, a typically juvenile tumor. A mathematical evaluation initially also included differentiation (!?), intercellular mucoid material, necrosis, and mitoses. In addition, tumor size was also evaluated as well as the type of surgical treatment – either (a) radical operation or amputation; or (b) less than (a).

In contrast to previous studies the grading parameters were not grouped a priori (as, for instance, mitoses over ten, tumor diameter over 5 cm), but objectively divided into the "most discriminating categories." Statistically significant differences as to the rate of metastases and survival were found for tumors showing (1) 0–2; (2) 3–20; and (3) over 20 mitoses/ten high power fields ($= 1.5 \, mm^2$). Mitotic activity turned out to be the most signi-

ficant single prognostic parameter! Distinction of less than 10% and over
10% necrosis did not show any significance in prognosis. Only the absence
or presence of necrosis was significant and only with sarcomas exhibiting
mitotic activity of over 20 mitoses per ten high power fields. Thus, by
counting mitoses and registering the absence or presence of necrosis three
risk groups with distinctly separate curves regarding risk of metastases and
survival became evident. Curve I is compatible with low malignancy – G1,
curve II with G2, and curve III with G3/4, i.e., high-grade malignancy.
Regarding tumor size, a diameter over 8 cm showed no significant differences
in the metastatic risk, but it did in survival! Incorporating tumor size and
two types of surgical treatment resulted in four distinctly separate survival
groups, which may be essential in therapeutic planning.

The findings of the EORTC study group are impressive on account of
their mathematical accuracy on the one hand, and the simplicity of reproducible evaluation of prognostic parameters on the other. These results
can serve very well as a basis for a grading system, which is already being
done in a German coordinated Study of Soft Tissue Sarcomas in Adults
(Adult CWS Study; MEISTER 1992) (Table 4). The authors mention that
their results apply to all soft tissue sarcomas regardless of type. In this
context it has to be pointed out that especially "childhood" sarcomas such
as rhabdomyosarcoma were either underrepresented (with only 3%), or
missing all together, for example, as Ewings sarcoma. Particularly these two
tumors seem to follow their own rules which are different from, for instance,
leimyosarcoma or adult fibrosarcoma. Notoriously low in mitotic activity,
they have to be graded as G3, i.e., high-grade malignant, as has previously
been pointed out (COSTA et al. 1982; ENZINGER and WEISS 1988). For the
entire group of "small blue round cell tumors" including rhabdomyosarcoma, Ewing's sarcoma, primitive neuroectodermal tumour and others,
decisive differences in prognosis are known in relation to localization and, to
lesser degree, also to age. The EORTC study included adult patients with a

Table 4. Proposal for grading based on survival curves (EORTC
experience; VAN UNNIK et al. 1987)

Mitotic score	Necrosis	Grade of malignancy
0	0	Curve I ~ G1 (30 patients)
0	1	low-grade malignancy
1	0	Curve II ~ G2 (107 patients)
1	1	intermediate grade
2	0	malignancy
2	1	Curve III ~ G3 (28 patients) high-grade malignancy

Mitotic score: 0 = 0–2/10 HPF, 1 = 3–20/10 HPF, 2 = over
20/10 HPF.
Necrosis: 0 = absent, 1 = present.

mean age of 41 years, the oldest being 70, the youngest 16 years of age. Thus, the results of simplified, mathematically accurate grading may be effective not only for soft tissue sarcomas as a group, but also for individual tumors especially, for example, leiomyosarcomas in the adult age group. Different rules become effective for juvenile sarcomas (ENZINGER and WEISS 1988).

Again, it has to be stressed that even this grading scheme can only be applied after consideration of various parameters, especially type of sarcoma, size of tumor and its localization, and also the age of the patient (SULSER 1978; SCHMIDT et al. 1986; HAWKINS and COMACHO-VELASQUEZ 1987).

3 Discussion of Grading Parameters

3.1 Counting of Mitoses

A grading system based chiefly on counting mitoses is asking for a discussion and exact definition or recognition of mitotic figures and on how to count them. Factors which may influence the presence or recognition of mitoses have to be considered. Reduction of number of mitotic figures had been reported with late fixation of tissue specimens and possible autolysis (DALLENBACH 1979; GRAEM and HELWEG-LARSEN 1979; CROSS et al. 1990; DONHUIJSEN et al. 1990). This problem, however, turned out to be negligible. As a rule, mitoses remain demonstrable as "frozen figures," even after several hours. Obviously, proliferation continues during that time without tissue fixation (DONHUIJSEN et al. 1988, 1990). The distinction from pyknosis is important in exact definition of mitotic figures. Criteria of mitoses are the lack of a nuclear membrane, hairy chromatin, and basophilic cytoplasm in contrast to increased eosinophilia with pyknosis (BAAK and OORT 1983). The number of mitoses counted in a given area of tumor tissue depends on (a) cellular density; and (b) thickness of histologic sections (SADLER and COGHILL 1989). Regarding cellular density, a standardization of cutting histologic sections with an exact thickness of $3\,\mu m$ should be aimed for. Regarding the thickness of histologic sections, the procedure of counting mitoses has to be standardized. It is advisable to start the count in an area with the highest cellularity, with subsequent evaluation of randomly selected areas with equally or similarly high cellularity. For the evaluated high power fields the exact dimensions have to be given in square millimeters. The determination of the percentage of mitoses per given number of cells, for instance, for 1000 cells, would be more exact, resulting in a mitotic index, or volume-corrected index (HAAPSALO-PESONEN 1989; DONHUIJSEN et al. 1990).

This procedure, however, is very time consuming, even if simplified. Moreover, there is a bias in relation to varying cellular densities (THAM

1992; HILSENBECK and ALLRED 1992; SIMPSON et al. 1992). Heterogeneity, more so in sarcomas than in carcinomas, has to be considered in the evaluation of the number of mitoses.

Sufficient tumor tissue has to be examined to guarantee that the material is representative. Moreover, local and temporary changes in proliferative activity in relation to supply of oxygen and growth factors have to be respected (RABES and MEISTER 1979; KATENKAMP and RAIKHLIN 1985; KATENKAMP 1988; KILLION and FIDLER 1989). These factors deserve consideration when evaluating the results of a mitoses count, but they are not a strong argument against doing so.

3.2 Immunohistochemical Demonstration of Proliferation Markers

Additional more sophisticated methods such as immunohistochemical marking of proliferative markers, e.g., Ki-67 or PCNA, have shown trends which could be applied to achieve more exact results than by a simple count of mitoses in routinely stained sections (SILVESTRINI et al. 1988; GARCIA et al. 1989; EILBER et al. 1990; STENFERT KROESE et al. 1990; ZEHRER et al. 1990). New methods, however, also create their own methodologic problems which may be misleading. Initially Ki-67 antibody required unfixed material, which might not have been representative of the whole tumor because of selection beforehand. Later a Ki-67-associated antibody became commercially available which could also be used on paraffin-embedded material (MiB 1). Nevertheless, recognition of the G phases, especially because of the varying duration of G1, still complicates the evaluation of proliferative activity by this method (GERDES et al. 1992; KEY et al. 1992). PCNA, on the other hand, appears to be less specific as a proliferation marker (WAASEM and LANE 1990; HALL et al. 1990). Discrepancies between Ki-67 and PCNA values may be explained by their expression during different phases, which is maximal for G2 and initial G1, with Ki-67 and concerns the S phase for PCNA (LANDBERG et al. 1990). Nevertheless, promising results were found in special problems, such as, for instance, correlation of a low PCNA index with better prognosis in malignant fibrous histiocytoma, especially the low malignancy myxoid variant (IWASAKI et al. 1987). Possibly additional application of DNA analysis may offer more precise information about prognosis in soft tissue sarcomas.

3.3 DNA Analysis

DNA analysis by flow cytophotometry has been applied in the attempt to predict the outcome of a variety of tumors. In soft tissue tumors it was found helpful to separate benign, low-grade and/or high-grade malignant behavior of certain given tumor types which had only given the impression of a "gray zone" with a potential, but not calculable malignancy by routine histologic examination (KREICBERG et al. 1980; KIYABU et al. 1988; BECKER et al. 1991). Some of the results are encouraging. Thus, in one study (STENFERT KROESE et al. 1990) the DNA index, calculated from the ratio of the G1 peak of tumor cells to that for regulary present normal cells, was apparently not dependent on sarcoma type, but was in general associated with the presence and grade of malignancy, as 14% of benign, 25% of G1, 42% of G2, and 86% of G3 sarcomas showed a DNA index over 1! However, it has to be stressed, that simple answers, i.e., benign or malignant, cannot be expected for the entirety of soft tissue tumors using this method. Sometimes "unexpected" results show up, such as aneuploidy for benign and diploidy for (highly) malignant tumors (EL-NAGGAR and GARCIA 1992). In addition to the extra expenditure, there are methodologic shortcomings such as evaluation of small samples with the associated problem of their being representative. Moreover, there is the handicap of not having optical control of the evaluated tissue samples (STENFERT KROESE et al. 1990). Nevertheless, the initial restriction to fresh tissue sample has in the meantime been overcome, as paraffin-embedded material can also be used for DNA analysis (HEDLEY et al. 1983, 1985; SCHUTTE et al. 1985).

As the flow-cytometric system of DNA analysis became convincing due to its precision, the static or image system, i.e., "image DNA analysis," allows, on the other hand, histologic control and morphologic orientation of a special site to be evaluated, also on paraffin-embedded, for instance, archival, material (AUER et al. 1989). The application of a proposed algorithm for grading malignancies as a result of flow and/or image cytometry needs further study, especially in the evaluation of soft tissue tumors (BÖCKING et al. 1984; KREICBERG et al. 1987; SAPI et al. 1989; BÖCKING 1990; ETO et al. 1992). A review of 26 studies (conducted between 1984 and 1992) dealing with DNA analysis in soft tissue tumors in general or with individual tumor types revealed a correlation between ploidy and prognosis in 13 cases. Five times no such correlation was found. In 8 studies the results were inconclusive (BAUER et al. 1991; BARETION 1993, personal communication). Also, the application of DNA analysis in monitoring therapeutic success is imaginable (BÖCKING et al. 1984).

Especially the combination of DNA analysis and determination of the proliferative index showed promising results with G1 sarcomas being predominantly diploid with low Ki-67 values, G3 sarcomas predominantly aneuploid with high Ki-67. It is very important that in this study G2 sarcomas could be divided into two groups, either revealing the characteristics of G1 or of G3 sarcomas, with corresponding differences in prognosis and therapeutic consequences (STENFERT KROESE et al. 1990; VAN HAELST-PISANO et al. 1991).

4 Conclusions

4.1 Grade, Type, and Therapy

For practical purposes, counting mitoses on routine paraffin sections with a standardized thickness of $3\,\mu$m appears to be a good method for grading soft tissue tumors, with the additional consideration of the presence or absence of necrosis (MEISTER 1992). This concept is mathematically/statistically supported by results of the EORTC study (VAN UNNIK et al. 1987). Nevertheless, exact typing is a prerequisite for grading, as grading criteria such as mitoses and necrosis may show differences for given tumor types regarding their weighing. As a principle, certain tumor types should be graded as highly malignant (G3/4) and treated accordingly by (neoadjuvant) chemotherapy; this includes rhabdomyosarcomas, Ewing's sarcoma, and primitive neuroectodermal tumors (SCHMIDT et al. 1986; HAWKINS and CAMOCHO-VELASQUEZ 1987). This does not rule out the fact that even with these tumors shades of different grades of malignancy may exist, for instance, rhabdomyosarcoma containing even a single small focus of an alveolar pattern, with a consequently poorer prognosis, regardless of mitotic activity and necrosis (SCHMIDT et al. 1986).

Most important for therapeutic planning is a distinction between (a) low-grade sarcomas, with chiefly local aggressive growth and a high risk for local recurrence, but hardly ever showing any considerable risk for metastases (G1 sarcomas!); and (b) fully malignant "true" sarcomas with varying, albeit considerable risk for metastases (G2 sarcomas? G3/4 sarcomas!). In the first group, complete surgical removal of the tumor is essential and as a rule often curative; for the second group, chemo- and radiotherapy, or increasingly neoadjuvant chemotherapy are indicated. Here, surgery only helps in local tumor control (MEISTER 1988).

Finally, it has to be emphasized that a pathologist should not and indeed can not give an optimal prognosis on a soft tissue tumor on its histomorphologic appearance alone. What is generally true for neoplastic processes is especially the case for soft tissue tumors, which are notorious for their heterogeneity, regarding not only the presence of grading parameters, but also differentiaton features i.e., typing. This fact has been known in routine hemotoxylin and eosin-stained sections, and is even more the case with special stains such as van Gieson, PAS and Ag, etc. and is highest for immunohistochemical expressions which may frequently appear to be "aberrant" – or at least unexpected!

4.2 Proliferation Markers, DNA Analysis, and Therapy

Sophisticated methods such as immunohistochemical marking of proliferative markers, DNA analysis (by flow photocytometry or image cytometry), together with the incorporation of proliferative markers, may, without doubt, give new insight into tumor biology, also with respect to locally and chronologically changing proliferative activity. For soft tissue tumors as a whole, with their notorious heterogeneity in contrast to the more homogeneous carcinomas, the handicap of nonrepresentative selection has to be considered. Moreover, more precise flow photocytometry without optical control has to be contrasted with less precise but controllable image cytometry. Depending on each individual case, either method may be better suited for the study of precise questions in tumor cell proliferation.

With an increasing number of more complicated methods, an increase in methodologic errors and artifacts can also be expected, as can higher material and personnel costs.

Whereas DNA analysis may be helpful in the distinction between benign or malignant behavior in given tumor types, immunohistochemical evaluation of tumor proliferation markers may possibly assist in grading generally. There are already indications of a possible distinction within the largest group with G2 classification between cases which are closer to either G1 – low-grade malignancy – or G3/4 – high grade malignancy; this is a result of applying Ki-67 markers in combination with DNA analysis (STENFERT KROESE et al. 1990). Thus, a division of soft tissue sarcomas into two groups is the aim, with either chiefly surgery, or chemo-radiotherapy as treatment modalities (MEISTER 1988) (Fig. 9). Moreover, correlation between high Ki-67 index and response to chemotherapy is apparent.

Future hopes, chiefly regarding typing, but also interrelated with grading or prognosis, stem from the investigation of cytogenetic changes and

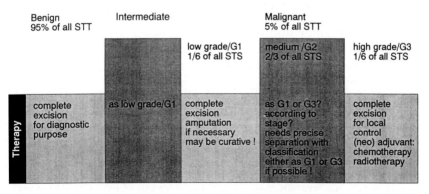

Fig. 9. Dignity of soft tissue tumors. Percentage of soft tissue tumors (*STT*) according to MEISTER et al. (1988); fractions of soft tissue sarconas (*STS*) according to VAN UNNIK et al. (1987)

molecular biologic features (oncogenes), whereby new insights in tumor pathogenesis may also be obtained (IWASAKI et al. 1987).

4.3 Grading Criteria in Pseudosarcoma

It should not be overlooked that in the majority of cases "accepted grading parameters" are applied to soft tissue tumors which already have an established malignancy. Criteria, mainly atypia and mitoses, have been evaluated for the distinction between benign and malignant only for some tumor types such as smooth muscle tumors (SILVERBERG 1976). On the other hand, tumor-like lesions such as "pseudosarcomatous" nodular fasciitis or proliferative myositis may show massive expression of "accepted criteria of malignancy," e.g., cellular atypia, number and even atypia of mitoses, without any risk for metastases, typically also with a lack of local aggressive growth, and mostly showing regression even after only partial removal without any risk of recurrence. Such criteria, which may be helpful for the prognosis of sarcomas, have to be evaluated for their significance in often reactive tumor-like lesions, i.e., "pseudosarcomas."

Thus once more it is important to emphasize the inclusion of all possible histomorphologic and clinical parameters into the evaluation of tumors in general so as not to depend on one "prognostic criterion" alone which may become a "diagnostic pitfall."

References

Altmannsberger M, Alles J, Fitz H, Jundt G, Osborn M (1986) Mesenchymale Tumormarker. Verh Dtsch Ges Pathol 72: 150–163
Appelman H (1986) Smooth muscle tumors of the gastrointestinal tract. Am J Surg Pathol 10(Suppl 1): 83–99
Baak J (1990) Mitosis counting in tumors. Hum Pathol 21: 683–684
Baak J, Oort J (1983) A manual of morphometry in diagnostic pathology. Springer, Berlin Heidelberg New York
Bauer H, Kreisberg A, Tribukait B (1991) DNA content prognosis in soft tissue sarcoma. Acta Orthop Scand 62: 187–194
Becker R, Venzon D, Lack E et al. (1991) Cytometry and morphometry of malignant fibrous histiocytoma of the extremities. Am J Surg Pathol 15: 957–964
Böcking A (1990) DNA-Zytometrie und Automation in der klinischen Diagnostik. Verh Dtsch Ges Pathol 74: 176–185
Böcking A, Adler C, Common H et al. (1984) Algorithm for a DNA-cytophotometric diagnosis and grading of malignancy. Anal Quant Cytol 30: 1–8
Broders A, Hargrave R, Meyerding H (1939) Pathological features of soft tissue fibrosarcoma: with special reference to the grading of its malignancy. Surg Gyneco Obstet 69: 267–280
Brooks J (1982) Immunohistochemistry of soft tissue tumors. Hum Pathol 13: 969–974
Brooks J (1986) The significance of double phenotypic pattern and markers in human saracomas. Am J Pathol 125: 113–123

Brooks J (1989) Disorders of soft tissue. In: Sternberg S (ed) Diagnostic surgical pathology. Raven, New York

Brown D, Theaker J, Banks P, Gatter K, Mason D (1987) Cytokeratin expression in smooth muscle tumors. Histopathology 11: 477–486

Castro E, Hajdu S, Fortner J (1973) Surgical therapy of fibrosarcoma of extremities: a reappraisal. Arch Surg 107: 284–286

Coindre J, de Marscarel A, Trojani M, de Mascarel I, Pages A (1988a) Immunohistohemical study of rhabdomyosarcoma. Unexpected staining with S 100 protein and cytokeratin. J Pathol 155: 127–132

Coindre J, Bui N, Bonichon F et al. (1988b) Histopathologic grading in spindle cell soft tissue sarcomas. Cancer 61: 2305–2309

Costa J, Wesley R, Glatstein E, Rosenberg S (1984) The grading of soft tissue sarcomas. Cancer 53: 530–541

Cross S, Start R, Smith J (1990) Does delay in fixation affect the number of mitotic figures in processed tissue? J Clin Pathol 43: 597–599

Dallenbach F (1979) Das sogenannte Leiomyosarkom in situ des Uterus. Verh Dtsch Ges Pathol 63: 633–640

Donhuijsen K (1986) Reproducibility and significance in grading of malignancy. Hum Pathol 17: 1122–1125

Donhuijsen K, Budach V, van Beuningen D, Schmidt U (1988) Instability of xenotransplanted soft tissue sarcomas. Cancer 61: 68–75

Donhuijsen K, Schmidt U, Hirche H et al. (1990) Changes in mitotic rate and cell cycle fractions caused by delayed fixation. Hum Pathol 21: 709–714

Eilber F, Huth J, Mirra J, Rosen G (1990) Progress in the recognition and treatment of soft tissue sarcomas. Cancer 65: 660–666

El-Naggar, Garcia G (1992) Epitheloid sarcoma. Flow cytometric study of DNA content and regional DNA heterogeneity. Cancer 69: 1721–1728

Enzinger F, Weiss S (1988) Soft tissue tumors, 2nd edn. Mosby, St Louis

Enzinger F, Winslow D (1962) Liposarcoma: a study of 103 cases. Virchows Arch 335: 361–388

Erlandson R (1984) Diagnostic immunohistochemistry of human tumors. An interim evaluation. Am J Surg Pathol 8: 615–624

Eto H, Toiyam K, Tsuda N, Tagawa Y, Itakura H (1992) Flow cytometric DNA analysis of vascular soft tissue tumors, including African endemic-type Kaposi's sarcoma. Hum Pathol 23: 1055–1060

Evans H (1979) Liposaracoma: a study of 55 cases with reassessment of its classification. Am J Surg Pathol 3: 507–523

Evans H, Soule E, Winkelman R (1979) Atypical lipoma, atypical intramuscular lipoma, and well differentiated retroperitoneal liposarcoma. Cancer 43: 574–584

Fidler I (1978) Tumor heterogeneity and the biology of cancer invasion and metastasis. Cancer Res 38: 2651–2660

Garcia R, Coltrera M, Gown A (1989) Analysis of proliferative grade using anti-PCNA/cyclin monclonal antibodies in fixed, embedded tissues: comparison with flow cytometry analysis. Am J Pathol 134: 733–739

Gerdes J, Becker M, Key G, Cattoretti (1992) Immunhistological detection of tumor growth factor (Ki-67 antigen) in formalinfixed and routinely processed tissue. J Pathol (in press)

Graem N, Helweg-Larsen K (1979) Mitotic activity and delayed fixation of tumor tissue. Acta Pathol Scand [A] 87: 375–378

Haapsalo H, Pesonen E (1989) Volume corrected mitotic index (M/V-Index). Pathol Res Pract 185: 551–554

Hajdu S (1979) Pathology of soft tissue tumors. Lea and Febiger, Philadelphia

Hall P, Levison D, Woods A et al. (1990) Proliferating nuclear antigen (PCNA) immunolocalisation in paraffin sections. J Pathol (in press)

Haukins H, Camacko-Velasquez J (1987) Rhabdomyosarcoma in children. Am J Surg Pathol 11: 531–542

Hedley O, Friedlander M, Taylor I et al. (1983) Methods for analysis of cellular DNA content of paraffin-embedded pathological material using flow cytometry. J Histochem Cytochem 31: 1333

Hedley O, Friedlander M, Taylor I (1985) Application of DNA flow cytometry of paraffin-embedded archival material for the study of aneuploidy and its clinical significance. Cytometry 6: 327–333

Hermanek P, Scheibe O, Spiessl B, Wagner G (1987) TNM-Klassifikation maligner Tumoren, 4th edn. Springer, Berlin Heidelberg New York

Hilsenbeck S, Allred D (1992) Improved method of estimating mitotic activity in solid tumors. Hum Pathol 23: 601–602

Iwasaki H, Isayama T, Johzaki K, Kikuchi M (1987) MFH: evidence of perivascular mesen-chymal cell origin. Am J Pathol 128: 528–537

Katenkamp D (1988) Cellular heterogeneity. Explanation of changing of tumor phenotype and biologic behaviour in soft tissue sarcomas. Pathol Res Pract 183: 698–705

Katenkamp D, Raikhlin (1985) Stem cell concept and heterogeneity of malignant soft tissue tumors. Exp Pathol 28: 3–11

Katenkamp D, Stiller D (1990) Weichgewebstumoren. Barth, Jena

Key G, Becker M, Baron B et al. (1992) Preparation and immunobiochemical haracterization of Ki-67 equivalent murine antibody (MIB 1–3) generated against recombinant parts of the Ki-67 antigen (to be published)

Killion J, Fidler I (1989) The biology of tumor metastasis. Sem Oncol 16: 106–115

Kiyabu M, Bishop B, Parker J et al. (1988) Smooth muscle tumors of the gastrointestinal tract. Flow cytometric quantitation of DNA and nuclear antigen content and correlation with histologic grade. Am J Surg Pathol 12: 954–960

Kreicberg A, Söderberg A, Zetterberg A (1980) The prognostic significance of nuclear DNA-content in chondrosarcoma. Anal Quant Cytol 4: 271

Kreicberg A, Tribukeit B, Willem J et al. (1987) DNA flow analysis in soft tissue tumors. Cancer 59: 128–133

Landberg G, Tan E, Roos G (1990) Flow cytometric multiparameter analysis of cell nuclear antigen/cyclin and Ki-67 antigen. Exp Cell Res 187: 111–118

Mackenzie D (1964) Fibroma: a dangerous diagnosis. Br J Surg 51: 607–612

Meister P (1988) Weichgewebssarkome. Klassifizierung oder Graduierung? Zentralbl Allg Pathol Pathol Anat 134: 355–362

Meister P (1992) Weichgewebssarkome. I. Allgemeines. Fortbld Aktuel Krebsdiagn Ther 60/61: 29–34

Miettinen M, Lehto V, Badley R, Virtanen I (1982) Expression of intermediate filaments in soft-tissue sarcomas. Int J Cancer 30: 541–546

Myhre-Jensen O, Kaae O, Madsen E et al. (1983) Histopathological grading in soft tissue tumors. Acta Pathol Scand [A] 91: 145–150

Perrone T, Dehner L (1988) Prognostically favorable "mitotically active" smooth-muscle tumors of the uterus. Am J Surg Pathol 12: 1–8

Pritchard D, Soule E, Taylor W, Ivins J (1974) Fibrosaroma. Cancer 33: 888–897

Quinn C, Wright N (1990) The clinical assessment of proliferation and growth in human tumors. J Pathol 160: 93–102

Rabes H, Meister P (1979) Analysis of proliferative compartments in human tumors. Cancer 44: 799–813

Russel W, Cohen J, Enzinger F et al. (1977) A clinical pathological staging system for soft tissue sarcomas. Cancer 40: 1562–1570

Sadler D, Coghill S (1989) Histopathologists, malignancies and undefined high-power fields. Lancet 333: 785–786

Sapi Z, Bodo M, Sugar J (1989) DNA cytometry of soft tissue tumors with TV image analysis. Pathol Res Pract 185: 363–367

Schmidt D, Reimann O, Treuer J, Harms D (1986) Cellular differentiation and prognosis in embryonal rhabdomyosarcoma. Virchows Arch 409: 183–194

Schutte B, Reynder M, Bosman F et al. (1985) Flow cytometric determination of DNA ploidy level in nuclei isolated from paraffin-embedded material. Cytometry 6: 26–30

Scott S, Reiman H, Pritchard D, Ilstrup DC (1989) Soft tissue fibrosarcoma. Cancer 64: 925–931

Silverberg S (1976) Reproducibility of the mitotic count in the histologic diagnosis of smooth muscle tumors of the uterus. Hum Pathol 7: 451–454

Silvestrini R, Costa A, Veneroni S et al. (1988) Camparative analysis of different approaches to investigate cell kinetics. Cell Tissue Kinet 21: 123–131

Simpson J, Dutt P, Page D (1992) Expressions of mitoses per thousend cells and cell density in breast carcinoma. Hum Pathol 23: 608–611

Stenfert Kroese M, Rutgeres D, Wils I et al. (1990) The relevance of the DNA index and proliferation rate in the grading of benign and malignant soft tissue tumors. Cancer 65: 1782–1788

Sulser H (1978) Das Rhabdomysarkom. Virchows Arch 379: 35–71

Swanson S, Brook G (1990) Proliferation markers Ki-67 and p104 in soft tissue lesions. Am J Pathol 137: 1491–1500

Takafumi U, Katsuyuki A, Masahiko T (1989) Prognostic significance of Ki-67 reactivity in soft tissue sarcomas. Cancer 63: 1607

Tham K (1992) Estimation of mitotic count in tumors. Hum Pathol 23: 1313–1314

Van Haelst-Pisani C, Buckner J, Reiman H, Schaid D, Edmonson J, Hahn R (1991) Does histologic grade in soft tissue sarcoma influence response rate to systemic chemotherapy? Cancer 68: 2354–2358

Van Unnik J, Coinder J, Contesso G et al. (1987) Grading of soft tissue sarcomas. In: Ryan JR, Baker LO (eds) Recent concepts in sarcoma treatment. Kluwer, Utrecht

Waaseem N, Lane D (1990) Monoclonal antibody analysis of the proliferating cell nuclear antigen (PCNA). J Cell Sci 90: 121–129

Weiss S (1993) Histological typing of soft tissue tumors, 2nd edn. Springer, Berlin Heidelberg New York

Weiss S, Bratthauer G, Morris P (1988) Postirradiation malignant fibrous histiocytoma expressing cytokeratin. Am J Surg Pathol 12: 554–558

Zehrer R, Bauer T, Marks K, Weltevreden A (1990) Ki-67 and grading of malignant fibrous histiocytoma. Cancer 66: 1984–1990

Fibrous Tumors and Tumor-like Lesions of Childhood: Diagnosis, Differential Diagnosis, and Prognosis

D. Schmidt

1 Introduction

The most important group of lesions among the fibrous tumors of childhood are the fibromatoses. These are rare, non-metastasizing (myo-)fibroblastic tumor-like lesions of unknown etiology with the following characteristic features:

1. They tend to invade the surrounding tissue more or less aggressively.
2. They tend to recur after incomplete excision.
3. Some types may regress spontaneously, and regression may be complicated by contraction.
4. They never metastasize.
5. Certain fibromatoses may be either solitary or multiple.
6. Most types occur in very young age groups and can appear as congenital tumors.
7. The biologic behavior, particularly the risk of recurrences, correlates partially with the histological subtype, i.e., some fibromatoses tend to recur only rarely, while others, especially desmoid-type fibromatoses, show high recurrence rates.

Several classification schemes have been proposed for this group of disorders (ALLEN 1977; ROSENBERG et al. 1978; ENZINGER and WEISS 1988).

Current Topics in Pathology
Volume 89, Eds. D. Harms/D. Schmidt
© Springer-Verlag Berlin Heidelberg 1995

They are by no means uniform, since they are based on different criteria of varying importance. Thus, comparison is difficult. The following criteria are usually applied for characterization of the various entities: histological appearance, localization, degree of aggressiveness, tendency to recur, number of lesions, time of manifestation (congenital, infantile, juvenile, etc.), and familial occurrence. The most widely accepted classification scheme of the "fibrous proliferations of infancy and childhood" is that proposed by ENZINGER and WEISS (1988). This classification scheme has also been adopted at the Kiel Pediatric Tumor Registry (KPTR) and forms the basis of the current investigation of 134 cases of fibromatosis.

2 Incidence of Fibromatoses

Among the fibrous tumors of childhood the fibromatoses are most frequent. Despite the vast number of studies on the different clinicopathologic aspects of fibromatoses, it is difficult to obtain a clear picture of the relative incidence of the various subtypes. One reason for this is the lack of a uniform classification system. Recently, COFFIN and DEHNER (1991) analyzed their material on fibroblastic and myofibroblastic tumors in children and compared the relative incidence of the different subtypes of fibromatoses with that from four published series. It became readily apparent that great differences exist in the relative incidence. The most frequent subtype in the COFFIN and DEHNER series was infantile myofibromatosis, accounting for 22%, followed by desmoid fibromatosis (20%). In previous investigations desmoid fibromatosis was very rare (7%) and was not even mentioned as an entity in two of the publications (ROSENBERG et al. 1978). The frequency distribution in our comparatively unselected material is quite different from the data reported in the literature. In contrast to all other series, we found a clear predominance of desmoid fibromatosis which accounted for 60.6% of all cases (Table 1). The next most frequent types were infantile

Table 1. Relative frequency of fibromatoses in the KPTR

Type	Number (n)	Percent (%)
Desmoid fibromatosis	100	60.6
Infantile myofibromatosis	21	12.8
Fibrous hamartoma	21	12.8
Fibromatosis colli	8	4.8
Fibromatosis palmaris and plantaris	8	4.8
Infantile digital fibromatosis	4	2.4
Calcifying aponeurotic fibroma	2	1.2
Unclassified	1	0.6
	165	

myofibromatosis and fibrous hamartoma of infancy, accounting for 12.8% each. In a previous study (SCHMIDT and HARMS 1985), which included 59 cases from this institution, we noted an incidence of 27% for desmoid fibromatosis. At present, we cannot offer an explanation for this discrepancy as the number and types of soft tissue tumors regularly sent to the KPTR have not changed in essence over the years. It is curious, however, that during the last year alone we have encountered six cases of infantile myo-fibromatosis, as many as occurred in the period 1977–1990. These most recent cases are not included in Table 1.

In the following, the pertinent clinical and pathologic features essen-tial to the diagnosis, differential diagnosis, and prognosis in each of the fibromatosis subtypes will be discussed.

3 Special Types of Fibromatoses

3.1 Desmoid Fibromatosis

In contrast to abdominal desmoid fibromatosis, which shows a strong female predominance, extra-abdominal desmoid fibromatosis is more frequent in males. The male-to-female ratio in our series was 2:1 which is identical to that reported by COFFIN and DEHNER (1991). The median age of our 100 patients was 5 years (range: 0–336 months); 7% of the cases were con-genital, and 30% occurred in infants younger than 1 year. Thus, the patients in our series were considerably younger than those reported by COFFIN and DEHNER (1991). All age groups taken together, desmoid fibromatosis has a peak incidence in the second and third decade (cf. CHUNG et al. 1991). The main localizations in our material were the head and neck region with 24.4% of the cases and the extremities representing 21% of the cases. Next in frequency were the trunk (16.3%), the shoulder girdle (12.7%), the hip (11.6%), and the abdominal or retroperitoneal regions (10.5%). It is noteworthy that three cases (3.5%) presented with multiple lesions since desmoid fibromatosis is generally thought to occur as a single lesion. Exceptions have been familial cases, cases associated with Gardner's syn-drome, and intra-abdominal fibromatosis (cf. CHUNG et al. 1991).

Desmoid fibromatosis showed an infiltrative though not destructive growth pattern, especially into surrounding skeletal muscle tissue. Thin fibrous projections were often seen at the periphery of the lesions, despite the occasional deceptive macroscopic appearance of a well-demarcated tumor. These projections are the main source of relapse after incomplete or marginal excision. The cellularity of the lesions varied considerably. They consisted of bundles of slender, uniform, spindle-shaped cells with indistinct cytoplasm. In immature cases, it was very difficult and sometimes even

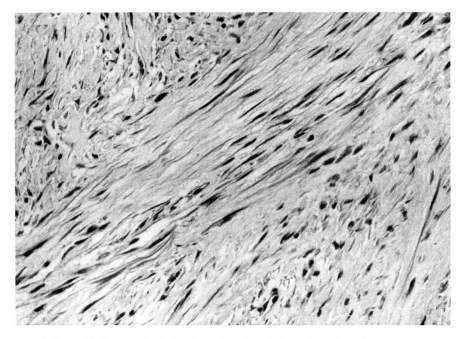

Fig. 1. Desmoid fibromatosis. Lesion is moderately cellular and consists of slender fibroblasts and myofibroblasts. H&E, ×350

impossible to distinguish between an immature, cellular form of desmoid fibromatosis and infantile fibrosarcoma, particularly in small biopsy specimens. In general, fibrosarcoma presents with higher mitotic activity, areas of necrosis, and less collagen production, while foci of mucoid degeneration do not occur. This contrasts with fibromatosis, in which at least small mucoid areas are not uncommon. The more mature variants of desmoid fibromatosis in children are collagen rich and less cellular, and are thus identical to adult desmoid fibromatosis (Fig. 1).

Previous ultrastructural (NAVAS-PALACIOS 1983) and immunohistochemical investigations (HASEGAWA et al. 1990) as well as our own studies on 48 cases (Table 2) demonstrate that the proliferating cells in desmoid fibromatosis are fibroblasts and myofibroblasts. Depending on the definition of a myofibroblast, one could even argue that desmoid fibromatosis represents a pure proliferation of myofibroblasts with different degrees of differentiation. This conclusion can be drawn from the finding that myofibroblasts may assume four main phenotypes (ROCHE 1990; SAPPINO et al. 1990). Vimentin is constantly found (Fig. 2), whereas the expression of desmin and muscle-specific actin varies. In our series, 32/48 (66%) cases reacted with a monoclonal antibody against muscle-specific actin, and 21/48 (44%) cases were desmin positive. Expression of more than one type of intermediate filament protein is a common finding. Thus, 21/48 (44%) cases

Table 2. Results of immunohistochemical reactions in desmoid fibromatosis

Antigen	Number (n)	Percent (%)
Vimentin	48/48	100
Actin	32	66
Desmin	21	44
Protein S-100	27	56
Vimentin only	11	23
Vimentin + actin	14	30
Vimentin + desmin	2	4
Vimentin + actin + desmin	21	43

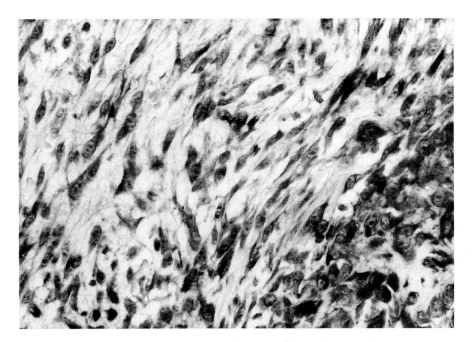

Fig. 2. Desmoid fibromatosis. Many cells are positive for vimentin. ×350

presented with expression of vimentin, muscle-specific actin, and desmin while 14 cases (30%) expressed vimentin and muscle-specific actin. Only two cases exhibited positivity for vimentin and desmin, without expression of muscle-specific actin. Although double or triple stainings were not performed, these immunohistochemical findings are strongly consistent with myofibroblastic proliferations. Neural markers were also found. They included the expression of neuron-specific enolase and protein S-100 in about 50% of the cases.

Follow-up data on desmoid fibromatosis show that recurrence and morbidity rates vary widely mainly depending on the anatomical site. This also influences the type of treatment which usually consists of an attempt at complete removal of the lesion, but may also include radiation therapy (WALTHER et al. 1988), chemotherapy (RANEY et al. 1987), and hormonal therapy (KINZBRUNNER et al. 1983) in those patients in whom complete excision is not feasible. These therapeutic strategies were also employed in the patients of our series, sometimes in various combinations. Despite adjuvant treatment many of the patients developed local recurrences, sometimes more than one. Interestingly, no regressive changes were noted in the primary lesions or recurrences which could be investigated after irradiation, chemotherapy, or hormonal therapy. Overall, the recurrence rate in our series was 56.8% with a median interval of 24 months between primary operation and first relapse. Two patients died, one from edema of the brain after resection of a fibromatosis of the neck, another from generalized disease.

Until recently, all attempts to establish a relationship between histomorphological features and the tendency of local recurrence had failed. However, in 1989 YOKOYAMA et al. pointed out that lesions presenting with a large number of small, slit-like blood vessels ($<20\,\mu$m in diameter) in the

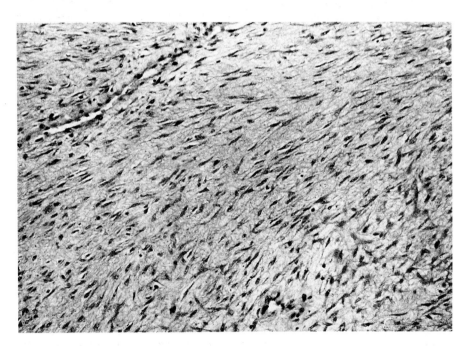

Fig. 3. Desmoid fibromatosis. Slit-like blood vessel is present (*left upper corner*). This finding is associated with the likelihood of recurrence if present in great numbers in the center of the lesion. H&E, ×140

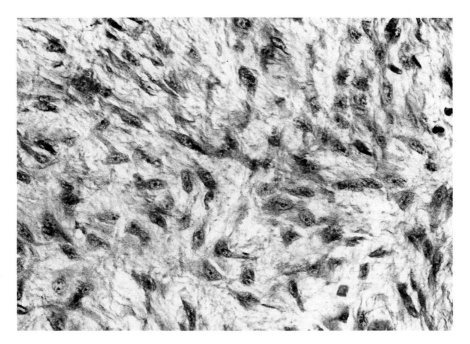

Fig. 4. Desmoid fibromatosis. Area consisting of immature cells (myofibroblasts). Lesions containing large quantities of these cells are prone to recur, especially if slit-like blood vessels are present concurrently. H&E, ×350

center of the tumors (Fig. 3) and with plump, stellate-shaped cells (Fig. 4) and/or myxomatous foci showed a higher recurrence rate than lesions without these features. In a study of 82 cases of desmoid fibromatosis we could confirm and extend these findings (SCHMIDT et al. 1991). Lesions which contained only low numbers of these peculiar blood vessels did not recur, while, in contrast, highly vascular tumors recurred in 11 of 14 cases. Lesions with an intermediate (moderate) number of vessels (six to nine vessels per $6.25 \, \text{mm}^2$) relapsed in ten of 15 cases. This moderately vessel-rich group of tumors could be further divided into two prognostically different subgroups: a high number of so-called undifferentiated cells (immature myofibroblasts) were associated with a high recurrence rate, while a low number of such cells indicated a more favorable prognosis. No correlation could be found between the number and size of the nucleolar organizer regions (AgNORs) (Fig. 5) and the clinical course in desmoid fibromatosis. EGAN et al. (1987) demonstrated previously that it was even possible to differentiate fibromatosis from fibrosarcoma using this method. It was expected that tumors with recurrent disease would be characterized by large numbers of small AgNORs, and nonrecurrent tumors by small numbers of large AgNORs. Interestingly, however, when desmoid fibromatosis was compared with fibromatosis subtypes which are not prone to recurrence, a

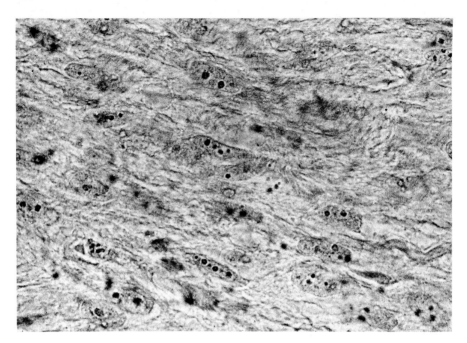

Fig. 5. Desmoid fibromatosis. A small number of nucleolar organizer regions (AgNORs) is found in this particular case. ×560

statistically significant difference in AgNOR numbers could be demonstrated (SCHMIDT et al. 1991).

3.2 Infantile Myofibromatosis

Infantile myofibromatosis was diagnosed in 21 cases accounting for 12.8%. Thus, its frequency in our material is much lower than in the series of COFFIN and DEHNER (1991). However, the incidence of multicentric growth is almost identical, since three of our patients (14.3%) and three of 20 patients (15%) in the series of COFFIN and DEHNER (1991) presented with multiple lesions. Two cases which we recently encountered, but which are not included among the other cases, are noteworthy. A newborn child presented with a tumor of the uterus, which was highly reminiscent of a leiomyosarcoma because of the mitotic activity and the presence of necrosis. Soon after the first operation, the girl developed several lytic lesions of the spine, and the diagnosis of multicentric infantile myofibromatosis was eventually established. The other case stemmed from our autopsy material. This patient presented with numerous tumor nodes in the soft tissues and many internal organs, including the heart. In general, lung, myocardium, and gastrointestinal tract are the most common sites when visceral organs are involved. Most of the cases in our material were located in the dermis and subcutis, whereas one was found in the soft palate, and another one occurred in the right atrium of the heart with extension into the right ventricle. The patients included ten boys and 11 girls. Four tumors presented at birth, the oldest patient was 13 years old. However, it must be emphasized that myofibromatosis does not only occur in childhood, but may also be encountered in adult patients (DAIMARU et al. 1989), frequently presenting as a solitary lesion (myofibroma) (WOLFE and COOPER 1990). In infancy, it is supposed to be the most common fibrous tumor (WISWELL et al. 1988).

Histologically, infantile myofibromatosis showed a characteristic zonal phenomenon, as described by CHUNG and ENZINGER (1981). At the periphery, bundles of plump to spindle-shaped cells with eosinophilic to pale cytoplasm were discernible (Fig. 6). Often, a small pale perinuclear halo was visible. In the center of the lesion, solid sheets of more primitive cells predominated, and a hemangiopericytomatous pattern of the blood vessels was frequently noted. If only small biopsies are available, such areas can be indistinguishable from hemangiopericytoma in conventional stains, even in reticulin stains. Thus, the diagnostic clue is the combination of a leiomyomatous aspect of the lesion at the periphery and a hemangiopericytomatous pattern in the central parts. The presence of necrosis, sometimes with extensive calcification, should not be misinterpreted as a

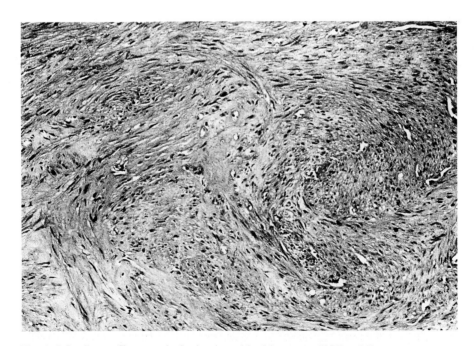

Fig. 6. Infantile myofibromatosis. Lesion resembles leiomyoma. H&E, ×350

sign of malignancy since regressive changes are commonly noted (FLETCHER et al. 1987). In one of our cases, areas of necrosis with calcification covered more than 50% of the section. Immunohistochemically, all four cases studied expressed vimentin and muscle-specific actin, three out four were positive for desmin. Thus, the muscle markers actin and desmin seemed to be more frequently positive in infantile myofibromatosis than in desmoid fibromatosis. None of our cases recurred, which is in accordance with findings from the literature.

3.3 Fibrous Hamartoma of Infancy

Twenty-one cases in our material corresponded to this type of fibromatosis accounting for 12.8%. There was a male predominance with a male-to-female ratio of 2:1. The median age at presentation was 12 months, and 75% of cases occurred in infants younger than 1 year. Four cases (19%) were diagnosed at birth. In accordance with findings of other investigators we found a predominance of lesions in the shoulder girdle (77.8%). Other locations were the trunk and the inguinal region. In only one case was a

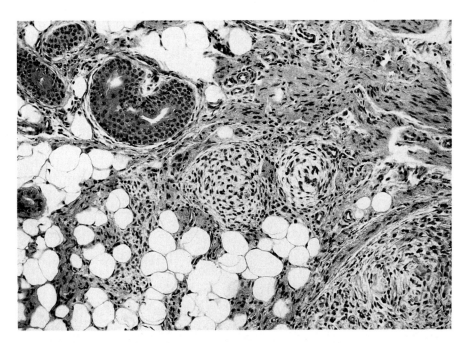

Fig. 7. Fibrous hamartoma of infancy. Lesion consists of mature fat cells, groups of immature cells, and trabeculae of fibroblasts. H&E, ×350

multicentric growth noted in the axilla and in proximity to the scapula. Histologically, fibrous hamartoma shows three components: mature fibrous trabeculae, loosely arranged, more immature-appearing cellular areas, and islets of mature, univacuolar adipose tissue (Fig. 7). The relative proportion of these components varied. In addition to these components, a collagen-rich, spindle-cellular component with a neuroid appearance may occur. Immunohistochemically, the fibroblastic components reacted with antibodies against vimentin and muscle-specific actin. Interestingly, they did not react for desmin – this in contrast to other types of fibromatosis which frequently show variable expressions of vimentin, muscle-specific actin, and desmin. Recurrences are usually encountered at the site of the previous excision. In our material, none of the seven cases for which we had follow-up information recurred.

3.4 Fibromatosis Colli

Fibromatosis colli represented the third largest group in our material accounting for eight cases (4.8%). Males clearly predominated (male-to-female ratio: 7:1). In three patients, the lesions presented 3 weeks after birth, while in the remaining patients they were encountered within the first 2–3 months. All lesions occurred in the sternocleidomastoid muscle without predilection for one side as has been reported by others (cf. ENZINGER and WEISS 1988). Histologically, there was an intimate relationship between proliferating spindle cells and skeletal muscle fibers which frequently appeared to be atrophic and formed myogenic giant cells. Immunohistochemically, the spindle cells reacted positively for vimentin in all cases, whereas they were positive for muscle-specific actin in three lesions and for desmin in two cases. None of the lesions recurred.

3.5 Fibromatosis Palmaris and Plantaris

This diagnosis was rendered in eight cases of our material accounting for 4.8% of the cases. The patients included one male and seven females. The median age at diagnosis was 103 months (range: 72–127 months). All lesions presented in the hands. Histologically, they consisted of interlacing bundles of spindle cells with round to oval nuclei in a collagenous background. Some cases demonstrated poorly cellular areas with collagenization and hyalinization. Two cases demonstrated an infiltration of the subcutaneous fatty tissue. One patient had tuberous sclerosis. Another patient developed a recurrence 3 months after the first operation.

3.6 Infantile Digital Fibromatosis

A diagnosis of infantile digital fibromatosis (inclusion body fibromatosis) was rendered in four cases accounting for 2.4%. The median age of the patients was 8.5 months (range: 9–78 months). Two out of the four cases occurred during the first year of life, but none was identified at birth as is known to occur in about one third of the cases. The patients included one male and three females. Two tumors each were found on the digits of the hands and feet. In one of the four cases multiple lesions were present on the digits of one hand. None of our cases presented in extradigital sites as has been reported in some cases in the literature (PURDY and COLBY 1984; VIALE et al. 1988). Histologically, the lesions were ill defined and located in the dermis extending upwards to the epidermis and downwards to the sub-cutaneous tissue. They consisted of interlacing fascicles of spindle cells corresponding to fibro- and myofibroblasts set in a dense collagenous background. Mitoses were rare. All cases revealed the characteristic in-tracellular globular inclusions which varied in size and distribution and were therefore sometimes difficult to find (Fig. 8). When these inclusions were studied immunohistochemically, they did not react with a monoclonal anti-muscle-specific actin antibody. By contrast, the cytoplasm of these cells was

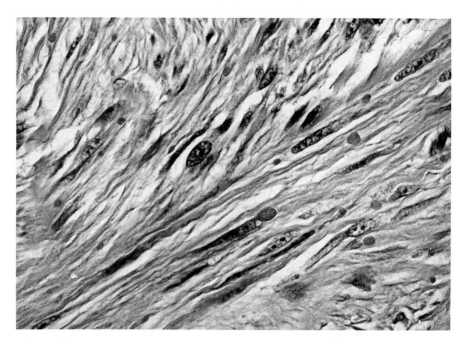

Fig. 8. Infantile digital fibromatosis. Several cells contain intracytoplasmic globular inclusions. H&E, ×560

clearly positive. Positive reactions were also obtained for vimentin and desmin attesting to the myofibroblastic nature of many of the spindle cells. The nature of the inclusions has been a matter of debate for some time. Some investigators were able to identify actin in these inclusions (IWASAKI et al. 1983; FRINGES et al. 1986), but this finding was contradicted by others (VIALE et al. 1988). Most recently, MUKAI et al. (1992) sought clarity by using different fixatives and types of enzymatic pretreatment. Using a combination of KOH in 70% alcohol and trypsin for formalin-fixed tissue specimens they were indeed able to demonstrate actin in these inclusions. In one of the two cases for which we had follow-up information several recurrences occurred, but the tumor growth eventually ceased. This is in accordance with reports from the literature which cite a recurrence rate of up to 75% (ALLEN 1977), but nevertheless an excellent outcome.

3.7 Calcifying Aponeurotic Fibroma

Calcifying aponeurotic fibroma occurred in two patients of our series accounting for 1.2% of the cases. The age of the two patients was 31 and 34 months, respectively. Both were males. In one patient the tumor was

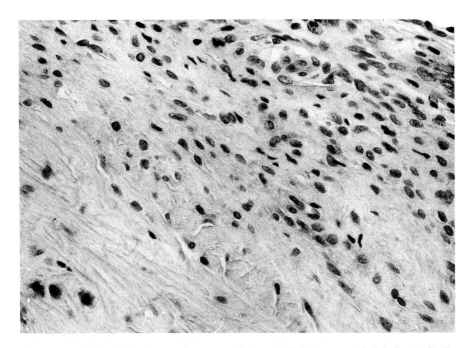

Fig. 9. Calcifying aponeurotic fibroma. Area with chondroid appearance. Nuclei of several cells are positive for protein S-100. ×560

located on the dorsum of the foot, in the other patient it presented between the fourth and fifth fingers of one hand. These are the most common locations, but calcifying aponeurotic fibroma has also been described in sites other than the extremities including the supraclavicular region and the paravertebral fascia (KEASBEY 1953). It has also been identified in adult patients (GOLDMAN 1970), but children and adolescents are more commonly affected. Histologically, the lesions consisted predominantly of spindle cells with plump, round to oval nuclei, and ill-defined cytoplasm. Between the cells a large number of collagen fibrils were present. Small areas had a chondroid appearance, and foci with hyalinization were also seen. Calcification was not found, but the absence of calcification does not militate against the diagnosis, since calcifying aponeurotic fibromas in small children may lack calcification, in contrast to those of older patients. In one case the differential diagnosis from desmoid-like fibromatosis was facilitated by the demonstration of protein S-100 in small groups of cells which had a chondroid appearance (Fig. 9). Recurrences are frequent in this type of fibromatosis with up to 50% of the cases, and one of our two patients also developed several recurrences which were reexcised.

3.8 Unclassified Fibromatosis

One tumor could not be assigned to any of the known fibromatosis categories. This tumor presented in the neck of a 13-year-old boy. Histologically, it consisted of fascicles of spindle-shaped cells and aggregates of rather plump cells.

4 Giant Cell Fibroblastoma

Only one case in our series corresponded to the recently described entity of giant cell fibroblastoma (SHMOOKLER and ENZINGER 1982). Since registration of this case we have only seen two further cases which attests to the rarity of this lesion. Extensive reports on this type of tumor have been published by DYMOCK et al. (1987) and FLETCHER (1988). The male patient in the current series presented with a subcutaneous tumor of the lower leg at age 24 months. This age is typical, since most lesions appear in children younger than 5 years. In contrast to the current case, however, the typical location is the trunk. Other locations include the inguinal region, forearm, and abdominal wall. Microscopically, the tumor was poorly demarcated and showed two histologic patterns. One revealed irregularly branching spaces and clefts which were lined by bizarre giant cells with hyperchromatic and moderately irregularly shaped nuclei showing no mitotic activity (Fig. 10).

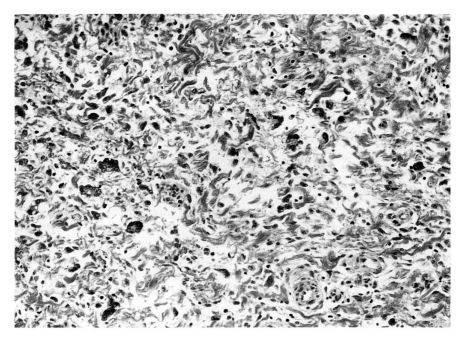

Fig. 10. Giant cell fibroblastoma. Lesion is composed of small cells and floret-type giant cells. Goldner trichrome stain; ×350

Immunohistochemically, these mono- and multinuclear giant cells were negative for factor VIII-related antigen and did not react with a monoclonal anti-endothelial antibody (BMA 120). Thus, immunophenotypically the lining cells do not correspond to endothelial cells, and the spaces are not blood vessels. This conclusion is supported by the finding that the slits contain mucinous material which reacts metachromatically in Giemsa stain. The second component consisted of loosely arranged, plump to spindle-shaped cells with elongated, partially wavy nuclei. In places, a myxoid ground substance was noted between the cells. Other areas were highly collagenized. A considerable number of mast cells was found in the myxoid areas. Mitotic activity was low.

In differential diagnosis, a neurogenic tumor must be excluded. Unlike neurogenic tumors the solid part of giant cell fibroblastoma shows – mostly in a focal arrangement – a second type of multinuclear giant cell with floret-like arrangement of the hyperchromatic nuclei. Thus, two kinds of giant cells occur: (a) multinucleated giant cells incompletely lining the angiectoid spaces; and (b) multinucleated floret-like giant cells in the solid component of the tumor. The histogenesis of this very distinctive fibroblastic tumor is unknown, but arguments have been made favoring a relationship to dermatofibrosarcoma protuberans (SHMOOKLER et al. 1989). This hypothesis

was supported by a recent report of ALGUACIL-GARCIA (1991) describing a
case of dermatofibrosarcoma protuberans in which, during the course of
disease, the tumor developed the appearance of a giant cell fibroblastoma.
Recurrences are frequent in this type of tumor with up to 50% of the cases.
In our patient no recurrence was observed within a period of 1 year after
diagnosis.

5 Conclusion

The different subtypes of fibromatosis display a characteristic histologic,
cytologic, and immunohistochemical profile. Some lesions are more fibroblastic, others myofibroblastic, and thus reflect the "continuum" between
fibroblasts and leiomyocytes. Prognostically, they can be separated into two
groups: with and without tendency of recurrence. With regard to the former
group, the clinical behavior of desmoid fibromatosis can now be better
predicted.

References

Alguacil-Garcia A (1991) Giant cell fibroblastoma recurring as dermatofibrosarcoma pro-
    tuberans. Am J Surg Pathol 15: 798–801
Allen PW (1977) The fibromatoses: a clinicopathologic classification based on 140 cases, part 1.
    Am J Surg Pathol 1: 255–270
Chung EB, Enzinger FM (1981) Infantile myofibromatosis. Cancer 48: 1807–1818
Chung EB, Cavazzana AO, Fassina AS, Ninfo V (1991) Fibrous and fibrohistiocytic tumors and
    tumorlike lesions. In: Ninfo V, Chung EB, Cavazzana AO (eds) Tumors and tumorlike
    lesions of soft tissue. Churchill Livingstone, New York, pp 11–66
Coffin CM, Dehner LP (1991) Fibroblastic-myofibroblastic tumors in children and adolescents:
    a clinicopathologic study of 108 examples in 103 patients. Pediatr Pathol 11: 559–588
Daimaru Y, Hashimoto H, Enjoji M (1989) Myofibromatosis in adults (adult counterpart of
    infantile myofibromatosis). Am J Surg Pathol 13: 859–865
Dymock RB, Allen PW, Stirling JW, Gilbert EF, Thornbery JM (1987) Giant cell fibro-
    blastoma. A distinctive, recurrent tumor of childhood. Am J Surg Pathol 11: 263–271
Egan MJ, Raafat F, Crocker J, Smith K (1987) Nucleolar organizer regions in fibrous prolifera-
    tions of childhood and infantile fibrosarcoma. J Clin Pathol 41: 31–33
Enzinger FM, Weiss SW (1988) Fibrous proliferations of infancy and childhood. In: Enzinger
    FM, Weiss SW (eds) Soft tissue tumors. Mosby, St Louis, pp 164–200
Fletcher CDM (1988) Giant cell fibroblastoma of soft tissue: a clinicopathological and im-
    munohistochemical study. Histopathology 13: 499–508
Fletcher CDM, Achu P, Van Noorden S, Mckee PH (1987) Infantile myofibromatosis: a light
    microscopic, histochemical and immunohistochemical study suggesting true smooth muscle
    differentiation. Histopathology 11: 245–258
Fringes B, Thais H, Böhm N, Altmannsberger M, Osborn M (1986) Identification of actin
    microfilaments in the intracytoplasmic inclusions present in recurring infantile digital
    fibromatosis (Reye tumor). Pediatr Pathol 6: 311–314
Goldman RL (1970) The cartilage analogue of fibromatosis (aponeurotic fibroma). Further
    observations based on seven new cases. Cancer 26: 1325–1328

Hasegawa T, Hirose T, Kudo E, Abe JI, Hizawa K (1990) Cytoskeletal characteristics of myofibroblasts in benign neoplastic and reactive fibroblastic lesions. Virchows Arch [Pathol Anat] 416: 375–382

Iwasaki H, Kikuchi M, Ohtsuki I, Enjoji M, Suenaga N, Mori R (1983) Infantile digital fibromatosis: identification of actin filaments in cytoplasmic inclusions by heavy meromyosin binding. Cancer 52: 1653–1661

Keasbey LE (1953) Juvenile aponeurotic fibroma (calcifying fibroma). Cancer 6: 338–345

Kinzbrunner B, Ritter S, Domingo J, Rosenthal J (1983) Remission of rapidly growing desmoid tumors after tamoxifen therapy. Cancer 52: 2201–2204

Mukai M, Torikata C, Iri H, Hata J, Naito M, Shimoda T (1992) Immunohistochemical identification of aggregated actin filaments in formalin-fixed, paraffin-embedded sections. I. A study of infantile digital fibromatosis by a new pretreatment. Am J Surg Pathol 16: 110–115

Navas-Palacios JJ (1983) The fibromatoses. An ultrastructural study of 31 cases. Pathol Res Pract 176: 158–175

Purdy LJ, Colby TV (1984) Infantile digital fibromatosis occurring outside the digit. Am J Surg Pathol 8: 787–790

Raney B, Evans A, Granowetter L, Schnaufer L, Uri A, Littman P (1987) Nonsurgical management of children with recurrent or unresectable fibromatosis. Pediatrics 79: 394–398

Roche WR (1990) Editorial. Myofibroblasts. J Pathol 161: 281–282

Rosenberg HS, Stenback WA, Spjut HJ (1978) The fibromatoses of infancy and childhood. Perspect Pediatr Pathol 4: 269–348

Sappino AP, Schürch W, Gabbiani G (1990) Biology of disease. Differentiation repertoire of fibroblastic cells: expression of cytoskeletal proteins as markers of phenotypic modulations. Lab Invest 63: 144–161

Schmidt D (1985) Fibromatosis of infancy and childhood. Histology, ultrastructure and clinicopathologic correlation. Z Kinderchir 40: 40–46

Schmidt D, Klinge P, Leuschner I, Harms D (1991) Infantile desmoid-type fibromatosis. Morphological features correlate with biological behaviour. J Pathol 164: 315–319

Shmookler BM, Enzinger FM (1982) Giant cell fibroblastoma. A peculiar tumor of childhood (abstract). Lab Invest 46: 76A

Shmookler BM, Enzinger FM, Weiss SW (1989) Giant cell fibroblastoma. A juvenile form of dermatofibrosarcoma protuberans. Cancer 64: 2154–2161

Viale G, Doglioni C, Iuzzolino P, Bontempi L, Colombi R, Coggi G, Dell'Orto P (1988) Infantile digital fibromatosis-like tumour (inclusion body fibromatosis) of adulthood: report of two cases with ultrastructural and immunocytochemical findings. Histopathology 12: 415–424

Walther E, Hünig R, Zalad S (1988) Behandlung der aggressiven Fibromatose (Desmoid). Verringerung der Rezidivrate durch postoperative Bestrahlung. Orthopäde 17: 193–200

Wiswell TE, Davis JD, Cunningham BE, Solenberger R, Thomas PJ (1988) Infantile myofibromatosis: the most common fibrous tumor of infancy. J Pediatr Surg 23: 314–318

Wolfe JT, Cooper PH (1990) Solitary cutaneous "infantile" myofibroma in a 49-year-old woman. Hum Pathol 21: 562–564

Yokoyama R, Shinohara N, Tsuneyoshi M, Masuda S, Enjoji M (1989) Extra-abdominal desmoid tumors: correlations between histologic features and biologic behavior. Surg Pathol 2: 29–42

Malignant Fibrous Histiocytoma: A "Fibrohistiocytic" or Primitive, Fibroblastic Sarcoma

P. Meister

> The question of more practical importance is whether the concept of malignant fibrous histiocytoma is a useful one. (Weiss 1982)

1 Definition of Malignant Fibrous Histiocytoma

Synchronously with the acceptance of fibrohistiocytic tumors, especially of malignant fibrous histiocytoma (MFH) as a tumor type in the second edition of the WHO classification of soft tissue tumors (Weiss 1993), there is increasing criticism of MFH as an entity (Donhuijsen et al. 1987; Dehner 1988; Fletcher 1992). MFH of the bone was questioned as an entity already years ago (Dahlin et al. 1977). MFH as a sarcoma type became popular during 1960s among Stout and his co-workers (Ozello et al. 1963; O'Brien and Stout 1964; Stout and Lattes 1967). MFH was described as being characteristically composed of two cell types: (a) roundish or polygonal – histiocyte-like; and (b) spindly – fibroblast-like. Varying number of multinucleated giant cells, with or without atypia, may be admixed. Collagenous or mucoid intercellular substances vary intralesionally and interlesionally. A whorly cellular arrangement, called "storiform pattern," was thought to be

Current Topics in Pathology
Volume 89, Eds. D. Harms/D. Schmidt
© Springer-Verlag Berlin Heidelberg 1995

an important differential diagnostic criterion for MFH – even if not ubiquitous (MEISTER et al. 1979; ENZINGER 1986).

The result of studying cell cultures of MFH was interpreted as evidence for MFH being actually derived from histiocytes, which may act as facultative fibroblasts (OZELLO et al. 1963). Thus, the presence of histiocyte-like and fibroblast-like cells was explained and the term "malignant histiocytoma" proposed in the Armed Forces Institute of Pathology (AFIP) umor fascicle (STOUT and LATTES 1967). During a discussion of the question whether benign fibrous histicytomas may ever become malignant fibrous histiocytomas, the currently preferred term MFH was initially applied for dermal tumors. The revised second edition of the AFIP fascicle (LATTES 1982) still emphasized the term "malignant histiocytoma," but included synonyms such as malignant xanthoma or xanthofibroma, respectively xanthofibrosarcoma, malignant giant cell tumor of soft tissue, also the contemporary term of MFH (KOBACK and PERLOW 1949). The variety of terms is also reflected in publications concerning the subject of MFH until the 1980s (ENZINGER 1969). Several types of dermal tumors such as fibrous xanthoma, giant cell tumor of soft tissue, villonodular synovialitis and dermatofibrosarcoma protuberans were grouped under the term of "fibrous histiocytomas" (EKFORS and RANTAKOKKO 1978; LATTES 1982a). The concept of "fibrohistiocytic tumors," including former fibrous and xanthomatous skin tumors (TEN SELDAM and HELWIG 1974), was also introduced into the second edition of the WHO classification of soft tissue tumors (WEISS 1993). Fibrohistiocytic tumors were divided into three prognostic groups: (a) benign – "dermatofibroma"; (b) intermediate, only exceptionally metastasizing – dermatofibrosarcoma and newly angiomatoid fibrous histiocytoma; and finally (c) fully malignant with considerable risk of metastases – MFH. However, the latter do show differences in degree of malignancy or histological subtypes.

2 Subtypes of MFH

In agreement with a proposal by Enzinger and Weiss (WEISS and ENZINGER 1978; WEISS 1982; ENZINGER 1986; ENZINGER and WEISS 1988), the following subtypes of MFH can be distinguished: (a) myxoid, if at least half of the total tumor is myxoid; (b) classical storiform/pleomorphic; (c) giant cell variant (malignant giant cell tumor of soft tissue); and (d) inflammatory, or xanthomatous, MHF with sheets of "foam cells" and admixture of different kinds of inflammatory cells (MILLER et al. 1980). Angiomatoid fibrous histiocytoma, formerly listed as a fifth subtype was recently redefined as an intermediate fibrohistiocytic tumor (WEISS 1993). However, not only a relatively good prognosis is peculiar for this tumor; other peculiarities are also found, such as histologically chiefly cells of histiocytic type, even reportedly with immunhistochemical expression of histiocyte/macrophage markers

(LEU and MAKEK 1986; WEGMANN and HEITZ 1985; SMITH et al. 1991), and classical occurrence during childhood, occasionally accompanied by general clinical symptoms as fever and leukocytosis (ENZINGER 1979).

In the four remaining subtypes of MFH significant prognostic differences are evident for the myxoid variant, which can also be graded as G1 – low-grade malignant as a result of mitotic activity and activity of proliferative markers (WEISS and ENZINGER 1977; ENZINGER and WEISS 1983; IWASAKI et al. 1992). From experience, storiform/pleomorphic MFH is considered in general to be a high-grade malignant tumor (WEISS 1982; ENZINGER and WEISS 1988). Evaluation of histologic grading parameters such as mitotic activity is controversial. Even using sophisticated methods, trends for grading these tumors either as G2 or G3 show up (ZEHER et al. 1990; BECKER et al. 1991; IWASAKI et al. 1992). For giant cell type there is a trend to a worse prognosis than with the majority of the storiform/pleomorphic type (ENZINGER and WEISS 1988; BROOKS 1989). Inflammatory or xanthomatous MFH was originally thought to do especially poorly. This is mirrored in reports about overall survival, which for inflammatory MFH may reach zero (!) (BROOKS 1989). There were also proposals to subtype MFH according to the prevalence of cell types, i.e., (a) chiefly histiocytic; (b) chiefly fibroblastic; and (c) mixed (HADJU 1979; MEISTER et al. 1980a). This approach is worthwhile in pointing out the range of intralesional heterogeneity, especially with storiform/pleomorphic MFH. Prognostic significance, however, did not become evident for these subtypes. Nevertheless, it has been claimed that a pronounced storiform pattern may be associated with a worse prognosis (ENJOJI et al. 1980). A storiform pattern in MFH is not found ubiquitously. It is not specific, but typical for MFH. In reconstructive studies, a storiform pattern turned out to result from peripheral overlap of adjacent compartments with perivascular, primitive fibroblastic proliferation (MEISTER et al. 1979).

3 "Histogenesis" of MFH

The presence of two cellular phenotypes is still a reason for a discussion of "histogenesis" – or rather differentiation of MFH. The initial concept of MFH as a histiocytic neoplasia with facultative fibroblasts gave the basis for a unitarian concept of this cytologically biphasic tumor (OZELLO et al. 1963; WEISS 1982). A later concept was based on MFH as a biphasic, biclonal neoplasia, with histiocytes on the one hand and fibroblasts on the other (MERKOW et al. 1971). Especially with the introduction of new methods into the study of MFH, such as electron microscopy and immunohistochemistry, interest was directed towards noncommitted pluripotential stem cells, which may show trends of differentiation towards histiocytic and/or fibroblastic features. These observations served to conceive the idea of MFH as primitive, mesenchymal neoplasia which may – in varying proportions – develop histiocytic and/or fibroblastic features (FU et al. 1975; TAXY and BATTIFORA 1977; ALGUACIL-GARCIA et al. 1977, 1978; LIMACHER et al. 1978; REDDICK et al. 1979; LAGACE et al. 1979; SOULE and ENRIQUEZ 1979; HARRIS 1979; TSUNEYOSHI et al. 1981; MEISTER and NATHRATH 1980; DuBOULAY 1982; NATHRATH and MEISTER 1982; KINDBLOM et al. 1982; MERCK et al. 1983; BROOKS 1986; WÜNSCH and DUBRAUSZKY 1987; MIETTINEN and SOINI 1989; HIROSE et al. 1989).

As most immunohistochemical studies did not prove any markers for bone marrow – derived histiocytes/macrophages in the histiocytic component (STRAUCHEN and DIMITRIU-BONA 1986; SMITH et al. 1991; IWASAKI et al. 1992; MIETTINEN and SOINI 1992) and also further cell culture and multiparameter cell biologic studies showed evidence of primitive (perivascular) mesenchymal cell and partial fibroblastic differentiation, the unitarian concept of MFH as a primitive sarcoma gained momentum (ROHOLL et al. 1985a,b; WOOD et al. 1986; IWASAKI et al. 1987, 1991; ENZINGER and WEISS 1988). Some of the tumor cells may show fine-structural evidence of histiocytic differentiation such as lysosomes and immunohistochemical functional markers, which is, however, not restricted to MFH (HOFFMAN and DICKERSIN 1983). This phenomenon could also be explained as a loss of supression because of anaplasia (DENK 1988; KATENKAMP 1988; LLOMBART-BOSCH et al. 1988; HASHIMOTO et al. 1990; IWASAKI et al. 1991). Consecutively with dedifferentiation, and also unexpectedly, formerly called "aberrant" antibody expression could be explained, especially keratin as an epithelial marker in Ewing's sarcoma and MFH (MOLL et al. 1987; WEISS et al. 1988) as well as desmin and S-100 in MFH (BROOKS 1986; DONHUIJSEN et al. 1988). Smooth muscle antigen can be expected to be positive in MFH, as myofibroblasts had already been recognized as a constituent part by electron microscopy (CHURG and KAHN 1977). Unexpected antibody expression in scattered cells in MFH has to be distinguished from focal expression of markers of higher differentiation, or miscellaneous features of higher differentiation, compatible with lipoblasts, rhabdo- or leiomyoblasts, Schwann cells in soft tissue tumors, and osteoblasts or chondroblasts especially in bone tumors. This phenomenon can either be interpreted as being metachronous, with dedifferentiation of previously higher differentiated sarcomas, as is especially well known with secondary MFH in dedifferentiated liposarcoma and chondrosarcoma (EVANS 1979; WICK et al. 1987; KATENKAMP 1988; KATENKAMP and NEUPERT 1988; HASHIMOTO et al. 1990). Dedifferentiation may occur spontaneously or after radio- or chemotherapy (KATENKAMP 1988; WEISS et al. 1988). Moreover, MFH-like focal features do not necessarily express "dedifferentiation." The concept of MFH as neoplasia of primitive mesenchymal cells would allow the explanation of these undifferentiated areas as expressing an arrest in differentiation, side by side with areas which have succeeded in higher differentiation (WEISS 1982; MEISTER 1988). Thus, fibrohistiocytic foci can also be imagined in benign tumors such as, for instance, in lipoma (ALLEN 1990).

In general, cytology and histology of fibrohistiocytic tumors as a group, including MFH, could be compared with normal loose, areolar fibrous connective tissue (KRETZSCHMAR 1984; MEISTER 1988). With both, varying amounts of mucoid and/or nonfasciculated collagenous intercellular substance are present. "Histiocytes" are mentioned as tissue constituent second only to fibroblasts in standard histology texts (MAXIMOV 1927; BUCHER 1980). The exact type of these histiocytes is open to discussion, especially whether they are of a bone marrow-derived histiocytic/macrophage nature or not. Controversial reports regarding the presence of histiocytic markers in MFH (STRAUCHEN and DIMITRIU-BONA 1986; SOINI and MIETTINEN 1992) may find some explanation in the concept of fixed tissue histiocytes, or noncommitted pluripotential cells or mesenchymal cells, which can become histiocytes – or also fibroblasts (BUCHER 1980). Differentiation to histiocytes may be induced by colonization by a few bone marrow-derived histiocytes. This idea of colonization and induction of fixed cells to function as macrophages is well known in Kupffer cells in the liver (WISSE and KNOCK 1977; HOWARD 1979).

4 Immunohistochemical Markers in MFH

Immunohistochemical studies not only of MFH, but also of soft tissue tumors in general, previously emphasized observed features of heterogeneity in routinely stained sections (KATENKAMP 1988; LLOMBART-BOSCH et al. 1988; BROOKS 1986, 1989; HIROSE et al. 1989; SOINI and MIETTINEN 1989). As muramidase (lysocyme) expression was thought to be typical for histiocytes, this antibody was tested in MFH, where only a minority of (questionable) tumor cells were found to react. Also, additionally applied antibodies to alpha 1-antitrypsin and antichymotrypsin did not ubiquitously decorate tumors cells, moreover, the problem arose of how to distinguish histiocytic tumors cells from interspersed reactive histiocytes (DUBOULY 1982; MEISTER and NATHRATH 1980; NATHRATH and MEISTER 1982). Expression of markers of muscular differentiation, especially smooth muscle actin, signified myofibroblastic differentiation in MFH (CHURG and KAHN 1977; BROOKS 1986, 1989; WÜNSCH and DUBRAUSZKY 1987). On the other hand, it has to be stressed that there is no single immunohistochemical marker being typical or proof for MFH (ENZINGER and WEISS 1988; MEISTER 1988). Nevertheless, alpha 1-antitrypsin and antichymotrypsin expression may be of help to accentuate histiocytic features in some cases of MFH. A similar indication is given by hemosiderin in tumor cells in iron stains. Moreover, both antibodies exhibit a similar pattern as apparently comparable cells in normal loose areolar fibrous connective tissue (MEISTER 1988). As loose areolar fibrous connective tissue could be compared to MFH, dense, tendinous fibrous connective tissue, lacking expression of the three antibodies mentioned above, would compare with fibrosarcoma as its neoplastic counterpart (MEISTER 1988).

Finally, numerous unexpected antibody expressions observed during differential diagnostic work-up of various soft tissue tumors were initially often called and thought of as being "aberrant" (BROOKS 1989). Not only confusion, but also insight into tumor biology were gained, especially regarding heterogeneity, and various cellular phenotypes – synchronous or metachronous, the latter especially with regard to spontaneous dedifferentiation or as an effect of therapy. These morphologic changes may be associated with such in biologic behavior (KATENKAMP 1988). Changes comparable to the in vivo relationship with the course of time where also found experimentally with an increasing number of cell passages (KATENKAMP and NEUBERT 1982; KATENKAMP 1988; LLOMBART-BOSCH et al. 1988; KOSSMEHL et al. 1990; HASHIMOTO et al. 1990). Unexpected immunohistochemical markers may differ from case to case, either pointing to a more highly differentiated tumor, for example, leiomyosarcoma or even melanoma or carcinoma, with similarities leading to the false diagnosis of MFH, or they may actually mean a focal lack of higher differentiation; or tumors may predominantly consist of undifferentiated, pluripotential cells. Conventionally these tumors could then be classified as MFH (WÜNSCH and DUBRAUSZKY 1987; MEISTER 1988; ENZINGER and WEISS 1988).

5 Grading of MFH

In addition to a distinction of subtypes, grading of MFH is controversial (DONHUIJSEN et al. 1986; ENZINGER and WEISS 1988). Myxoid variants usually also show corresponding low mitotic activity compatible with grade G1 – low-grade malignancy (IWASAKI et al. 1992). The majority of classical storiform/pleomorphic MFH have to be classified either as G2 or G3, with equivocal opinions as to the grading parameters (DONHUIJSEN et al. 1986). Other prognostic parameters such as tumor size and superficial localization were given priority in prognosis (RYDHOLM and SYK 1986; ENZINGER and WEISS 1988). Nevertheless, the mathematically evaluated material of 169 soft tissue sarcomas of the EORTC included 23% MFH, whereby the number of mitoses was found to be the most important (significant) prognostic parameter (VAN UNNIK et al. 1987). Moreover, in correlation with immunohistochemical typing of individual cell constituents of MFH, the proliferative capacity of the individual cell constituents was investigated (IWASAKI et al. 1991). With classical storiform/pleomorphic MFH, polygonal histiocyte-like cells, fibroblast-like spindle cells, as well as atypical multinucleated giant cells expressed similar proliferation markers, with 70% of these cells being decorated by PCNA! In contrast, multinucleated giant cells of the osteoclast type not only lacked the proliferative marker PNCA, but were also distinguished from atypical giant cells by decoration by macrophage/histiocyte markers (HAM 56, CD 68). Semiquantitative evaluation revealed a marked (+ + +) expression of PCNA in 50% of the cells in storiform/pleomorphic MFH – albeit in only 12.5% of myxoid MFH which was significantly lower! Thus, findings similar to empirically known differences in the grade of malignancy between these two subtypes were observed, albeit handicapped by the small number of myxoid MFH (IWASAKI et al. 1992). Especially interesting are the investigations into the nature of osteoclast-type giant cells with atypical giant cell variants and foamy histiocytic elements with inflammatory, xanthomatous MFH. The former, i.e., osteoclast-like giant cells, again show histiocytic markers and lack proliferative markers. In the latter some of the apparently histiocytic elements show evidence of being reactive, whereas others appear to be neoplastic, without unequivocal distinction between these two cell types in routine stains.

6 Clinicopathologic Aspects of MFH

6.1 Incidence

MFH is frequently listed as the most common soft tissue sarcoma (RUSSELL et al. 1977; WEISS and ENZINGER 1978; HAJDU 1979; KEARNY and SOULE 1980; ENJOJI et al. 1980; MEISTER et al. 1980a,b). Lately some decrease in incidence, or reduction in diagnosis, of MFH has been noted. Using not only immunohistochemical means, but also with a better understanding of histologic patterns in hemotoxylin and eosin stains in the differential diagnosis of myxoid spindle cell tumors and storiform, pleomorphic tumors, chiefly liposarcomas, leimyosarcomas, rhabdomyosarcomas, and malignant peripheral nerve sheath tumors are recognized as such (MEISTER 1984; ENZINGER and WEISS 1988; FLETCHER 1992). After inflammatory MFH, inflammatory variants have also been reported for fibro- and liposarcoma (ENZINGER and WEISS 1988; MEIS and ENZINGER 1991). Thus an inflammatory component does not imply the diagnosis of MFH. Foci of apparently reactive osteoclast-type giant cells may also occur with a variety of sarcomas and carcinomas.

6.2 Age and Sex Distribution

Like most soft tissue sarcomas, for example, liposarcoma, leiomyosarcoma, and classical, non-juvenile fibrosarcoma, the peak age for MFH is in the sixth and seventh decades. The mean age among our patients was 58 years (ENZINGER and WEISS 1988; MEISTER et al. 1980). Even after consideration of a classical report on MFH in childhood, the age group below 20 years is only rarely involved (KAUFFMAN and STOUT 1961). Regarding secondary MFH with dedifferentiated liposarcoma, as well as osteosarcoma, it can be expected that the peak is skewed to the upper range of the usual age group (ENZINGER and WEISS 1988; WICK et al. 1987). As with many other soft tissue sarcomas, with the exception of few like angiosarcoma, there is a slight male predeliction of 4:3 (HAJDU 1979).

6.3 Localization

MFH is found chiefly in the lower extremities, especially the thighs, often with extension into the buttocks. This is controversial with regard to class-ification as localization in the trunk. Results are comparable with most soft tissue sarcomas, such as liposarcoma which can be found in the region with the largest soft tissue mass, i.e., the thigh (HAJDU 1979; MEISTER 1984; ENZINGER and WEISS 1988; BROOKS 1989). The calves are less frequently involved. In second place MFH is found in the trunk, especially the retro-peritoneal area. This is the most common localization for inflammatory MFH, which had been historically described in this area as "retroperitoneal xanthogranuloma" (OBERLING 1935).

6.4 Prevalence of Subtypes

Classical storiform/pleomorphic MFH is the most common. Intralesional and interlesional variations exist in pleomorphism, storiform pattern, and collagenous and mucoid intercellular substances (MEISTER 1988; ENZINGER and WEISS 1988; BROOKS 1989). By definition, for myxoid MFH, myxoid appearance is required in one half of the total tumor (WEISS and ENZINGER 1978; LAGACE et al. 1979; MERCK et al. 1983). Storiform/pleomorphic MFH makes up about 60%, myxoid 25%, giant cell variants 10% (usually with only focal expression), and inflammatory/xanthomatous variants and un-determined types the remaining 5% (ENZINGER and WEISS 1988; BROOKS 1989). Giant cell variants, are not only characterized by osteoclast-type giant cell, but also by high vascularity, typically correlated with areas rich in giant cells and distinct micronodular pattern (GUCCION and ENZINGER 1972; ANGERVALL et al. 1981). Inflammatory/xanthomatous MFH is the rarest variant, often showing only focally typical features of classical MFH. Its special role is also underlined by occasional general symptoms as leuco-cytosis and/or eosinophilia (KOBACK and PARLOW 1949; KYRIAKOS and KEMPSON 1976; KAHN 1973; KAY 1978; ROGUES et al. 1979; MERINO and LiVOLSI et al. 1980; MILLER et al. 1980; VILANOVA et al. 1980).

7 Macroscopical Features

Dependent on subtypes, myxoid MFH also grossly shows a myxoid or mucoid appearance. The storiform/pleomorphic type reveals, in relation to a high collagen content, either a firm whitish or, with a predominance of fat storing histiocytic, multinucleated elements, a soft yellowish appearance. The giant cell type may also grossly express high vascularity by reddish areas. The inflammatory/xanthomatous type with sheets of fatty foam cells typically presents as a yellow, soft tumor (ENZINGER and WEISS 1988).

8 Microscopical Features

Mesenchymal tumors are notoriously heterogenious. This is especially true for MFH, which may be focally expressed not only in a number of different types of sarcomas, but also in melanomas and even in undifferentiated carcinoma (KATENKAMP and RAIKHLIN 1985; WEISS 1982; FLETCHER 1992). Heterogeneity is also observed concerning association of various subtypes of MFH. A classical storiform/pleomorphic pattern can quite frequently be found side by side with at least small areas of a myxoid variant (ENZINGER and WEISS 1988; WEISS et al. 1988).

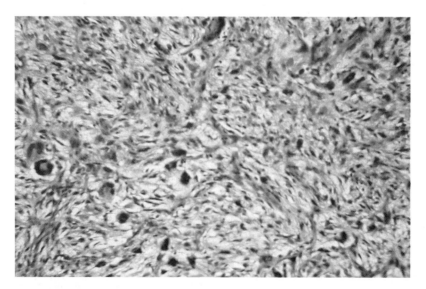

Fig. 1. Storiform/pleomorphic MFH: typical histology with mononucleated and multinucleated histiocystic elements and fibroblastic spindle cells exhibiting a storiform pattern. Moderate cellularity. H&E

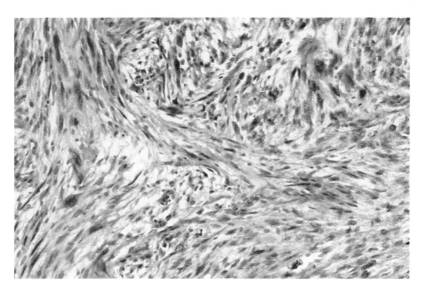

Fig. 2. Storiform/pleomorphic MFH, with a predominantly fibroblastic storiform area. H&E

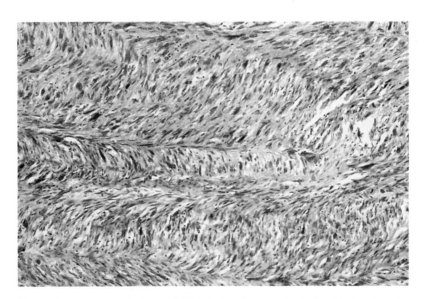

Fig. 3. Same tumor as in Fig. 2, with fibroblastic component showing transition to fascicles, i.e., features compatible with fibrosarcoma. H&E

Areas of different appearance may be observed in separate adjacent nodules. Or there may be a zone of transition from one to an other appearance of MFH. Exact criteria for subtyping were only proposed for the myxoid subtype, whereby half of the tumor has to be myxoid. Correspond-

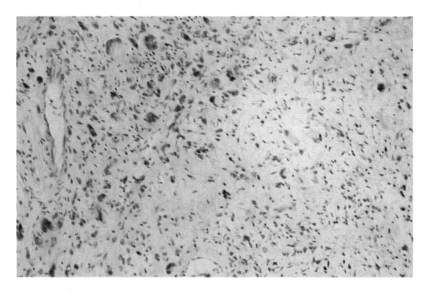

Fig. 4. Storiform/pleomorphic MFH with gradual transition to a hypocellular myxoid area, still containing multinucleated giant cells. H&E

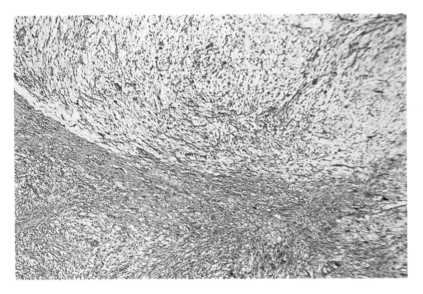

Fig. 5. Storiform/pleomorphic MFH with a rather well-defined hypocellular, myxoid nodule. H&E

ing criteria are not given for giant cell variants with only focal expression, or for the inflammatory/xanthomatous type. Nevertheless, for the latter a predominance of tumor areas with foamy histiocytes and interspersed inflammatory cells should be present.

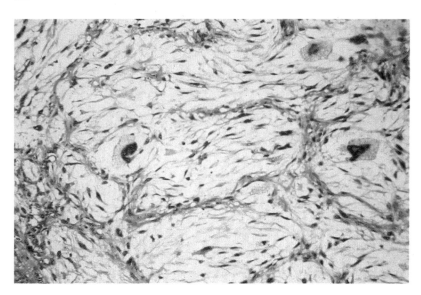

Fig. 6. Myxoid MFH with tupical low cellularity, lacking marked cellular atypia. Prominent arcuate vasculature with perivascular cell condensation. H&E

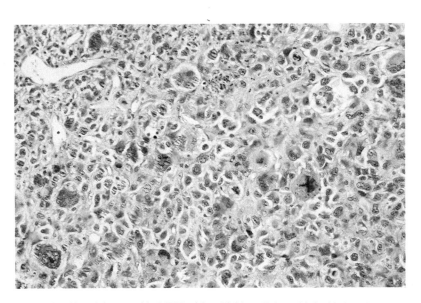

Fig. 7. Storiform/pleomorphic MFH with a highly cellular, chiefly histiocytic area containing numerous giant cells and prominent blood vessels. Focally inflammatory cells. However, no features typical for giant cell or inflammatory/xanthomatous variant. H&E

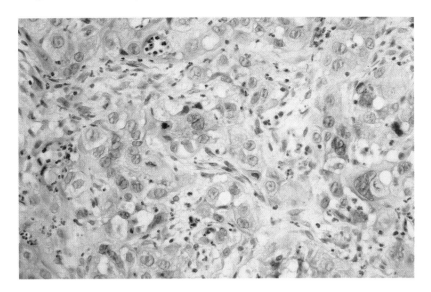

Fig. 8. Anaplastic tumor resembling MFH in Fig. 7. However, it is not MFH but undifferentiated portion of otherwise better differentiated carcinoma with cytokeratin expression even in the depicted area. PAP, cytokeratin

Small areas with xanthomatous, foamy cells intermingled with different types of inflammatory cells, also in the absence of tumor necrosis and detectable reason for inflammatory reaction or single cells of osteoclast-type, are, however, no exception especially with storiform/pleomorphic MFH (Figs. 1–8).

9 Differential Diagnosis of MFH

Differential diagnosis is very much dependent on different subtypes and their histologic features described above. Regarding differentiation of myxoid MFH from other myxoid benign or malignant tumors, distinction from myxoid liposarcoma may be problematic, especially if based on conventional examination, however, also when applying immunohistochemistry (TSUNEYOSHI et al. 1983; ENZINGER and WEISS 1988). Cytoplasmic vacuoles containing mucoid or fatty material may be present with both. Multinucleated giant cells are usually absent in myxoid liposarcoma. However, occasionally a few floret-type multinucleated cells may be observed. Characteristic multivacuolar tumor lipoblasts are quite frequently missing in myxoid liposarcoma. Both tumors may be lobular. Finally, the low-power pattern of a tumor with peripherally delineated lobules, a branching vascular pattern, and irregular foci of necrosis with torn appearance is decisive in the diagnosis of myxoid liposarcoma. Even more difficult may be the differential diagnosis between myxoid MFH and spindle cell lipoma, which is (by definition) lacking atypical lipoblasts, but may show pleomorphism and hemangiopericytoma-like areas. Quite commonly, spindle cell lipoma looks grossly like a lipoma. Lipoma-like areas have to be looked for. Benign and malignant peripheral nerve sheath tumors typically exhibit, even if small, short, wavy bundles of spindle cells with indented or vacuolated nuclei. Focally vascularity may be high, but without branching or arcuate pattern. Vascular walls often appear to be hyalinized. Neurofibroma may exhibit alternating myxoid and fibrous areas.

Neurinomas typically reveal alternating hypocellular and hypercellular areas, the latter often with palisading. With degenerative changes cellular pleomorphism may be marked with benign peripheral nerve sheath tumors ("ancient neurinoma"). Often the combination of mitotic activity and infiltrative growth helps to recognize malignancy. Myxoid leio- or rhabdomyosarcomas lack the typical arcuate vascular network of myxoid MFH. Because of interlacing bundles it is easier to recognize leiomyosarcoma by pattern than rhabdomyosarcoma. Brick-red ameboid cells may lead to the false diagnosis of rhabdomyosarcoma in MFH and liposarcoma. For identification of muscular tumors, expression of the typical intermediary filament desmin is most helpful. Last but not least, tumor-like lesion can be very hard to distinguish from myxoid MFH. This is especially true for nodular fasciitis if the characteristic context with subcutaneous fascia is not recognizable and a focal storiform pattern is present. Also in these cases the search for the typical pattern is most helpful, which implies work-up of the specimen by numerous sections and, if necessary, complete embedding.

The storiform/pleomorphic type also has as its main competitor in differential diagnosis a liposarcoma, i.e., the pleomorphic type. The latter typically contains large multivacuolated tumor lipoblasts with atypical, deformed, or impressed nuclei. MFH may also show fat-containing atypical cells. Vice versa, pleomorphic liposarcoma may present markedly eosinophilic brick-red giant cells without cytoplasmic vacuoles, which not only remind one of MFH, but also of the rare adult pleomorphic rhabdomyosarcoma. Again, desmin expression is a very helpful tool in recognition of rhabdomyosarcoma (ALTMANNSBERGER et al. 1985). Occurrence of MFH-like areas, for instance, with dedifferentiation of liposarcoma, rhabdomyosarcoma, leiomyosarcoma, and also malignant peripheral nerve sheath tumor should be always kept in mind as pitfalls in differential diagnosis (KATENKAMP 1988; HASHIMOTO et al. 1990). Moreover, MFH-like areas deserve attention, also in metastatic melanoma or undifferentiated, for instance, renal, carcinomas (ENZINGER and WEISS 1988; FLETCHER 1992). Recently attention has also been drawn to malignant lymphoma presenting as soft tissue tumors, sometimes with the impression of a myxoid round to spindle cell tumor, which can also be recognized immunohistochemically in most cases (LANHAM et al. 1989; MEISTER 1992). Differential diagnosis of non-Hodgkin and Hodgkin lymphoma are the main concern with inflam-matory/xanthomatous MFH. A host of other possibilities has to be included in differential diagnosis of this subtype as myelosarcoma, especially in the presence of occasional leukemoid reaction (VILANOVA et al. 1980; ROGUES et al. 1979), malignant histiocytosis, histiocytosis X (eosinophilic granuloma) on the one hand, and xanthogranulomatous inflammatory reaction on the other hand (compare "retroperitoneal xanthogranulomatosis"!) (ENZINGER and WEISS 1988). The decision as to whether the tumor is benign or malig-nant may also be hard with the giant cell variant of MFH, which at least focally may resemble pigmented villonodular synovialitis. On the other hand, chondro- or osteoplasia may be found with the giant cell variant more frequently than with storiform/pleomorphic MFH, thus including ex-traskeletal chondro-, or osteosarcoma in the differential diagnosis (BHAGAVAN and DORFMAN 1982; BROOKS 1989). Again, sampling of sufficient tissue for diagnosis has to be emphasized as the most effective "special method" in the diagnosis of soft tissue tumors, especially with regard to their notorious heterogeneity.

10 Prognosis in MFH

Morphologically the distinction of different subtypes of MFH is important in differential diagnosis and recognition of a given sarcoma as MFH. Another aspect of distinguishing between subtypes concerns possible differences in biologic behavior, prognosis, and consequently therapy planning (ENZINGER and WEISS 1988; BROOKS 1989). Specified according subtypes, differences are most impressive and significant for myxoid MFH (metastatic rate 23%; 5-year survival rate 66%), versus storiform/pleomorphic MFH (metastatic rate 42% – almost twice as high; 5-year survival rate 30%, maximally 42%) (ENZINGER and WEISS 1988; BROOKS 1989). Surprising is a reported higher recurrence rate for myxoid MFH, which could be explained by initial un-derestimation of these tumors resulting in insufficient surgery. No significant differences are known for the giant cell variant, which in general appears to fall into the high-risk area of the prognosis given for storiform/pleomorphic MFH.

Inflammatory/xanthomatous MFH has originally thought to be of espe-cially high-grade malignancy (KYRIAKOS and KEMPSON 1976; ENZINGER and WEISS 1988). But there is no significantly higher metastatic risk. However, there is a higher risk of local recurrences, which could be due to two factors: (a) misdiagnosis as a reactive inflammatory process without surgery in toto; and (b) late detection and large tumor size on initial diagnosis because of retroperitoneal localization, which also often means limited surgery. Thus the 5-year survival rate ranges from 30% down to 0%(!), with 100% dying of disease, irrespective of length of time (BROOKS 1989).

Beside the biologic differences regarding subtypes, evaluation of single histologic parameters, such as counting mitoses in routinely stained sections or immunohistochemical evaluation of proliferations markers such as PCNA and KI-67, as well as the addition of and comparison with DNA analysis shows at least trends as to clinicopathologic correlation for the individual subtypes on the one hand and for MFH as a whole on the other hand (ENZINGER and WEISS 1988; BECKER et al. 1991; IWASAKI et al. 1992; ZEHER et al. 1990).

For the sake of completeness atypical fibroxanthoma (AFX) should also be mentioned (TEN SELDAM and HELWIG 1974). In some classifications AFX is conceived of as superficial MFH of the storiform/pleomorphic type (ENZINGER and WEISS 1988; BROOKS 1989). In general, better prognosis of soft tissue tumors restricted to cutis and/or subcutis is emphasized (HAJDU 1979). Especially for MFH an increase of the metastatic rate from 10% with only subcutaneous infiltration to 37% with fascial and 43% with muscular invasion has been reported (ENZINGER and WEISS 1988). However, there are also reports that AFX can be distinguished from MFH of soft tissues by a cutaneous localization and good prognosis with only rare metastases. Immunohistochemical investigations of AFX revealed, in contrast to MFH, frequent expression of S-100 and corresponding fine-structural evidence of Langerhans granules (ALGUACIL-GARCIA et al. 1977; ENZINGER and WEISS 1988). AFX is possibly a different tumor from MFH, arising typically in sun-damaged skin.

11 Conclusions

1. The concept of fibrohistiocytic tumors in general, and MFH especially, appears to be useful (WEISS 1993). It has also been introduced into the second edition of the standardized classification of soft tissue tumors by the WHO (WEISS et al. 1993).
2. Nevertheless, criticism on overdiagnosis of MFH, especially of the storiform/pleomorphic type as well as of the myxoid type, has to be taken seriously (FLETCHER 1992). Better understanding of the nature of MFH as a primitive mesenchymal neoplasia, with a phenotype which may be focally expressed in various soft tissue tumors and moreover in neoplasias in general also helps in differential diagnostic evaluation (KATENKAMP 1988). A comparable development has also been observed with hemangiopericytoma which, after its first description, became a very popular diagnosis (STOUT and MURRAY 1942). Recognition of a hemangiopericytoma pattern in various soft tissue tumors reduced the number of "true" hemangiopericytomas; however, it did not abolish the concept of hemangiopericytoma as a tumor type (TSUNEYOSHI et al. 1984).

3. Newer investigations, in vivo and in vitro, show evidence of MFH being a neoplasia of chiefly undifferentiated, primitive perivascular mesenchymal cells (Roholl et al. 1985b; Iwasaki et al. 1987, 1992). Most commonly, if there is any differentiation, features of fibroblasts and histiocytes can be detected. Apparently, in general no features of bone marrow-derived histiocytes/macrophages can be demonstrated in these "facultative histiocytes." Moreover, these primitive neoplastic cells, retaining pluripotentiality, may also be differentiated otherwise, or may reappear during dedifferentiation of originally higher differentiated sarcomas (Hashimoto et al. 1990).
4. As the accent in terminology was originally on the histiocytic part (Ozello et al. 1963), according to above, it should actually be shifted to the fibrous or fibroblastic component of MFH. Nevertheless, there is no strong argument against the concept that MFH truly is a "fibrohistiocytic" neoplasia. For clinicopathologic correlation it would be advantageous if the term "sarcoma" would appear in the diagnosis – which was the case in apparently one of the first published cases when the term "fibroxanthosarcoma" was proposed (Nöthen 1920).
5. Modern cell biologic or molecular biologic (Roholl et al. 1985) and cytogenetic (Molenaar et al. 1989) methods gain weight in the characterization of soft tissue tumors in general. Using these methods there was evidence for two cell lines in MFH, albeit in the presence of a wide range of karyotypic abnormalities – which again would relate to the marked heterogeneity generally seen in MFH (Hecht et al. 1983; Mandahl et al. 1985; Bridge et al. 1987; Mandahl et al. 1989; Heppner 1989; Genberg et al. 1989). On the other hand, a common chromosomal marker in these two cell lines pointed to a common stem cell (Genberg et al. 1989; Iwasaki et al. 1991). Even subtypes of MFH may be identified cytogenetically (Mandahl et al. 1989).
6. This does not exclude other directions of differentiation in some MFH, ranging from evidence of frequently smooth, rarely striated muscle cells to epithelial features. Thus, a distribution pattern may be present which reminds one of an experimental model in the modern "science of chaos" (fractional geometry). Here, globules of different colors, which could represent cells with varying differentiation, appear singly or in small groups against a background of chiefly white globules when mixed inadvertently. The white globules are comparable to the predominantly undifferentiated mesenchymal or primitive fibroblastic population in MFH. Different colors, on the other hand, would represent varying higher (or aberrant) differentiations. On the other hand, for instance, leiomyosarcoma (which may show close relations to MFH) would thus be characterized by a white background of predominantly leiomyoblasts, with only scattered elements of fibroblastic or histiocytic differentiation – the latter showing a focally typical MFH pattern.

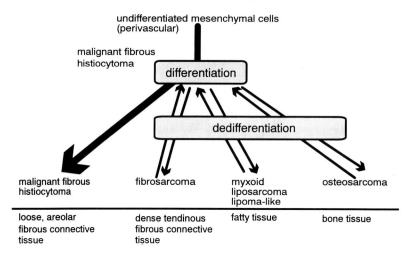

Fig. 9. Differentiation of MFH ("histogenesis")

7. The role of MFH as "the" primitive sarcoma is underlined by experimental sarcomas, often presenting the morphology of MFH – even after possible previous higher differentiation (KATENKAMP and NEUPERT 1982). Fibrosarcomas with increasing number of cell passages may develop similar histiocytoid cells to MFH. Moreover, sarcomas induced by foreign material or irradiation frequently reveal an MFH pattern (HARDY et al. 1980; WEISS 1982; LEE et al. 1984).
8. The concept of differentiation ("histogenesis") of MFH (Fig. 9) should show MFH as a *primitive, "embryonal" fibrosarcoma*.

References

Alguacil-Garcia A, Unni K, Goellner J (1977) Atypical fibroxanthoma of the skin. Cancer 40: 1471

Alguacil-Garcia A, Unni K, Goellner J (1978) MFH: an ultrastructural analysis of six cases. Am J Clin Pathol 69: 121–129

Allen P (1990) "Dedifferentiated" pleomorphic lipoma. Case presentation. IAP Congress, Buenos Aires

Altmannsberger M, Weber K, Droste R, Osborn M (1985) Desmin is a specific marker for rhabdomyosarcomas of human and rat origin. Am J Pathol 118: 85–95

Angervall L, Hagmar B, Kindblom L, Merck C (1981) Malignant giant cell tumor of soft tissues. Cancer 47: 736–747

Becker R, Venzon D, Lack E et al. (1991) Cytometry and morphometry of MFH of the extremities. Am J Surg Pathol 15: 957–970

Bhagavan B, Dorfman H (1982) The significance of bone and cartilage formation in MFH of soft tissue. Cancer 49: 480–488

Bridge J, Sanger W, Shaffer B, Neff J (1987) Cytogenetic findings in MFH. Cancer Genet Cytogenet 29: 97–102

Brooks J (1986) The significance of double phenotypic patterns and markers in sarcomas. Am J
    Pathol 125: 113–123
Brooks J (1989) Disorder of soft tissue. In: Sternberg S (ed) Diagnostic surgical pathology.
    Raven, New York
Bucher O (1980) Cytologie, Histologie und mikroskopische Anatomie des Menschen, 10th edn.
    Huber, Bern
Churg A, Kahn L (1977) Myofibroblasts and related cells in malignant fibrous and fibrohistio-
    cytic tumors. Hum Pathol 8: 205–218
Dahlin D, Unni K, Matsumo T (1977) Malignant (fibrous) histiocytoma of bone-fact or fancy?
    Cancer 39: 1508–1516
Dehner L (1988) MFH: nonspecific morphologic pattern, specific entity, or both? Arch Pathol
    Lab Med 112: 236–237
Denk H (1988) Immunohistologic heterogeneity of malignant tumors. Pathol Pract Res 183:
    693–697
Donhuijsen K, Kroll M, Krause U (1986) MFH: prognostische Bedeutung der histologischen
    Befunde. DMW 111: 46–51
Donhuijsen K, Schmidt U, Metz K, Leder L (1987) MFH: hotch-potch or entity? Blut 55: 365
Donhuijsen K, Metz K, Leder L (1988) Desmin- und S-100-protein positive MFH. Pathologe 9:
    261–267
Du Bonley (1982) Demonstration of alpha-1-antitrypsin and alpha-1-antichymotrypsin in
    fibrous histiocytomas using immunoperoxidase technique. Am J Surg Pathol 6: 559–564
Ekfors T, Rantakokko V (1978) An analysis of 38 MFH in the extremities. Acta Pathol Scand
    [A] 86: 25–35
Enjoji M, Hashimoto H, Tsuneyoshi M, Iwasaki H (1980) MFH: a clinicopathologic study of
    130 cases. Acta Pathol Jpn 30(5): 727–741
Enzinger F (1969) Histological typing of soft tissue tumors. WHO, Geneva
Enzinger F (1979) Angiomatoid malignant fibrous histiocytoma. Cancer 44: 2147–2157
Enzinger F (1986) MFH 20 years after Stout. Am J Surg Pathol 10: 43–53
Enzinger F, Weiss S (1988) soft tissue tumors, 2nd edn. Mosby, St Louis
Evans H (1979) Liposarcoma: a study of 55 cases with reassessment ofits classification. Am J
    Surg Pathol 3: 507–523
Fletcher C (1982) Pleomorphic MFH: fact or fiction? Am J Surg Pathol 16: 213–228
Fu Y, Gabbiani G, Kay G, Lattes R (1975) Malignant soft tissue tumors of probable histiocytic
    origin (MFH). Cancer 35: 176–198
Genberg M, Mark J, Hakelius L et al. (1989) Origin and relationship between different cell
    types in MFH. Am J Pathol 135: 1185–1196
Guccion J, Enzinger F (1972) Malignant giant cell tumor of soft parts. Cancer 29: 1518–1529
Hajdu S (1979) Pathology of soft tissue tumors. Lea and Febiger, Philadelphia
Hardy T, An T, Brown P, Tertz J (1980) Postirradiation sarcoma (MFH) of axilla. Cancer 42:
    118–124
Harris S (1979) The ultrastructure of benign and malignant fibrous histiocytoma. Histo-
    pathology 4: 29–44
Hashimoto H, Daimuru Y, Tsuneyoshi M, Enjoji M (1990) Soft tissue sarcomas with additional
    anaplastic components. Cancer 66: 1578–1586
Hecht F, Berger C, Hecht B, Speiser B (1983) Fibrous histiocytoma stem line. Cancer Genet
    Cytogenet 8: 359–362
Heppner (1989) Tumor cell societies. J Natl Cancer Inst 81: 648–649
Hirose T, Kudo E, Hasegawa T, Abe J, Hizawa K (1989) Expression of intermediate filaments
    in MFH. Hum Pathol 20: 871–877
Hoffman M, Dickersin G (1983) MFH. An ultrastructural study of eleven cases. Hum Pathol
    14: 913–922
Howard J (1979) The origin and immunological significance of Kupffer cells. In: Furth R (ed)
    Mononuclear phagocytes. Blackwell, Oxford
Iwasaki H, Isayam T, Johzaki K, Kikuchi M (1987) MFH. Evidence of perivascular mesen-
    chymal cell origin. Am J Pathol 128: 528–537
Iwasaki H, Isayama T, Ohjimi Y et al. (1991) MFH. A tumor of facultative histiocytes showing
    mesenchymal diferentiation in cultured cells. Cancer 69: 4337–4447
Iwasaki H, Yoshitake K, Ohjimi Y et al. (1992) MFH: proliferative compartment and hetero-
    geneity of "histiocytic" cells. Am J Surg Pathol 16: 735–745

Kahn L (1973) Retroperitoneal xanthogranuloma and xanthosarcoma (malignant fibrous xanthoma). Cancer 14: 411–422

Katenkamp D (1988) Cellular heterogeneity. Explanation for changing of tumor phenotype and biological behaviour. Pathol Res Pract 183: 698–705

Katenkamp D, Neupert G (1982) Experimental tumors with features of MFH. Exp Pathol 22: 11–27

Katenkamp D, Raikhlin (1985) Stem cell concept and heterogeneity of malignant soft tissue tumors. Exp Pathol 28: 3–11

Kauffmann F, Stout A (1961) Histiocytic tumors (fibrous xanthoma and histiocytoma) in children. Cancer 14: 496–482

Kay S (1978) Inflammatory fibrous histiocytoma (xanthogranuloma). Am J Surg Pathol 2: 313–319

Kearny M, Soule E (1980) MFH. A retrospective study of 167 cases. Cancer 45: 167–178

Kindblom L, Jacobsen G, Jacobsen M (1982) Immunohistochemical investigations of tumors of supposed fibrohistiocytic origin. Hum Pathol 13: 834

Koback M, Perlow S (1949) Xanthomatous giant cell tumor arising in soft tissues. Arch Surg 59: 909–916

Kosmehl H, Langbein L, Katenkamp D (1990) Experimental rhabdomyosarcoma with regions like malignant fibrous histiocytoma (MFH). J Pathol 160: 135–140

Kretzschmar H (1984) Quantitative immunohistochemische Untersuchungen zur Histogenese der malignen fibrösen Histiocytome. Dissertation, Munich

Kyriakos M, Kempson R (1976) Inflammatory fibrous histiocytoma. Cancer 37: 1584–1606

Lagace R, Delage C, Seemayer T (1979) Myxoid variant of MFH: ultrastructural observations. Cancer 43: 526–534

Lanham G, Weiss S, Enzinger F (1989) Malignant lymphoma. A study of 75 cases presenting in soft tissue. Am J Surg Pathol 13: 1–10

Lattes R (1982a) MFH. A review article. Am J Surg Pathol 6: 761–772

Lattes R (1982b) Tumors of soft tissue. Fasc 1, ser 2, revised. AFIP, Washington

Lee Y, Pho R, Nather A (1984) MFH at site of metal implant. Cancer 54: 2286–2289

Leu H, Makek M (1986) Angiomatoid MFH. Arch Pathol Lab Med 110: 467

Limacher J, Delage C, Lagace R (1978) MFH: clinicopathologic and ultrastructural study of 12 cases. Am J Surg Pathol 2: 265–274

Llombart-Bosch A, Carda C, Boix J, Pellin A, Peydro-Olaya A (1988) Value of nude mice xenografts in the expression of cell heterogeneity of human sarcomas of bone and soft tissue. Pathol Res Pract 183: 683–692

Mandahl N, Heim S, Kristofferson U et al. (1985) Telomeric association in a MFH. Hum Genet 71: 321–324

Mandahl N, Heim S, Willen H et al. (1989) Characteristic anomalies identify subtypes of MFH. Genes Chrom Cancer 1: 9–14

Maximov A (1927) Bindegewebe und blutbildendes Gewebe. In: Von Möllendorff W (ed) Handbuch der mikroskopischen Anatomie, vol II. Springer, Berlin

Meis J, Enzinger F (1991) Inflammatory fibrosarcoma of the mesentery andretroperitoneum. Am J Surg Pathol 15: 1146–1156

Meister P (1984) Tumoren und tumorförmige Veränderungen des Weichgewebes. In: Aufdermaur M, Baur E, Fassbender HG et al. (eds) Pathologie der Gelenke und weilteichtumoren. Springer, Berlin Heidelberg New York (Spezielle pathologische Anatomie, vol 18/2)

Meister P (1988) Malignant fibrous histiocytoma. History, histology, histogenesis. Pathol Res Pract 183: 1–7

Meister P (1992) Malignant lymphomas of soft tissues. Verh Dtsch Ges Pathol 76: 140–145

Meister P, Nathrath W (1980) Immunohistochemical markers of histiocytic tumors. Hum Pathol 11: 300–301

Meister P, Höhne M, Konrad E, Eder M (1979) Fibrous histiocytoma: an analysis of storiform patter. Virchows Arch [A] 383: 31–41

Meister P, Konrad E, Nathrath W, Eder M (1980a) MFH: histological patterns and cell types. Pathol Res Pract 168: 193–212

Meister P, Wünsch P, Konrad E, Kirchner T (1980b) Tumoren und tumorförmige Veränderungen des Weichgewebes. Pathologe 2: 19–30

Merck C, Angervall L, Kindblom S, Oden A (1983) Myxofibrosarcoma: a malignant soft tissue tumor of fibrohistiocystic origin. Acta Pathol Scand [A] 282[Suppl:]91

Merino M, LiVolsi V (1980) Inflammatory MFH. Am J Clin Pathol 73: 276–281

Merkow L, Frich J, Sliekin M et al. (1971) Ultrastructure of fibroxanthosarcoma (malignant fibroxanthoma). Cancer 28: 372–383

Miettinen M, Soini Y (1989) MFH. Heterogenous patterns of intermediate filament proteins by immunohistochemistry. Arch Pathol Lab Med 113: 1363–1366

Miller R, Kreutner A, Kurtz S (1980) Malignant inflammatory histiocytoma (inflammatory fibrous histiocytoma). Cancer 45: 179–187

Molenaar W, DeJong B, Buist J et al. (1989) Chromosomal analysis and classification of soft tissue sarcomas. Lab Invest 60: 266–274

Moll R, Lee I, Gould V et al. (1987) Immunohistochemical analysis of Ewing's tumors. Am J Pathol 127: 288–304

Nathrath W, Meister P (1982) Lysozyme (muramidase) and alpha-1-antichymotrypsin as immunohistochemical tumor markers. Acta Histochem 71[Suppl 25]: 69–72

Nöthen F (1920) Ein Fall von Fibroxanthosarkom. Frankf Z Pathol 23: 471

Oberling C (1935) Retroperitoneal xanthogranuloma. Am J Cancer 23: 477

O'Brian, Stout A (1964) Malignant fibrous xanthoma. Cancer 17: 1445–1458

Ozello L, Stout A, Murray M (1963) Cultural characteristic of malignant histiocytomas and fibrous xanthomas. Cancer 16: 331

Reddick R, Michelitch H, Triche T (1979) Malignant soft tissue tumors (MFH, pleomorphic liposarcoma, and pleomorph rhabdomyosarcoma): an electron microscopic study. Hum Pathol 10: 327–343

Rogues A, Horton L, Leslie J, Buxton-Thomas M (1979) Inflammatory fibrous histiocytoma in the left upper abdomen with leukemoid blood picture. Cancer 43: 1800–1804

Roholl P, Kleijne J, van Basten C et al. (1985a) A study to analyse the origin of tumor cells in MFH. Cancer 56: 2809–2815

Roholl P, Kleijne J, van Unnik J (1985b) Characterisation of tumor cells in MFH, in comparison with malignant histiocytes. Am J Pathol 121: 269–274

Russell W, Cohen J, Enzinger F et al. (1977) A clinical and pathological staging system for soft tissue sarcomas. Cancer 40: 1562–1570

Rydholm A, Syk I (1986) MFH of soft tissue. Correlation between clinical variables and histologic malignancy grade. Cancer 57: 2323–2324

Smith M, Costa M, Weiss S (1991) Evaluation of CD68 and other histiocytic antigens in angiomatoid malignant fibrous histiocytoma. Am J Surg Pathol 15: 757–763

Soule E, Enriquez P (1979) Atypical fibrous histiocytoma, malignant fibrous histiocytoma, malignant histiocytoma and epitheloid sarcoma. Cancer 30: 128–143

Stout A, Murray M (1942) Hemangiopericytoma. A vascular tumor featuring Zimmermann's pericytes. Ann Surg 116: 26

Stout A, Lattes R (1967) Tumors of soft tissue. Fasc 1, ser 2. AFIP, Washington

Strauchen J, Dimitriu-Bona A (1986) MFH: expression of monocyte/macrophage differentiation antigens detected with monoclonal antibodies. Am J Pathol 124: 303–309

Taxy J, Battifora H (1977) MFH: a clinicopathologic and ultrastructural study. Cancer 40: 254–267

Ten Seldam R, Helwig E (1974) Histological typing of skin tumors. WHO, Geneva

Tsuneyoshi M, Enjoji M, Shinchara N (1981) MFH. An electromicroscopic study of 17 cases. Virchows Arch [A] 394: 135–145

Tsuneyoshi M, Hashimoto H, Enjoji M (1983) Myxoid MFH versus myxoid liposarcoma. Virchows Arch [A] 400: 187–199

Tsuneyoshi M, Daimuru Y, Enjoji M (1984) Malignant hemangiopericytoma and other sarcomas with hemangiopericytomalike pattern. Pathol Res Pract 178: 446–453

Van Unnik J, Coindre J, Contesso G et al. (1987) Grading of soft tissue sarcoma. In: Ryan JR, Baker LO (eds) Recent concepts in sarcoma treatment. Kluwer, Utrecht

Vilanova J, Burgos-Bretones J, Simon R, Rivera-Pomar J (1980) Leukaemoid reaction an eosinophilia in inflammatory fibrous histiocytoma. Virchows Arch [A] 388: 237–243

Wegmann W, Heitz P (1985) Angiomatoid malignant fibrous histiocytoma. Virchows Arch [A] 406: 59–66

Weiss S (1982) MFH. A reaffirmation. Am J Surg Pathol 6: 773–784

Weiss S (1993) Histological typing of soft tissue tumors. Springer, Berlin Heidelberg New York

Weiss S, Enzinger F (1977) Myxoid variant of MFH. Cancer 39: 1672–1685

Weiss S, Enzinger F (1978) MFH: an analysis of 200 cases. Cancer 41: 2250–2266

Weiss S, Bratthauer G, Morris P (1988) Postirradiation MFH expressing cytoceratin. Am J
    Surg Pathol 12: 534–558
Wick M, Siegel G, Mills S et al. (1987) Dedifferentiated chondrosarcoma of bone. Virchows
    Arch [A] 441: 23–32
Wisse E, Knook D (1977) Kupffer cells and other liver sinusoidal cells. Elsevier, Amsterdam
Wood G, Beckstead J, Turner R et al. (1986) MFH tumor cell resemble fibroblasts. Am J Surg
    Pathol 10: 323–335
Wünsch P, Dubrauszky V (1987) MFH. Klinische Pathologie, Immunhistologie und Enzymhis-
    tochemie. Verh Dtsch Ges Pathol 71: 349
Zeher R, Bauer T, Marks K, Weltevreden A (1990) Ki-67 and grading of MFH. Cancer 66:
    1984–1990

Recent Advances in Tumors of Adipose Tissue

P.W. ALLEN

1 Introduction

The introduction of the modern organ imaging techniques, magnetic resonance imaging (MRI) and computerized tomography (CT), has been the most important recent practical advance in the diagnosis and management of soft tissue tumors. In my experience, fine needle aspiration cytology investigation of soft tissue tumors presently results in an unacceptably high level of false-negative results. In my opinion, it should only be performed as a research procedure, and then only in tandem with the safer and more reliable core biopsy handled by urgent processing and paraffin sectioning of the tissue core. A false-negative report based on the interpretation of an aspiration cytology smear by a cytopathologist inexperienced in the aspiration cytology of an uncommon or rare soft tissue tumor, as is usually the case, may not only delay treatment but may even precipitate litigation.

At The Queen Elizabeth Hospital, deep soft tissue tumors are investigated by MRI and CT scanning. After the radiology has been jointly reviewed by both the radiologist and the surgeon, a fine needle core biopsy is performed under X-ray guidance by an experienced radiologist with a high positive "strike" rate. The biopsy site is placed so that the tract can be excised en bloc with the tumor if the histology is malignant. Additional core needle biopsy material can be taken for cytogenetics and electron

Current Topics in Pathology
Volume 89, Eds. D. Harms/D. Schmidt
© Springer-Verlag Berlin Heidelberg 1995

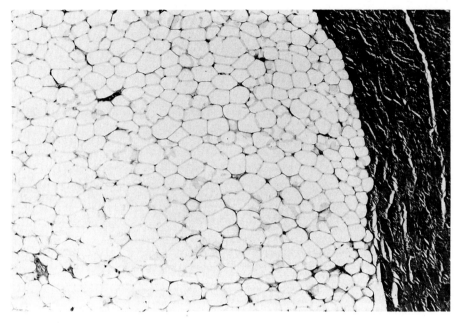

Fig. 1. Madelung's disease (benign symmetric lipomatosis). Histologically bland mature adipose tissue lies adjacent to voluntary muscle fibers. A large unencapsulated mass of adipose tissue which extended from the base of the skull to the infraclavicular region was excised from a 68-year-old man for "cosmetic reasons." A diagnosis of well-differentiated liposarcoma was considered because of the massive size of the "tumor," which had been present for 10 years. The patient was a heavy drinker. Case referred by Dr. P. Storey, Brisbane, Australia

microscopy after a 1–2-cm core of macroscopically abnormal and viable tissue has been obtained for light microscopy. The biopsy histology result and all the clinical and imaging findings are discussed by the pathologist, radiologist and surgeon, and this consultation across the specialties usually results in a diagnosis that is sufficiently accurate to plan treatment. However, such detailed consultation is not a universally accepted practice, as the following recently referred case demonstrates.

A large fatty tumor measuring $20 \times 10 \times 5$ cm was excised from the neck of a male aged 60. The written clinical information accompanying the specimen indicated that the tumor had been present for 10 years and had been removed "mainly for cosmetic reasons". At operation, the tumor extended between the muscles of the neck and was so extensive that only one third could be removed. Histologically, totally mature fat was associated with a few voluntary muscle fibres which were scattered around the edges of some of the sections (Fig. 1). The large size suggested a diagnosis of liposarcoma so the pathologist advised organ imaging to ascertain the extent of the lesion and the tissue planes involved. He was promptly provided with a CT scan report dated 1 month earlier which described adipose tissue infiltrating virtually all the tissues of the neck from the base of the skull down to the infraclavicular region and also into the larynx. The radiologist had already made a diagnosis of benign symmetric lipomatosis (Madelung's disease) (REQUENA et al. 1992). Further inquiries revealed that the patient had been a heavy drinker for years. It is not clear whether the surgeon was aware of the CT scan results before the operation or whether he was familiar with Madelung's disease, but it is likely that a histological diagnosis of well-differentiated liposarcoma would have been made if the pathologist had not asked to see the CT report.

With the advent of MRI and CT scans, organ imaging has become as important in the diagnosis and treatment of deep soft tissue tumors as the plain X-Ray is for bone tumors. This case is an instructive example of the role of these investigations and the necessity for good communications between pathologist, surgeon and radiologist. It also draws attention to the lipomatoses, a poorly defined group of non-neoplastic lipomatous proliferations which includes Madelung's disease as well as the recently recognised Proteus syndrome.

2 Proteus Syndrome

This rare sporadic disease, which has its onset in early childhood, has been popularized by the recent motion picture "The Elephant Man." That case was originally thought to have been a variant of neurofibromatosis but is now regarded as one of the first accounts of Proteus syndrome (TIBBLES and COHEN 1986; COHEN 1988). The syndrome is characterized by multifocal skin and mesenchymal overgrowths involving almost any part of the musculo-skeletal system. Affected patients exhibit varying degrees of limb enlargement; macrocephaly with cranial exostoses; macrodactyly; deformities of the interphalangeal and metatarsal joints with peri-articular calcification, spurs and bony ankylosis; deeply rugose or cerebroid thickening of palms and soles; diffuse subcutaneous adipose and fibrous masses and linear skin lesions. About 60 cases have been described (SAMLASKA et al. 1989; LACOMBE et al. 1991; NAZARRO et al. 1991; BARMAKIAN et al. 1992; STRICKER 1992). The name is derived from the Greek god Proteus, who disguised himself by changing his shape. Skin and soft tissue lesions, which are usually apparent at birth, increase in size as the child develops and may assume tremendous proportions. Despite their grotesque appearance, patients are usually of normal intellect and usually have a normal life expectancy. In addition to neurofibromatosis, the disease has been confused with macrodystrophia lipomatosa (ALLEN 1981) and the fibromatoses, particularly those affecting the hands and the feet. Histologically, there is a diffuse proliferation of histologically bland fibro-fatty tissue.

Clinicians and pathologists should be aware of this condition when evaluating cases of macrodactyly. As Proteus syndrome may be manifest in many different forms, it is conceivable that some cases of isolated macro-dactyly and even lipomatous hamartoma of nerve may be formes frustes of Proteus syndrome. DESAI and STEINER (1990) included one case of Proteus syndrome amongst ten cases of macrodactyly, five of which had nerve involvement. Resolution of that possibility awaits the development of a specific diagnostic test for Proteus syndrome. HAPPLE (1987) has suggested that Proteus syndrome may result from a somatic mutation which is lethal in the non-mosaic state, an explanation which is supported by SCHWARTZ et al. (1991).

3 Bannayan-Zonana Syndrome

Synonyms include Bannayan syndrome; Riley-Smith-Rulvalcaba-Myhre syndrome; encephalocranio-cutaneus lipomatosis; familial macrocephaly syndrome; lipomatosis, angiomatosis and macrencephalia; and familial macrocephaly with mesodermal hamartomas. Bannayan originally described a single autopsy case of a 3-year-old child. The patient never regained full consciousness after an operation for removal of rapidly growing fatty tumors (BANNAYAN 1971). Other examples of similar conditions, which are now accepted as being the same disease (COHEN 1990; DILIBERTI 1992), have been published under a number of different names, most of which are listed as synonyms above. The presently recognized manifestations of the syndrome include symmetrical macrocephaly without ventricular enlargement; spinal canal enlargement; mild neurological dysfunction and post-natal growth deceleration; discrete, indolent, subcutaneous lipomas and hemangiomas; solitary or multiple, large, aggressively growing, infiltrating, fatty and vascular tumors in deep locations including bone (MILES et al. 1984; ALFONSO et al. 1986). Other minor features include down-slanting palpebral fissures; high palate; joint hyperextensibility; pectus excavatum; strabismus or amblyopia and prolonged drooling. Speech and motor delays are observed in all children but are usually well compensated by adulthood. There may be mild mental retardation (SAUL et al. 1982) and seizures, some of which are related to intracerebral hemorrhage from angiomas (MILES et al. 1984). Affected individuals may develop intracranial tumors (HIGGINBOTTOM and SCHULTZ 1982). When death occurs, it is usually the result of aggressively growing vascular or fatty tumors (OKUMURA et al. 1986; HAYASHI et al. 1992). The syndrome is inherited as an autosomal dominant with a male predominance (MILES et al. 1984) although the degree of expression in individuals varies (KLEIN and BARR 1990). It is not certain whether the basic defect is due to genetic heterogeneity or an autosomal dominant locus with at least two different allelic forms (MORETTI-FERREIRA et al. 1989). There is one report of an affected patient with a 16Y translocation (ISRAEL et al. 1991).

While most of the clinical features in each case are similar, a few patients exhibit combined features of Bannayan-Zonana and Proteus syndrome (BIALER et al. 1988), suggesting that the two disorders may represent distinct entities with overlapping manifestations (McCALL et al. 1992) or, alternatively, part of a phenotypic continuum shared by Proteus syndrome, Bannayan-Zonana syndrome and epidermal nevus syndrome. Some of the manifestations may be caused by a somatic mutation leading to variable patterns of mosaicism (EL SHANTI et al. 1992).

4 Lipomatous Hamartoma of Nerve

Benign fatty tumors of peripheral nerves can be subdivided into lumbosacral lipomas (KOMIYAMA et al. 1987; HIRSCH and PIERRE-KAHN 1988; TAVIERE et al. 1989), extraneural lipomas compressing a nerve, encapsulated intraneural lipomas (CHIAO et al. 1987), involvement of nerves by a lipomatosis (RAWLINGS et al. 1986; DE ROSA et al. 1987), and lipomatous hamartoma of nerve. Synonyms of lipomatous hamartoma include neural fibrolipoma, lipofibromatous hamartoma, fibrolipomatous hamartoma, neurolipomatosis, fibrolipoma of the median nerve, intraneural lipoma, fibro-fatty proliferation of the median nerve, fatty infiltration of the median nerve, and ossifying lipofibroma. This rare condition was apparently first mentioned by MASON (1953). Since then there have been a number of other papers (PALETTA and RYBKA 1972; LOUIS and DICK 1973; PALETTA and SENAY 1981; LOUIS et al. 1985; AYMARD et al. 1987; LANGA et al. 1987; AMADIO et al. 1988; HOUPT et al. 1989; OSTER et al. 1989; FEYERABEND et al. 1990; WALKER et al. 1991). The largest series consists of 26 cases from the Armed Forces Institute of Pathology (SILVERMAN and ENZINGER 1985). Seven of their 26 patients had an associated macrodactyly, most tumors were located in the hand in the territory of the median and occasionally, the ulnar nerve. Others have reported involvement of the ulnar nerve at the elbow (GOULDESBROUGH and KINNY 1989) and of the superficial branch of the radial nerve (JACOB and BUCHINO 1989). In cases without macrodactyly, lipomatous hamartoma of nerve usually affects the median nerve and rarely involves the radial or ulnar nerves. Nerves outside the arm do not seem to have been affected.

Half the lesions have been congenital or noted before the age of 2 (JOHNSON and BONFIGLIO 1969), and two thirds have come to medical attention in the second or third decade (SILVERMAN and ENZINGER 1985). Initial reviews suggested an equal sex incidence (ALLEN 1981) but the sex ratio in SILVERMAN and ENZINGER'S series was 12 males to seven females. Symptoms include a slowly enlarging soft tissue mass which may be associated with pain, paresthesiae, heaviness of the hand and varying degrees of motor and sensory dysfunction, including the carpal tunnel syndrome. The duration of history is usually longer than 2 years.

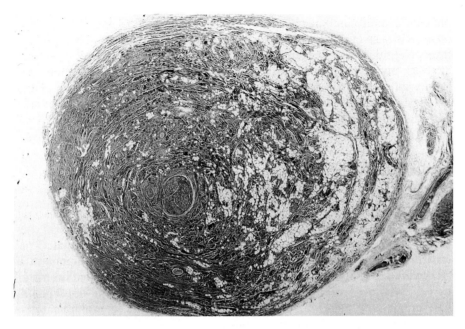

Fig. 2. Lipomatous hamartoma of nerve. Fibro-fatty tissue is expanding the area between the epineurium and the perineurium. Case referred by Dr. R. Sterling, Adelaide, Australia

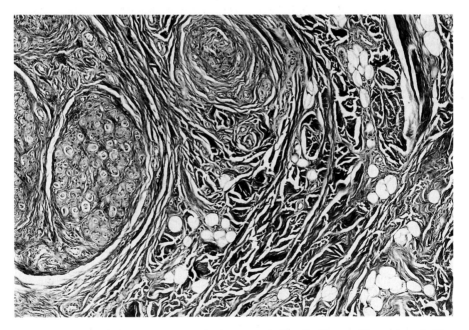

Fig. 3. Lipomatous hamartoma of nerve (same case as in Fig. 2). There is fibrous tissue inside the perineurium surrounding degenerating nerve fibers. Fat and fibrous tissue can be seen outside the perineurium

The affected nerve segment usually measures 3 or 4 cm in length but the process may extend from the distal end of a digital nerve up to within 4 or 5 cm of the elbow joint. Involved nerves have a well-encapsulated, worm or sausage-like appearance and do not adhere to the surrounding tissues, being confined by the epineurium.

Histologically, fibro-fatty tissue, small blood vessels and sometimes calcium and bone are found inside the epineurium but outside the perineurium (Figs. 2 and 3). The ratio of fibrous to fatty tissue varies from case to case and within different areas in the same tumor. Inside the perineurium, there is fibrous tissue proliferation, sometimes with interstitial myxoid change, and atrophy of the nerve fibres. Adipose tissue, calcium and bone apparently do not occur inside the perineural sheath.

SILVERMAN and ENZINGER regarded cases without macrodactyly to be essentially the same as those with enlargement of the fingers and intimated that the condition formerly known as macrodystrophia lipomatosa (fibro-fatty enlargement of the median nerve associated with bone overgrowth) was the same as lipomatous hamartoma with macrodactyly. They were unable to find any histological differences between their two groups, but it is not clear whether the fibro-fatty proliferation in those cases with macrodactyly was entirely within the perineurium or whether it also extended out extensively into the surrounding tissues. In one case at least, it appears that surrounding soft tissues were invaded.

Macrodactyly (KALEN et al. 1988; DESAI and STEINER 1990) has many causes including Maffucci's syndrome, Ollier's dyschondroplasia, neurofibromatosis, Klippell-Trenaunay-Weber syndrome, hemangiomatosis, lymphangiomatosis, arteriovenous fistulae, dysplasia epiphysialis hemimelica, melorheostosis, and Proteus syndrome (SAMLASKA et al. 1989). Some of these diseases are associated with adipose hyperplasia which may surround nerves, particularly in histological sections. BARSKY (1967) noted that some forms of macrodactyly are associated with overgrowth of the fatty tissues of the palm.

The prognosis of treated lipomatous hamartoma of nerve is excellent but there is some morbidity. SILVERMAN and ENZINGER obtained follow-up information from 12 patients treated by partial or complete excision. In two, sensory or motor changes remained. One had persistence and enlargement of the lesion without residual neurological findings. One patient with the carpal tunnel syndrome underwent carpal tunnel release with partial excision of the mass and experienced no further difficulty. In the eight patients without neurological symptoms for whom follow-up was available, four had no further difficulty and one had a persistent mass. In three patients the mass recurred repeatedly and in one, the recurrent mass was associated with sensory changes.

Paletta suggested that radical surgical excision in adults should only be performed in conjunction with nerve grafting (PALETTA and RYBKA 1972; PALETTA and SENAY 1981). Louis recommends that initial surgery should consist of biopsy and alleviation of any compression neuropathy. He believes that the role of microsurgical debulking procedures remains unclear (Louis and Dick 1973; Louis et al. 1985). Houpt et al. (1989) agree that in most cases, decompression of the nerve will suffice; resection by means of interfascicular dissection is rarely justified because of permanent loss of sensibility and motor function.

5 Cellular Subcutaneous Angiolipoma

Subcutaneous angiolipoma, the second most common type of fatty tumor seen by surgical pathologists, may be painful, multiple and familial, affects men more often than women, tends to occur on the extremities, and is rarely larger than 5 cm. In patients with multiple lesions, it is common to find that the ratio of small blood vessels to mature fat varies from lesion to lesion, and in some there may be virtually no vessels at all. The existence of the reverse situation, in which the fat is overwhelmed by large numbers of small blood vessels was not widely recognized and apparently did not cause practical difficulties until the AIDS epidemic. Some cellular angiolipomas,

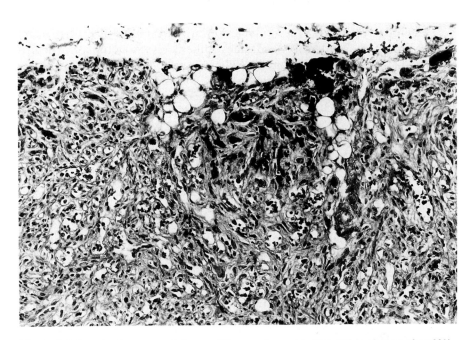

Fig. 4. Cellular subcutaneous angiolipoma. The vascular component makes up more than 90% of the tumor. There is a small amount of adipose tissue just under the capsule and fibrin thrombi are prominent inside some of the vessels. Case referred by Dr. C.P. Mason, Christchurch, New Zealand

particularly in young men with multiple lesions, have recently been confused with Kaposi's sarcoma. HUNT et al. (1990) have described three cellular angiolipomas in which the vascular component comprised more than 95% of each lesion (Fig. 4).

The differential diagnoses include spindle cell lipoma, Kaposi's sarcoma and spindle cell hemangioendothelioma. The most important features of cellular subcutaneous angiolipoma are the encapsulation, intravascular fibrin thrombi, septation, association with other more typical angiolipomas and occurrence in healthy individuals.

6 Periosteal and Parosteal Lipoma (Osteochondrolipoma of Soft Tissue)

Fatty tumors containing cartilage or bone have been described in the breast (LUGO et al. 1982; MARSH et al. 1989; METCALF and ELLIS 1985), the lung (pulmonary hamartoma or chondrolipoma), in pleomorphic adenomas of the salivary glands, in lipomatous hypertrophy of the median nerve and in osteochondrolipomas of soft tissues. There are two recent reviews of this last uncommon group of tumors (KATZER 1989; MILLER et al. 1992). On the basis of KATZER's four cases, it seems that cartilage or bone, often with hematopoietic marrow, may very rarely be found in subcutaneous lipomas but, in my experience, most benign chondrolipomatous tumors of soft tissue are located adjacent to bone. Conversely, the finding of bone or cartilage is common in periosteal and parosteal lipomas although the chondro and osseous components are not mentioned in the name. This has resulted in two separate bodies of literature about periosteal and parosteal lipomas on the one hand and chondrolipomas on the other, but they are both the same entity (ALLEN 1989). Periosteal tumors lie immediately beneath the periosteum while parosteal lipomas are situated in the soft tissues adjacent to the periosteum. MILLER et al. (1992) have analysed 14 cases from the files of the Armed Forces Institute of Pathology and reviewed the literature.

Periosteal and parosteal lipomas are found most frequently around the diaphysis of long bones, are larger than most lipomas and usually affect middle-aged patients. MILLER et al. suggested that periosteal lipomas start to grow beneath the periosteum and in time develop osseous and chondroid tissue from elements in the adjacent bone (Fig. 5). The metaplastic tissues continue to grow and may form a sessile attachment to the underlying bone. In other cases the tumor loses its bony attachment, resulting in a parosteal fatty tumor with multiple included islands of bone and cartilage (MILLER et al. 1992). Some parosteal tumors, particularly those in the forearm, may compress nerves and cause paresis of distal muscles. It seems likely that the tumor described as chondro-lipoangioma (MILCHGRUB et al. 1990) was a parosteal lipoma (osteochondrolipoma) with prominent blood vessels.

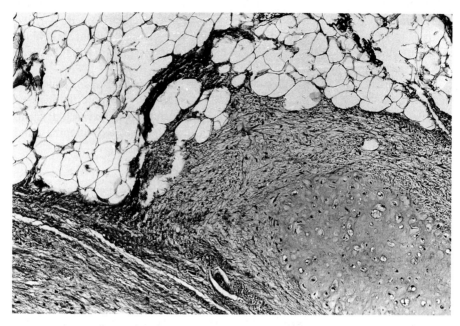

Fig. 5. Periosteal lipoma (osteochrondrolipoma of soft tissue). This tumor was loosely attached to the periosteum of the scapula. There is mature fibrous and fatty tissue and a group of mildly atypical cartilage cells. Bone was present elsewhere. This benign tumor should not be mis-diagnosed as a liposarcoma with chondroid metaplasia. Case referred by Dr. R. Pozzuoli, Faenza, Italy

Osteochondrolipomas have been called "mesenchymomas" or "hamar-tomas" because of their mixed mesenchymal differentiation. I personally prefer to avoid both terms because their promiscuous application to many unrelated mesenchymal tumors has resulted in clinicopathological impre-cision. Periosteal, parosteal and juxtacortical osteochondrolipomas do not recur locally (MILCHGRUB et at. 1990). There may be occasional binu-cleate cells in the chondroid component but the lack of cellular atypia in the adipose and fibrous areas distinguishes chondrolipoma from well-differentiated liposarcoma with osseous and cartilaginous metaplasia.

7 Myolipoma of Soft Tissue

Adipose metaplasia in smooth muscle tumors of the uterus (lipoleiomyoma) is comparatively common and has been recognized for many years as a change occurring in various kinds of Mullerian smooth muscle tumors (BRESCIA et al. 1989). At least two histologically similar tumors arising near the uterus had been reported (NUOVO et al. 1990) before MEIS and ENZINGER's recent paper on soft tissue lipoleiomyomas (MEIS and ENZINGER

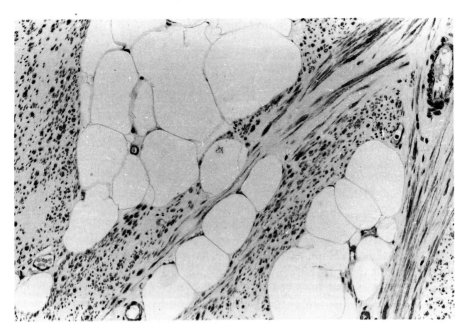

Fig. 6. Myolipoma of soft tissue which measured 15 × 3 × 6 cm and was located in the extra-peritoneal tissues near the umbilicus of a middle-aged female. Clinically it was thought to be a uterine fibroid. Mature fat and histologically bland smooth muscle bundles are present in approximately equal proportions. Desmin stain

1991). They described nine cases, mostly occurring in middle-aged females, usually in the abdomen in the same areas as parasitic fibroids are found. The three males in their series had lesions in the subcutis of the upper back, the fascia of the anterior abdominal wall and in the right inguinal canal. Most of the tumors were greater than 10 cm in size, consisted of approximately two thirds smooth muscle and one third of regularly interspersed adipose tissue (Fig. 6) which sometimes imparted a sieve-like appearance at low power. None of the tumors recurred.

I suspect that soft tissue myolipomas occurring in the pelvic or retro-peritoneal areas of women are related to uterine fibroids and could represent variants of so-called parasitic fibroids (ALLEN 1990). Although myolipomas are obviously different from chondrolipomas, they also have been called mesenchymomas, thus supporting my aversion to that imprecise and over-worked name. Myolipomas are sometimes confused with liposarcoma because of their large size but they exhibit no cellular or nuclear atypia. They are not related to well-differentiated liposarcomas with metaplastic smooth muscle (EVANS 1990).

8 Metastasizing Renal Angiomyolipoma

Angiomyolipomas usually arise in the kidney and, very occasionally, in the liver (NGUYEN and CATZAVELOS 1990; LINTON et al. 1991; WEEKS et al. 1991). Renal angiomyolipomas may have only an inconspicuous renal attachment with a massive retroperitoneal extension, which may be confused with liposarcoma (HRUBAN et al. 1989). Fewer than half are associated with tuberous sclerosis (BENDER and YUNIS 1982; TONG et al. 1990) and a very few are complicated by adenocarcinoma of the kidney, a combination which usually occurs in conjunction with tuberous sclerosis (LOWE et al. 1992). MUKAI et al. (1992) have recently described crystalloids in renal angiomyolipomas. Fine needle aspiration biopsy has been used diagnostically with some success (SANT et al. 1990) but should be unnecessary because of the diagnostic accuracy of modern CT scanning (TAKAYASU et al. 1987).

Renal angiomyolipomas may exhibit extreme pleomorphism and sometimes necrosis (Fig. 7), may invade vessels and even lymph nodes (BRECHER et al. 1986; WAISMAN 1987; RO et al. 1990; ANSARI et al. 1991), resulting in such misdiagnoses as renal cell carcinoma, liposarcoma or leiomyosarcoma of the kidney, but they virtually "never" metastasize. However, there have been two recent reports of unequivocal pulmonary metastases and death

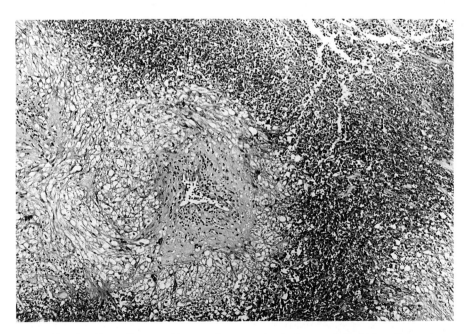

Fig. 7. Renal angiomyolipoma with extensive necrosis. A characteristic thick wall vessel associated with vacuolated smooth muscle cells lies adjacent to a large area of necrosis. Elsewhere, this tumor was histologically typical of a benign renal angiomyolipoma. Case referred by Dr. M. Wyche, Toowoomba, Australia

from bona fide metastasizing renal angiomyolipomas (FERRY et al. 1991; LOWE et al. 1992). Both papers review the one or two other previously reported possibly malignant cases. Most instances of supposed malignant transformation of angiomyolipomas merely reflect pathologists' misinterpretation of the histology rather than actual metastases and genuinely malignant behaviour. Renal angiomyolipoma is virtually "always" benign. Percutaneous transcatheter embolization has been employed therapeutically for benign angiomyolipomas (VAN BAAL et al. 1990).

9 Atypical Adipose Tumors and Liposarcomas

9.1 Definitions and General Considerations

There is still no general agreement on the definition, diagnostic criteria and classification of liposarcomas. In my experience, the signet ring and other "lipoblasts", which some have regarded as the essential diagnostic feature of liposarcoma (ORSON et al. 1987), are not specific enough to be used as the chief criterion. The statement that liposarcoma is the malignant tumor of lipoblasts (STOUT 1944) is generally true but is of minimal practical diagnostic value to surgical pathologists.

A reliable diagnosis of liposarcoma cannot always be made on histological grounds alone. Consideration must also be given to the tissue plane involved, the location and the patient's age. The tumor sometimes called well-differentiated lipoma-like liposarcoma (atypical lipoma) rarely recurs and virtually never metastasizes when located in the subcutis (EVANS et al. 1979; AZUMI et al. 1987; EVANS 1988). Histologically similar tumors located in voluntary muscle of the limbs frequently recur but probably do not metastasize before they have recurred repeatedly and undergone dedifferentiation (EVANS 1988). They rarely kill the patient. However, when seen in the retroperitoneum, the same histological picture indicates an 80%–90% death rate within 10 years (ALLEN 1981).

A liposarcoma is best defined as a tumor which differentiates as adipose tissue, frequently recurs locally, and metastasizes and kills in at least a small proportion of cases. On the other hand, a lipoma hardly ever recurs locally, does not metastasize and virtually never kills the patient.

9.2 Appearances and Unreliability of Lipoblasts

Lipoblasts can be recognized in an hematoxylin and eosin (H and E) stained section by the size and shape of their cytoplasmic lipid vacuoles, which usually indent the nuclei. Lipoblasts' nuclei are not always hyperchromatic

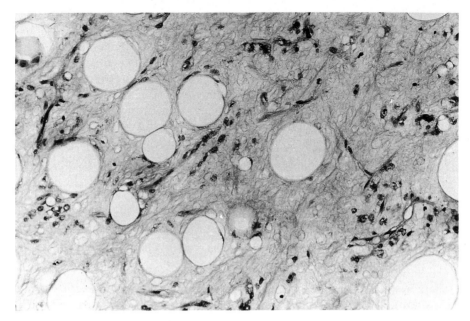

Fig. 8. Lipoblasts with round, clear vacuoles compressing nuclei in a myxoid liposarcoma which measured 13 × 6 × 3 cm from the peroneal compartment of the leg of a 39-year-old female. These genuine lipoblasts resemble the vacuolated fat cells in Figs. 10–13. This field is not particularly suggestive of myxoid liposarcoma although there is a suggestion of a plexiform capillary pattern on the right. Case referred by Dr. G. Hoffman, Perth, Australia

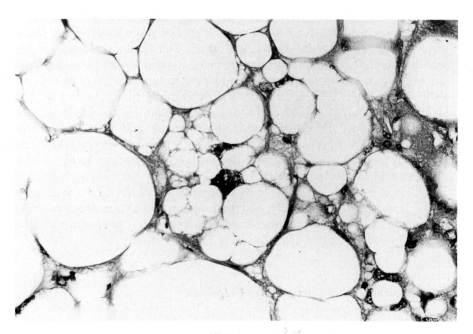

Fig. 9. Lipoblasts in a well-differentiated retroperitoneal liposarcoma from a 59-year-old man. There is a lipoblast with two atypical nuclei indented by multiple cytoplasmic lipid vacuoles in the centre of the field surrounded by histologically bland but biologically malignant adipose cells. The central cell is not much different from the multivacuolated cell in the lipoma illustrated in Fig. 13. Case referred by Dr. K. Mitchell, Perth, Australia

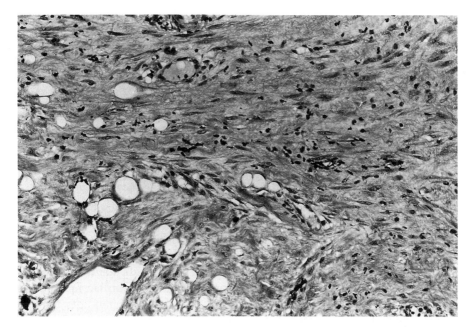

Fig. 10. Degenerating fat cells (pseudolipoblasts) in inflamed fat adjacent to the site of a previous excision biopsy of a breast carcinoma. The contracted, round, degenerating adipose cells resemble monovacuolated lipoblasts but they do not establish a diagnosis of liposarcoma

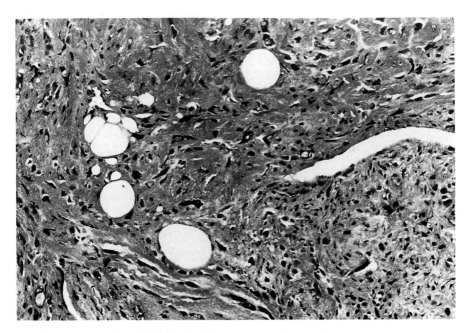

Fig. 11. Residual subcutaneous fat simulating lipoblasts. Section from the edge of a malignant fibrous histiocytoma. Contracted, residual subcutaneous fat cells resembling lipoblasts are surrounded by malignant fibrous histiocytoma tissue. Case referred by Dr. J. Cooper, Hong Kong

and atypical, particularly if they are compressed and indented, and they may be single or multiple. The vacuoles can be recognized as lipid in the same way as a normal fat cell is recognizable in an H and E section. The intracellular vacuoles are perfectly clear and transparent, there is not the slightest suggestion of intravacuolar mucin or other partially opaque non-lipid inclusions, the vacuoles are circular or oval in shape and their margins are sharply defined from the cytoplasm (Figs. 8 and 9). Fat stains are not necessary to prove the identity of mature fat cells in paraffin sections. The same principal applies to the identification of immature or otherwise ab-normal fat cells.

Cells closely resembling or indistinguishable from lipoblasts can be seen in degenerating fat in areas of inflammation or fat necrosis (Fig. 10); in residual, isolated, benign adipose tissue surrounded or infiltrated by a carcinoma or sarcoma (Fig. 11); in lipoblastoma and lipoblastomatosis; in subcutaneous pleomorphic lipomas (Fig. 12), in subcutaneous atypical lipomas, if one regards the last as separate from pleomorphic lipoma and spindle cell lipoma (Fig. 13). There are also a number of non-fatty tumors, both benign and malignant, which exhibit lipoblast-like cells (HUN et al. 1978; CHAN et al. 1986; LATTES and BIGOTTI 1991). Even if one proves that intracytoplasmic vacuoles consist of lipid, they are still not necessarily

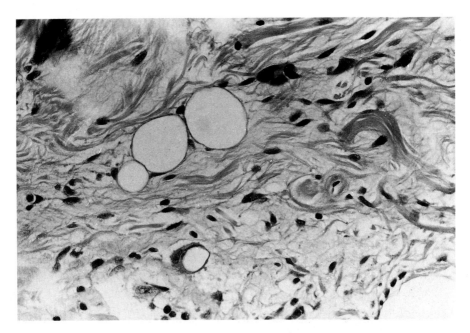

Fig. 12. Subcutaneous pleomorphic lipoma with a lipoblast. There are two floret cells, several twisted bands of dense collagen, three shrunken adipose cells and one cell with a single round lipid vacuole and a slightly atypical nucleus. This cell is indistinguishable from some forms of lipoblasts seen in liposarcomas. Case referred by Dr. R. Rowland, Adelaide, Australia

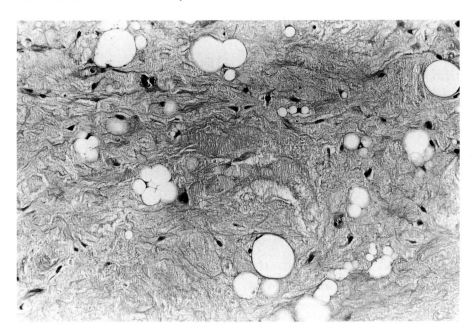

Fig. 13. Multivacuolated lipoblast in a benign subcutaneous tumor that otherwise resembled a spindle cell lipoma. Case referred by Dr. E. Slobedman, Adelaide, Australia

diagnostic of either neoplasia or of adipose differentiation. Hepatocellular carcinoma and adrenocortical carcinoma are two epithelial neoplasms which can produce lipid-rich cells indistinguishable from lipoblasts. Many of the foamy cells in malignant fibrous histiocytoma contain numerous, fine, intracytoplasmic lipid droplets. Convention alone dictates that such small lipid vacuoles in a tumor cell do not establish that it is a lipoblast. A rarely mentioned agreement almost of a gentlemanly nature, which is presently adhered to by most experienced surgical pathologists, decrees that adipose differentiation is indicated by large intracellular lipid droplets, in the order of 7-μm diameter, which usually indent the nucleus. Foamy macrophages are not lipoblasts.

Not only can lipoblast-like cells be seen in degenerating fat, benign fatty tumors and in carcinomas but lipoblasts may be absent in sections which are diagnostic of liposarcoma. Lipoblasts are not necessary to establish a diagnosis of either myxoid liposarcoma or sclerosing liposarcoma. Lipoblasts can nearly always be found in myxoid liposarcomas, provided that the biopsy is big enough, but it is possible to find areas which are free of lipoblasts in most myxoid liposarcomas (Fig. 14). This occasionally happens in small incisional or needle biopsies. In such cases, one can still make a firm diagnosis on the basis of a plexiform capillary pattern, mucinous pools, stellate and round stromal cells and a mucinous stroma, provided that well-

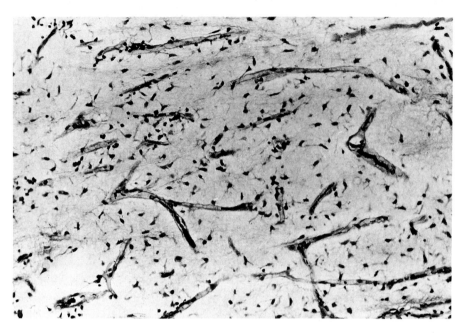

Fig. 14. Field of a myxoid liposarcoma with no lipoblasts. Despite the absence of lipoblasts and mucinous pools in this illustration, the characteristic plexiform capillaries and the moderately cellular background of stellate stromal cells should suggest myxoid liposarcoma and when taken in conjunction with a deep intramuscular location in a patient over the age of 10 years are virtually diagnostic. Lipoblasts were present elsewhere in this tumor. Case referred by Dr. R. Zito, Melbourne, Australia

interpreted organ imaging is available and one is aware of the patient's age and the tissue plane involved. Similarly, well-differentiated sclerosing liposarcoma may be bereft of recognizable lipoblasts so that, to the un-initiated, it resembles an atypical fibroblastic proliferation infiltrating apparently normal fat. A diagnosis of liposarcoma is made on the overall tumor pattern and on the tissue plane involved. Accordingly, the lipoblast cannot be regarded as the essential diagnostic criterion for liposarcoma in myxoid and sclerosing liposarcomas.

9.3 Classification of Liposarcomas

The most widely accepted classification of liposarcomas, as outlined in ENZINGER and WEISS' text book (1988) and confirmed by others (ORSON 1987; CHUNG 1990; CHUNG et al. 1991), implies that liposarcoma is one biological entity with four histological subtypes; (a) well-differentiated liposarcoma; (b) myxoid liposarcoma; (c) round cell liposarcoma; (d) pleomorphic liposarcoma. Well-differentiated liposarcoma is further sub-divided into lipoma-like, sclerosing, inflammatory and dedifferentiated liposarcoma. The classification of CHANG et al. (1989) is essentially the same as ENZINGER and WEISS' except for an additional subtype, fibroblastic liposarcoma, which probably corresponds to the dedifferentiated subtype of well-differentiated liposarcoma of ENZINGER and WEISS. These similar classifications have evolved from a number of large studies (ENTERLINE et al. 1960; ENZINGER and WINSLOW 1962; RESZEL et al. 1966; KINDBLOM et al. 1975; HASHIMOTO and ENJOJI 1982).

EVANS (1979) has stressed the histological and biological differences between myxoid liposarcoma and well-differentiated liposarcoma. The former occurs almost exclusively in muscle, mainly in the thigh, and is hardly ever located in the retroperitoneum, whereas well-differentiated liposarcoma frequently occurs in the retroperitoneum. EVANS excluded all subcutaneous and intramuscular tumors that histologically resembled well-differentiated liposarcoma from his series because he did not regard them as liposarcomas. He noted that dedifferentiation often occurred in well-differentiated liposarcoma. Dedifferentiation is a demonstrated or inferred histological change, usually occurring over a long period, from a well-differentiated to a less well-differentiated histological appearance. In well-differentiated liposarcoma, the dedifferentiated tissue usually resembles a malignant fibrous histiocytoma or fibrosarcoma. KINDBLOM et al. (1975) and HASHIMOTO and ENJOJI (1982) noted dedifferentiation in both myxoid and well-differentiated liposarcomas. Accordingly, pure myxoid lipo-sarcoma and pure well-differentiated liposarcoma should both be regarded as well-differentiated tumors. EVANS (1979) also proposed that round cell liposarcoma was merely a poorly differentiated cellular variant of myxoid liposarcoma. Only four of his 55 liposarcomas were pleomorphic lipo-sarcomas, all of them located in muscle.

The recent confirmation of the specific t(12:16) cytogenetic translocation in myxoid liposarcomas (PAULIEN et al. 1990; ENEROTH et al. 1990) adds additional support to the concept that myxoid liposarcoma is a biologically separate entity from well-differentiated lipoma-like or sclerosing lipo-sarcoma. Myxoid liposarcoma has a distinctive histological appearance characterized by large amounts of hyaluronidase-sensitive interstitial mucin often in "pools" or "lakes", a plexiform capillary pattern, stellate to round tumor cells and varying numbers of lipoblasts which are rarely bizarre or pleomorphic. Myxoid liposarcoma occurs almost exclusively in deep muscle groups, hardly ever involves the retroperitoneum, paratesticular region or larynx, has a local recurrence rate of approximately 50%, a metastasis rate of approximately 25%, a 5-year survival rate of approximately 70% and 10-year survival rate of approximately 50% (ALLEN 1981).

Myxoid change is not peculiar to myxoid liposarcoma. In fact, myxoid areas can nearly always be found in well-differentiated lipoma-like lipo-sarcomas, resulting in some being misdiagnosed as myxoid liposarcomas.

However, well-differentiated liposarcoma lacks the plexiform capillary pattern, mucinous pools and characteristic. stromal cells; is rather more fibroblastic; and tends to dedifferentiate as a fibrosarcoma or malignant fibrous histiocytoma rather than as a round cell tumor. Both myxoid liposarcoma and well-differentiated sarcoma may exhibit foci of chondroid and osseous metaplasia.

Thus myxoid liposarcoma stands apart from other fatty tumors whereas subcutaneous spindle cell lipoma (ENZINGER and HARVEY 1975; BEHAM et al. 1989; BOLEN and THORNING 1981; FLETCHER and MARTIN-BATES 1987; KITANO et al. 1979), subcutaneous pleomorphic lipoma (SHMOOKLER and ENZINGER 1981; BRYANT 1981; AZZOPARDI et al. 1983), subcutaneous atypical lipomas and atypical intramuscular fatty tumors (KINDBLOM et al. 1982; CUTRONA and GRECO 1981), well-differentiated retroperitoneal liposarcoma and dedifferentiating lipoma-like liposarcoma (EVANS et al. 1979) all share similar histological features and seem to be part of a continuous histological spectrum, with their behaviour being more dependent on the tissue plane involved than on their histological appearance.

The separate existence of pleomorphic liposarcoma is not certain. If one excludes all dedifferentiating liposarcomas, one is left with a small group, probably about 5%, of tumors, which resemble malignant fibrous histiocytomas but with large numbers of the pleomorphic vacuolated cells which are traditionally called lipoblasts. These vacuolated tumor cells have been assumed to indicate fatty differentiation. On the other hand, it is possible that the lipid droplets merely represent degenerative changes in high-grade undifferentiated sarcomas and may not be evidence of genuine adipose differentiation. Whatever the explanation, so-called pleomorphic liposarcoma comprises only a small percentage of liposarcomas and its prognosis is probably similar to high-grade malignant fibrous histiocytoma.

9.4 Liposarcoma in Children

Lipoblastoma and lipoblastomatosis can closely simulate a liposarcoma, with abundant cells indistinguishable from lipoblasts, and the lobulated tumor pattern may be the only histological indication of the correct diagnosis. Nowadays, few pathologists are likely to make a diagnosis of liposarcoma in a neonate and I am personally incredulous of reports of liposarcoma occurring in patients under the age of 10. SHMOOKLER and ENZINGER (1983) reported a series of liposarcomas in "children", but the youngest patient was about 10 years of age at presentation. All the others were in their early teens. A diagnosis of liposarcoma in a patient aged less than 5 years should always be greeted sceptically, if not with incredulity, and should not be accepted until all other possible diagnoses have been excluded.

Acknowledgments. I would like to thank all those who have referred cases to me personally or to the Australian Soft Tissue Tumor Registry over the last 25 years. The experience gathered mainly from those referred cases forms the basis of this article. The manuscript was typed by Ms. A.E. Clarke and the photomicrographs were printed by Mr. G. Garwood.

References

Alfonso I, Lopez PF, Cullen RF Jr, Martin-Jimenez R, Bejar RL (1986) Spinal cord involvement in encephalocraniocutaneous lipomatosis. Pediatr Neurol 2: 380–384

Allen PW (1981) Tumors and proliferations of adipose tissue. A clinicopathologic approach. Masson, New York

Allen PW (1989) Histopathology of rare chondroblastic metaplasia in benign lipomas. Letters to the case. Pathol Res Prac 184: 444

Allen PW (1990) Benign metastasizing Mullerian tumors and uterine sarcomas. Surg Pathol 3: 3–14

Amadio PC, Reimann H, Dobyns JH (1988) Lipofibromatous hamartoma of nerve. J Hand Surg [Am] 13: 67–75

Ansari SJ, Stephenson RA, Mackay B (1991) Angiomyolipoma of the kidney with lymph node involvement. Ultrastruct Pathol 15: 531–538

Aymard B, Boman-Ferrand F, Vernhes L, Floquet A, Floquet J, Morel O, Merle M, Delagoutte JP (1987) Hamartome lipofibromateux des nerfs peripheriques. Etude anatomo-clinique de 5 cas dont 2 avec etude ultrastructurale. Ann Pathol 7: 320–324

Azumi N, Curtis J, Kempson RL, Hendrickson MR (1987) Atypical and malignant neoplasms showing lipomatous differentiation. Am J Surg Pathol 11: 161–183

Azzopardi JG, Iocco J, Salm R (1983) Pleomorphic lipoma: a tumour simulating liposarcoma. Histopathology 7: 511–523

Bannayan GA (1971) Lipomatosis, angiomatosis, and macrencephalia. A previously undescribed congenital syndrome. Arch Pathol 92: 1–5

Barmakian JT, Posner MA, Silver L, Lehman W, Vine DT (1992) Proteus syndrome. J Hand Surg [Am] 17: 32–34

Barsky AJ (1967) Macrodactyly. J Bone Joint Surg 49A: 1255–1266

Beham A, Schmid C, Hodl S, Fletcher CD (1989) Spindle cell and pleomorphic lipoma: an immunohistochemicalstudy and histogenetic analysis. J Pathol 158: 219–222

Bender BL, Yunis EJ (1982) The pathology of tuberous sclerosis. Pathol Annu 17(1): 339–382

Bialer MG, Riedy MJ, Wilson WG (1998) Proteus syndrome versus Bannayan-Zonana syndrome: a problem in differential diagnosis. Eur J Pediatr 148: 122–125

Bolen JW, Thorning D (1981) Spindle-cell lipoma. A clinical, light and electron-microscopical study. Am J Surg Pathol 5: 435–441

Brecher ME, Gill WB, Straus FH (1986) Angiomyolipoma with regional lymph node involvement and long-term follow-up study. Hum Pathol 17: 962–963

Brescia RJ, Tazelaar HD, Hobbs J, Miller AW (1989) Intravascular lipoleiomyomatosis: a report of two cases. Hum Pathol 20: 252–256

Bryant J (1981) A pleomorphic lipoma in the scalp. J Dermatol Surg Oncol 7: 323–325

Chan JKC, Lee KC, Saw D (1986) Extraskeletal chondroma with lipoblast-like cells. Hum Pathol 17: 1285–1287

Chang HR, Hajdu SI, Collin C, Brennan MF (1989) The prognostic value of histologic subtypes in primary extremity liposarcoma. Cancer 64: 1514–1520

Chiao HC, Marks KE, Bauer TW, Pflanze W (1987) Intraneural lipoma of the sciatic nerve. Clin Orthop 221: 267–271

Chung EB (1990) Current Classification of soft tissue tumours. In: Fletcher CDM, Mckee PH (eds) Pathobiology of soft tissue tumors. Churchill Livingstone, Edinburgh, pp 43–81

Chung EB, Cavazzana AO, Fassina AS (1991) Tumors of adipose tissue. In: Ninfo V, Chung EB, Cavazzana AO (eds) Tumors and tumorlike lesions of soft tissue. Churchill Livingstone, New York, pp 67–89

Cohen MM (1988) Understanding Proteus syndrome, unmasking the elephant man, and stemming elephant fever. Neurofibromatosis 1: 260–280

Cohen MM (1990) Bannayan-Riley-Ruvalcaba syndrome: renaming three formerly recognised syndromes as one etiologic entity (letter). Am J Med Genet 35: 291–292

Cutrona D, Greco P (1981) Atypical subcutaneous lipoma, atypical intramuscular lipoma and well differentiated retroperitoneal liposarcoma. Pathologica 73: 579–588

De Rosa G, Cozzolino A, Guarino M, Giardino C (1987) Congenital infiltrating lipomatosis of the face: report of cases and review of the literature. J Oral Maxillofac Surg 45: 879–883

Desai P, Steiner GC (1990) Pathology of macrodactyly. Bull Hosp Jt Dis Orthop Inst 50: 116–125

DiLiberti JH (1992) Correlation of skeletal muscle biopsy with phenotype in the familial macrocephaly syndromes. J Med Genet 29: 46–49

El Shanti H, Bell WE, Waziri MH (1992) Epidermal nevus syndrome: subgroup with neuronal migration defects. J Child Neurol 7: 29–34

Eneroth M, Mandahl N, Heim S, Willen H, Rydholm A, Alberts KA, Mitelman F (1990) Localization of the chromosomalbreakpoints of t(12:16) in liposarcoma to subbands 12q13.3 and 16p11.2. Cancer Genet Cytogenet 48: 101–107

Enterline HT, Culberson JD, Rochlin DB, Brady LW (1960) Liposarcoma. A clinical and pathological study of 53 cases. Cancer 13: 932–950

Enzinger FM, Harvey DA (1975) Spindle cell lipoma. Cancer 36:1852–1859

Enzinger FM, Weiss SW (1988) Soft tissue tumors, 2nd edn. Mosby, St Louis

Enzinger FM, Winslow DJ (1962) Liposarcoma: a study of 103 cases. Virchows Arch [Pathol Anat] 335: 367–388

Evans HL (1979) Liposarcoma. A study of 55 cases with a reassessment of its classification. Am J Surg Pathol 3: 507–523

Evans HL (1988) Liposarcomas and atypical lipomatous tumors: a study of 66 cases followed for a minimum of 10 years. Surg Pathol 1: 41–54

Evans HL (1990) Smooth muscle in atypical lipomatous tumors: a report of three cases. Am J Surg Pathol 14: 714–718

Evans HL, Soule EH, Winkelmann RK (1979) Atypical lipoma, atypical intramuscular lipoma, and well-differentiated retroperitoneal liposarcoma: a reappraisal of 30 cases formerly classified as a well-differentiated liposarcoma. Cancer 43: 574–584

Ferry JA, Malt RA, Young RH (1991) Renal angiomyolipoma with sarcomatous transformation and pulmonary metastases. Am J Surg Pathol 15: 1083–1088

Feyerabend T, Schmitt R, Lanz U, Warmuth-Metz M (1990) CT morphology of benign median nerve tumors. Report of three cases and a review. Acta Radiol 31: 23–25

Fletcher CDM, Martin-Bates E (1987) Spindle cell lipoma: a clinicopathological study with some original observations. Histopathology 11: 803–817

Gouldesbrough DR, Kinny SJ (1989) Lipofibromatous hamartoma of the ulnar nerve at the elbow: bief report. J Bone Joint Surg [Br] 71: 331–332

Happle (1987) Lethal genes surviving by mosaicism: a possible explanation for sporadic birth defects involving the skin. J Am Acad Dermatol 16: 899–906

Hashimoto H, Enjoji M (1982) Liposarcoma. A clinicopathologic subtyping of 52 cases. Acta Pathol Jpn 32: 933–948

Hayashi Y, Ohi R, Tomita Y, Chiba T, Matsumoto Y, Chiba T (1992) Bannayan-Zonana syndrome associated with lipomas, hemangiomas, and lymphangiomas. J Pediatr Surg 27: 722–723

Higginbottom MC, Schultz P (1982) The Bannayan syndrome: an autosomal dominant disorder consisting of macrocephaly, lipomas, hemangiomas, and risk for intracranial tumors. Pediatrics 69: 632–634

Hirsch JF, Pierre-Kahn A (1988) Lumbosacral lipomas with spina bifida. Childs Nerv Syst 4: 354–360

Houpt P, Storm van Leeuwen JB, van den Bergen HA (1989) Intraneural lipofibroma of the median nerve. J Hand Surg [Am] 14: 706–709

Hruban RH, Belur BS, Epstein JI (1989) Massive retroperitoneal angiomyolipoma. A lesion that may be confused with well-differentiated liposarcoma. Am J Clin Pathol 92: 805–808

Hun K, Dorfman RF, Rappaport H (1978) Signet ring cell lymphoma. A rare morphologic and functional expression of nodular (follicular) lymphoma. Am J Surg Pathol 2: 119–132

Hunt SJ, Santa-Cruz DJ, Barr RJ (1990) Cellular angiolipoma. Am J Surg Pathol 14: 75–81

Israel J, Lessick M, Szego K, Wong P (1991) Translocation 19; Y in a child with Bannayan-Zonana phenotype. J Med Genet 28: 427–428

Jacob RA, Buchino JJ (1989) Lipofibroma of the superficial branch of the radial nerve. J Hand Surg [Am] 14: 704–706

Johnson RJ, Bonfiglio M (1969) Lipofibromatous hamartoma of the median nerve. J Bone Joint Surg 51: 984–990

Kalen V, Burwell DS, Omer GE (1988) Macrodactyly of the hands and feet. J Pediatr Orthop 8: 311–315

Katzer B (1989) Histopathology of rare chondroblastic metaplasia in benign lipomas. Pathol Res Prac 184: 437–443

Kindblom LG, Angervall L, Fassina AS (1982) Atypical lipoma. Acta Pathol Microbiol Scand [A] 90: 27–36

Kindblom LG, Angervall L, Svendsen P (1975) Liposarcoma. A clinicopathologic radiographic and prognostic study. Acta Pathol Microbiol Scand [A] 253[Suppl]: 3–71

Kitano M, Enjoji M, Iwasaki H (1979) Spindle cell lipoma: A clinicopathologic analysis of twelve cases. Acta Pathol Jpn 29: 891–899

Klein JA, Barr RJI (1990) Bannayan-Zonana syndrome associated with lymphangiomyomatous lesions. Pediatr Dermatol 7: 48–53

Komiyama M, Hakuba A, Inoue Y, Yasui T, Yagura H, Baba M, Nishimura S (1987) Magnetic resonance imaging: lumbosacral lipoma. Surg Neurol 28: 259–264

Lacombe D, Taieb A, Vergnes P, Sarlangue J, Chateil JF, Bucco P, Nelson JR, Battin J, Maleville J (1991) Proteus syndrome in 7 patients: clinical and genetic considerations. Genet Couns 2: 93–101

Langa V, Posner MA, Steiner GE (1987) Lipofibroma of the median nerve: a report of two cases. J Hand Surg [Br] 12: 221–223

Lattes R, Bigotti G (1991) Lipoblastic meningioma: "Vacuolated meningioma". Hum Pathol 22: 164–171

Linton PL, Ahn WS, Schwartz ME, Miller CM, Thung SN (1991) Angiomyolipoma of the liver: immunohistochemical study of a case. Liver 11: 158–161

Louis DS, Dick HM (1973) Ossifying lipofibroma of the median nerve. J Bone Joint Surg 55A: 1082–1084

Louis DS, Hankin FM, Greene TL, Dick HM (1985) Lipofibromas of the median nerve: long-term follow-up of four cases. J Hand Surg [Am] 10: 403–408

Lowe BA, Brewer J, Houghton DC, Jacobson E, Pitre T (1992) Malignant transformation of angiomyolipoma. J Urol 147: 1356–1358

Lugo M, Reyes JM, Putong PB (1982) Benign chondrolipomatous tumors of the breast (letter). Arch Pathol Lab Med 106: 691–692

Marsh WL, Lucas JG, Olsen J (1989) Chondrolipoma of the breast. Arch Pathol Lab Med 113: 369–371

Mason ML (1953) Presentation of cases. In: Proceedings of the American Society for Surgery of the Hand. J Bone Joint Surg 35A: 273–275

McCall S, Ramzy MI, Cure JK, Pai GS (1992) Encephalo-cranio-cutaneous lipomatosis and the Proteus syndrome: distinct entities with overlapping manifestations. Am J Med Genet 43: 662–668

Meis JM, Enzinger FM (1991) Myolipoma of Soft Tissue. Am J Surg Pathol 15: 121–125

Metcalf JS, Ellis B (1985) Choristoma of the breast. Hum Pathol 16: 739–740

Milchgrub S, McMurry NK, Vuitch F, Dorfman HD (1990) Chondrolipoangioma. A cartilage-containing benign mesenchymoma of soft tissue. Cancer 66: 2636–2641

Miles JH, Zonana J, Mcfarlane J, Aleck KA, Bawle E (1984) Macrocephaly with hamartomas: Bannayan-Zonana syndrome. Am J Med Genet 19: 225–234

Miller MD, Ragsdale BD, Sweet DE (1992) Parosteal lipomas: a new perspective. Pathology 24: 132–139

Moretti-Ferreira D, Koiffmann CP, Souza DH, Diament AJ, Wajntal AI (1989) Macrocephaly, multiple lipomas, and hemangiomata (Bannayan-Zonana syndrome): genetic heterogeneity or autosomal dominant locus with at least two different allelic forms? Am J Med Genet 34: 548–551

Mukai M, Torikata C, Iri H, Tamai S, Sugiura H, Tanaka Y, Sakamoto M, Hirohashi S (1992) Crystalloids in angiomyolipoma. A previously unnoticed phenomenon of renal angiomyo-lipoma occurring at a high frequency. Am J Surg Pathol 16: 1–10

Nazzaro V, Cambiaghi S, Montagnani A, Brusasco A, Cerri A, Caputo R (1991) Proteus syndrome. Ultrastructural study of linear verrucous and depigmented nevi. J Am Acad Dermatol 25: 377–383

Nguyen GK, Catzavelos C (1990) Solitary angiomyolipoma of the liver. Report of a case initially examined by fine needle aspiration biopsy. Acta Cytol 34: 201–204

Nuovo MA, Nuovo GJ, Smith D, Lewis SH (1990) Benign mesenchymoma of the round ligament. a report of two cases with immunohistochemistry. Am J Clin Pathol 93: 421–424

Okumura K, Sasaki Y, Ohyama M, Nishi T (1986) Bannayan syndrome-generalized lipomatosis associated with megalencephaly and macrodactyly. Acta Pathol Jpn 36: 269–277

Orson GG, Sim FH, Reiman HM, Taylor WF (1987) Liposarcoma of the musculoskeletal system. Cancer 60: 1362–1370

Oster LH, Blair WF, Steyers CM (1989) Large lipomas in the deep palmar space. J Hand Surg [Am] 14: 700–704

Paletta FX, Senay LC (1981) Lipofibromatous hamartoma of median nerve and ulnar nerve: surgical treatment. Plast Reconstr Surg 68: 915–921

Paletta FX, Rybka FJ (1972) Treatment of hamartomas of the median nerve. Ann Surg 176: 217–222

Paulien S, Turc-Carel C, Dal-Cin P, Jani-Sait S, Sreekantaiah C, Leong SP, Vogelstein B, Kinzler KW, Sandberg AA, Gemmill RM (1990) Myxoid liposarcoma with t(12:16)(q13:p11) contains site-specific differences in methylation patterns surrounding a zinc-finger gene mapped to the breakpoint region on chromosome 12. Cancer Res 50: 7902–7907

Rawlings CE, Bullard DE, Caldwell DS (1986) Peripheral nerve entrapment due to steroid-induced lipomatosis of the popliteal fossa. Case report. J Neurosurg 64: 666–668

Requena L, Hasson A, Arias D, Martin L, Barat-A (1992) Acquired symmetric lipomatosis of the soles. A plantar form of the Madelung-Launois-Bensaude syndrome. J Am Acad Dermatol 26: 860–862

Reszel PA, Soule EH, Coventry MB (1966) Liposarcoma of the extremities and limb girdles. A study of two hundred twenty-two cases. J Bone Joint Surg 48: 229–244

Ro JY, Ayala AG, el Naggar A, Grignon DJ, Hogan SF, Howard DR (1990) Angiomyolipoma of kidney with lymph node involvement. DNA flow cytometric analysis. Arch Pathol Lab Med 114: 65–67

Samlaska CP, Levin SW, James WD, Benson PM, Walker JC, Perlik PC (1989) Proteus syndrome. Arch Dermatol 125: 1109–1114

Sant GR, Ayers DK, Bankoff MS, Mitcheson HD, Ucci AA Jr (1990) Fine needle aspiration biopsy in the diagnosis of renal angiomyolipoma. J Urol 143: 999–1001

Saul RA, Stevenson RE, Bley R (1982) Mental retardation in the Bannayan syndrome. Pediatrics 69: 642–644

Schwartz CE, Brown AM, Der-Kaloustian VM, McGill JJ, Saul RA (1991) DNA fingerprinting: the utilization of minisatellite probes to detect a somatic mutation in the proteus syndrome. Experientia 58[Suppl]: 95–105

Shmookler BM, Enzinger FM (1981) Pleomorphic lipoma: a benign tumor simulating liposarcoma. A clinicpathologic analysis of 48 cases. Cancer 47: 126–133

Shmookler BM, Enzinger FM (1983) Liposarcoma occurring in children. An analysis of 17 cases and review of the literature. Cancer 52: 567–574

Silverman TA, Enzinger FM (1985) Fibrolipomatous hamartoma of nerve: a clinicopathologic analysis of 26 cases. Am J Surg Pathol 9: 7–14

Stout AP (1944) Liposarcoma – the malignant tumor of lipoblasts. Ann Surg 119: 86–107

Stricker S (1992) Musculoskeletal manifestations of Proteus syndrome: report of two cases with literature review. J Pediatr Orthop 12: 667–674

Takayasu K, Shima Y, Muramatsu Y, Moriyama N, Yamada T, Makuuchi M, Hirohashi S (1987) Imaging characteristics of large lipoma and angiomyolipoma of the liver: case reports. Cancer 59: 916–921

Taviere V, Brunelle F, Baraton J, Temam M, Pierre-Kahn A, Lallemand D (1989) MRI study of lumbosacral lipoma in children. Pediatr Radiol 19: 316–320

Tibbles JA, Cohen MM (1986) The Proteus syndrome: the Elephant Man diagnosed. Br Med J [Clin Res] 293: 683–685

Tong YC, Chieng PU, Tsai TC, Lin SN (1990) Renal angiomyolipoma: report of 24 cases. Br J Urol 66: 585–589

Van Baal JG, Lips P, Luth W, Bakker P, Davis G, Karthaus P, Voorwinde A, Dabhoiwala NF, Fleury P, Brummelkamp WH (1990) Percutaneous transcatheter embolization of symptomatic renal angiomyolipomas: a report of four cases. Neth J Surg 42: 72–77
Waisman J (1987) Additional cases of angiomyolipoma with regional lymph node involvement. Hum Pathol 18: 206
Walker CW, Adams BD, Barnes CL, Roloson GJ, FitzRandolph RL (1991) Case report 667. Fibrolipomatous hamartoma of the median nerve. Skeletal Radiol 20: 237–239
Weeks DA, Malott RL, Arnesen M, Zuppan C, Aitken D, Mierau G (1991) Hepatic angiomyolipoma with striated granules and positivity with melanoma-specific antibody (HMB-45): a report of two cases. Ultrastruct Pathol 15: 563–571

Classification of Rhabdomyosarcoma

W.A. Newton Jr.

1 Historical Development of Classification of Rhabdomyosarcoma

Lesions now classified as rhabdomyosarcoma (RMS) in children are as a rule comprised of very primitive cells which do not show obvious features of fully developed muscle. It is not surprising that the early attempts to classify this group of tumors focused upon tumors that showed some recognizable features of skeletal muscle such as cross-striations. STOUT (1946) gave credit to WEBER as the first to describe such a tumor in 1854 in his classical description of RMS of the skeletal muscles. WEBER described a patient who had a protruding tongue for several years that developed an obvious tumor mass about the size of a hand when it was removed at 21 years of age. The tissue consisted of small round or oval cells or nuclei with only scanty cytoplasm. A large proportion of the cells showed cross-striations. The conclusion of that author was that these cells were growing normal muscle fibers which were in different stages of development. He compared the microscopic appearance of these cells to those of a 4–5-month-old human embryo, but could not explain the tumor cells with scanty cytoplasm. He believed that these tumor cells developed out of inflammatory exudate which was found in the area of the excision. In retrospect, there can be little doubt that this was a neoplasm which would be diagnosed as an RMS today; it had enough

Current Topics in Pathology
Volume 89, Eds. D. Harms/D. Schmidt
© Springer-Verlag Berlin Heidelberg 1995

cross-striations present to recognize that the tumors cells had a skeletal muscle origin.

STOUT tabulated the cases reported in the world's literature as of 1946 which he considered to be RMS. He found 107 instances and added 14 of his own. All of these tumors were considered to have developed in or attached to skeletal muscle. One should contrast this number with the current data available about incidence of this group of tumors. A reasonable figure would be that there are approximated 300 new cases per year diagnosed in children and adolescents in the United States alone, and probably in the same rate elsewhere around the globe; origin in obvious muscle accounts for no more than a third of these lesions. Nonetheless, his work brought focus upon this type of cancer that has led to the further development of the current-day understanding of this tumor type. It is clear that the cases that he selected were those that had microscopic features which suggested a skeletal muscle origin. They consisted of cells that demonstrated either cross-striations, longitudinal myofibrils, or some vague suggestion of their formation in the majority of the cases. The tumor cells were either rounded, strap-shaped with two or more nuclei arranged in tandem, or racquet-shaped with a single nucleus on one expanded, rounded end with a tapering body extending outward from this for a variable distance. This publication emphasized these features as the basis of the diagnosis. It is not surprising that this diagnosis was not a common one for some time afterwards.

WOLBACH (1928) also emphasized the relationship between the appearance of these tumors and developing normal muscle. He described the morphology of a tumor that arose over the fifth and sixth dorsal vertebrae of a 4-year-old girl. His opening remark was that these lesions were sufficiently rare for the recording of each new example to be an obligation. Although his diagnosis was rhabdomyoma in this case, it should have been called an RMS. His report of the detailed morphology was published in an anatomic journal in 1928 describing for the first time evidence of myoblastic origin in the absence of cross-striations by the presence of centriole clusters and abortive fibril formation.

While the term embryonal had been used as early as 1892 (BERARD 1892), there was no attempt to subdivide RMS into subtypes. STOBBE and DARGEON (1950) were the first to draw attention to the embryonal subtype and to emphasize the fact that lesions consisting of more primitive-appearing cells were indeed tumors which could be called RMS, and because of their immaturity, or primitiveness, should be called embryonal RMS. Cross-striations were seen only occasionally. These tumors consisted of smaller, short, often spindled cells mixed with more rounded cells of various types. Giant cells, commonly present in the previously described tumors, were rarely encountered. All of their 15 cases developed in head and neck sites, often not in relation to obvious skeletal muscle.

Most authors credit RIOPELLE and THERIAULT (1956) with the coining of the term alveolar RMS. In fact, it was used earlier by BURGESS in 1914 and

PEYRON in 1929. These tumors consisted mainly of small, rounded, primitive-appearing cells which showed enough cytoplasmic changes to enable them to be considered RMS. The critical feature of this new subtype of RMS was the presence of structures resembling pulmonary alveoli in which tumor cell-lined spaces were either open or contained a varying number of similar-appearing cells. This subtype was one of the three major groups of RMS in the HORN and ENTERLINE (1958) classification. An extension of concept for alveolar RMS has proposed that the cellular constituents of this subtype are sufficiently recognizable that a tumor comprising these primitive small round cells can be identified as alveolar RMS, so-called "solid" alveolar RMS. A study of a group of patients considered to have this variant showed that this pattern predicted a poor outcome compared to other types of RMS (TSOKOS et al. 1984; TSOKOS and TRICHE 1986).

The third subtype included by HORN and ENTERLINE (1958) was called pleomorphic. The precise definition of this type is difficult to find. Even these authors did not describe it, but referred to the description by STOUT (1946). In fact, STOUT did not use the term pleomorphic, but rather gave a description for RMS generally as described above. The definitions given prior to the advent of successful immunohistochemistry describe a lesion similar to that seen in embryonal RMS in which the cells are larger and more variable. In recent years, with the recognition and more frequent diagnosing of malignant fibrous histiocytoma, pleomorphic RMS has almost disappeared in adults. A recent survey of all cases entered on the Intergroup Rhabdomyosarcoma Study (IRS) I–III demonstrated that this subtype was so rare that it is not even included in the current classification scheme being used for IRS IV.

If one would consider this very rare pleomorphic variant to be a subtype of embryonal RMS, there would be four subtypes for that category. The two most important would be the botryoid type and a newly defined group of tumors that are characterized by the dominance of spindle cells. Both subtypes have a clinically significant difference in survival as compared to all other types of RMS. The botryoid lesion has distinct gross and microscopic features which easily distinguish it from other embryonal RMS tumors. The tumor grows into a variety of open organs, i.e., bladder, vagina, bile duct, forming a grape-like appearance. Microscopically it has a loosely cellular, edematous stroma covered by an intact epithelial surface. Just below the epithelium one should be able to see a layer of similar myoblasts which is more concentrated producing the so-called cambium layer described by NICHOLSON (1952).

The spindle cell type, seen predominately in the paratesticular site, consists almost totally of spindle cells which may be separated by storiform bands of fibrous tissue, or almost no collagen between cells at all resembling a leiomyosarcoma. This subtype was first recognized by PALMER (PALMER et al. 1981) in his attempt to develop a cytohistologic classification for RMS, leading to a definitive study done on the IRS pathology database by I.

Leuschner et al. (1991, unpublished) and on German-Italian data by
CAVAZZANA (1992).

A modification of the HORN and ENTERLINE classification was utilized in
a study of therapy for childhood RMS by the International Society for
Pediatric Oncology (CAILLAUD et al. 1989; RODARY et al. 1988). Their thesis
was that were subgroups of embryonal and alveolar RMS that might show
a better or worse outcome than these subtypes as a whole. Tumors with a
greater degree of differentiation did better than the others. There was not a
significant correlation between their individual subtypes and prognosis.
While this study included data from 339 patients, the fact that there were
eight subtypes may not have allowed a large enough patient sample per
subtype for a statistically significant conclusion.

2 Why Subclassify RMS?

Most pathologists today subclassify RMS according to the HORN-ENTERLINE
classification system. One of the reasons is that there has been a general
belief that patients with the alveolar subtype did not survive as well as
patients with the other subtypes. There was not complete agreement with
this practice. In 1967, STOUT and LATTES lumped embryonal, botryoid, and
alveolar together into what they called juvenile RMS, and the other RMS
were known as pleomorphic or adult type. Their reason for this was that
there did not seem to be any difference in the survival of patients with the
three juvenile subtypes. That was unfortunately true at that time (LATTES
and STOUT 1982). Any series evaluating survival by subtype which includes
cases diagnosed before 1970 have come to same conclusion, primarily because
the recent changes in outcome produced by intensive combination therapy
were not evident in their data (BALE et al. 1983; HAJDU 1979). This may also
have been influenced by the small sample size of their patient population. In
order to properly evaluate survival in this highly variable group of tumors,
large numbers of patients are necessary to delineate the prognostic significance of factors such as extent of disease, site of primary tumor, age, and
sex, as well as histology.

The database that has been developed by the IRS Group has provided
an increasing number of patients and has made statistical evaluation of the
prognostic significance of these factors much more precise. The first review
of these data (GEHAN et al. 1981) showed that there as a striking decrease in
the survival rate of the patients with the alveolar subtype, most marked in
clinical groups I and IV, but overall for patients entered on IRS I (Fig. 1).
This was based on analysis of 554 patients treated in a common protocol
which did not take morphology into account when determining severity of
disease. The next study, IRS II, was designed to give more intensive therapy
to patients with the alveolar subtype, as well as to other groups that were

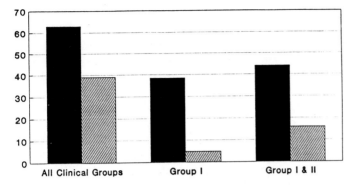

Fig. 1. Higher mortality rates of patients with alveolar (*solid columns*) compared to all other histologic subtypes (*hatched columns*) of RMS in all clinical groups of patients treated on IRS I

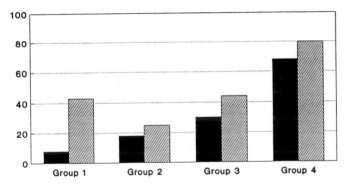

Fig. 2. Continuing differences in mortality rates of patients with alveolar RMS (*solid columns*) compared to embryonal RMS (*hatched columns*) by clinical group in IRS II

shown to have a less favorable outcome, i.e., parameningeal sites, and those with gross residual or metastatic disease present after diagnosis and initial surgery. A similar analysis done after IRS II continued to show a significantly decreased survival rate of patients with the alveolar subtype, particularly those with limited disease at diagnosis (CRIST et al. 1990) (Fig. 2). Other histologic subtypes were significantly different, with botryoid RMS having the most favorable, and embryonal RMS having an intermediate outcome rate. There were too few patients of the pleomorphic type to analyze.

A further analysis of patients on IRS I with alveolar subtypes (HAYES et al. 1977) clearly showed that alveolar subtype was associated with a number of unfavorable features. There was a higher mortality rate of 63% compared to 39% for all other histologic subtypes. This morphology was seen in fewer than 20% of the patients but accounted for greater than 29% of deaths ($p \leq 0.001$). It was also observed that patients with alveolar lesions showed increased local, regional, and distant metastases, particularly marked in clinical groups I and II. Those patients with grossly removed tumor had a 44% mortality compared to 16% for all others. There was double the mortality in the patients with lesions in the orbit, about the same on the head and neck, 65% versus 39% in the trunk, 60% versus 50% in the extremities, retroperitoneum 88.9% versus 54%, and the gastrointestinal tract 100% versus 75%. A review of the pathology of fatal RMS from IRS I and II showed a difference in the behavior of alveolar tumors (SHIMADA et al. 1987). Alveolar lesions had the highest rate of distant metastases and the lowest rate of local recurrences. A review of 79 embryonal and 24 alveolar RMS lesions in patients treated from 1970 to 1990 also demonstrated differences in the behavior of these two types of RMS (REILLY et al. 1991). Their conclusions were as follows: (a) the metastatic pattern of the histologic subtypes of RMS is different; (b) embryonal RMS metastasizes almost exclusively to lung; (c) no patient with embryonal RMS had marrow disease as the only site of metastasis.

A recent review of 34 patients with RMS of the extremities at Memorial Sloan-Kettering Hospital treated from 1970 to 1987 showed that the disease-free survival and overall survival were significantly affected by the histologic subtype with a 20% survival of patients with the alveolar type versus 70% of those with embryonal histology (GHAVIMI et al. 1989). A study of the factors predictive of mortality in this group showed that alveolar morphology was significant with a p value of < 0.001 (LAQUAGLIA et al. 1990). The patients with the alveolar subtype treated by the International Society for Pediatric Oncology (SIOP) from 1975 to 1984 also showed a poor survival rate of 33% in a group of 57 patients. Even those with nonmetastatic disease at diagnosis had a 40% chance of survival (REBOUL-MARTY et al. 1981).

Because of this obvious detrimental behavior of alveolar RMS, the IRS III study was designed to centrally review the histology at the time of diagnosis. Those with the alveolar subtype were given a more aggressive therapy program than those with other histologies. The clinical results of this treatment change are not yet known.

During the time of the IRS III study, an analysis of the prognostic significance of staging factors of patients with RMS was carried out using the International Union Against Cancer (UICC) Staging System on a limited group of IRS II patients. Histology was classified as unfavorable (alveolar RMS plus patients classified by PALMER et al. (1981) as monomorphous or anaplastic) versus favorable (all other subtypes). For some reason the survival rates of these two groups were not significantly different ($p = 0.25$). This led the authors to conclude that histology was not as important a prognostic factor as local invasiveness of the primary tumor, tumor size, clinical status of the regional nodes, and clinical or radiologic evidence of distant metastases. Reasons for the reduced importance of histology in this group of patients are not known. The size of the sample should have been adequate, but may not have been sufficient to demonstrate differences when other clinical factors may have skewed the outcome. It should be pointed out that the patients with alveolar RMS treated in IRS II had received more intensive therapy and perhaps had a better outcome.

In an attempt to better define the pleomorphic type in the IRS I–III case material, KODET has shown that patients whose lesions contain anaplastic cells have a poor survival rate, similar to that observed in patients with alveolar RMS (KODET et al. 1993). Anaplastic cells have been seen in both embryonal and alveolar RMS.

In addition to the fact that it is reasonable to classify RMS lesions because alveolar subtypes predict an unfavorable outcome, there are subtypes that predict a more favorable survival. The most notable of these is the botryoid variety of embryonal RMS which predicts a very high survival rate – from 95% to 100%. In addition, the newly defined spindle cell type of embryonal RMS is associated with an over 90% survival rate as well, particularly when seen in the paratesticular area (CAVAZZANA 1992; I. Leuschner et al. unpublished).

3 Classification of Tumors Entered on IRS I and II

The classification system utilized for the IRS I and II studies was that of HORN and ENTERLINE (1958). A review of the pathology findings at diagnosis of 1626 eligible patients, and the clinicopathologic correlation of these data have shown that this is a workable, prognostic system (LAWRENCE et al. 1987). These study diagnoses were the consensus of four or more pathologists experienced in the diagnosis of soft tissue tumors of children and adolescents. The committee diagnoses were embryonal in 877 (54%), alveolar in 343 (21%), botryoid in 88 (5%), and pleomorphic in 11 (1%). A comparison of their 3-year survival rates is shown in Fig. 3.

The decision was made by the IRS Committee that sarcomas which did not have cytologic features sufficient to make a specific histogenetic diagnosis and were in general comprised of primitive cells would be eligible for these studies. The term "sarcoma, type indeterminate" (STI) was used for these lesions. The survival rate for this group of patients was also reduced, similar to patients with alveolar RMS.

As these studies progressed, two new entities were separated out of this STI or undifferentiated cell category, namely those with extraosseous Ewing's sarcoma (SOULE et al. 1978; SHIMADA et al. 1988), and rhabdoid tumor of soft tissue (R. Kodet et al. unpublished). As these primitive cell lesions are better understood as to their biologic nature, additional entities will no doubt be identified.

In order to classify each lesion, those tumors that lacked adequate histologic material, or whose tissues were not interpretable because of poor preservation but were still felt to be a sarcoma, were diagnosed as sarcoma, NOS. This accounted for approximately 5% of all cases.

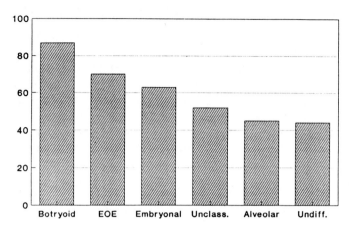

Fig. 3. Percentage 5-year survival of patients treated on IRS II by histologic subtype. *EOE*, extraosseous Ewings sarcoma

4 RMS Subtype Mixtures

Thus far, the discussions of classifications have assumed that· the subtypes exist as definitive entities consisting of similar cells and are separable from one another. In fact, this is not the case in many instances. For example, 10% of the lesions classified as embryonal on the IRS I–II studies were mixtures of embryonal and alveolar subtypes in which the embryonal component predominated. This raises some interesting questions about the histogenesis of these lesions, since we now know that these two subtypes have quite different natures based upon their different chromosomal changes. Alveolar RMS lesions have a 2,13 translocation, while embryonal RMS does not (LATTES and STOUT 1982). Embryonal lesions have been reported to have trisomy 2 (LATTES and STOUT 1982), and loss of constitutional heterozygosity for 11p (SCRABLE et al. 1989). Both subtypes demonstrate MyoD1 (SCRABLE et al. 1989).

5 Molecular Classification of RMS

As has been pointed out earlier, many of the soft tissue neoplasms in children consist of very primitive cells which may not have histologic features which would allow a specific histologic classification category. Similar-appearing neoplasms that are obviously forming primitive muscle cells may well have fundamental differences in their molecular structures. In other words, similar-appearing neoplasms could be called a phenotype of a particular category, while their molecular differences would constitute their specific genotype. A given subtype of RMS may in fact be a mixture of genotypes of a muscle-forming neoplasm, or may even be a mixture of muscle and other types of progenitor cells. The latter phenomenon of heterogeneity is probably the rule rather than the exception.

SCRABLE et al. (1989) have proposed a concept of molecular differential diagnosis for variations of RMS, while allowing separation of non-muscle-forming tumors in the process. This was a two-tiered approach: first, to separate tumors with and without muscle cells, and second, to separate the muscle-forming tumors into at least two subclasses. Hybridization of human MyoD1 cDNA to Northern blots of total RNA isolated from histologically diagnosed RMS resulted in a readily detectable amount of a 2-kb transcript irrespective of the individual variations in the histologic or clinical variations. Contrariwise, nonmuscle tumors such as fibrosarcoma, hepatoblastoma, osteosarcoma, and Wilms' tumors did not show this specific expression. This finding was consistent with all rhabdomyoblastomas tested.

The second level of separation of the muscle tumors was done by mapping the chromosome 11 from these tumors as well as on the patients leukocytes with a variety of probes to map the tumor genes. Loss of constitutional heterozygosity was demonstrated in all examples of embryonal RMS, but not in patients with alveolar RMS. Some of the latter demonstrated a t(2,13)(q37;q14) translocation.

The obvious use of this methodology is to separate those tumors that have a muscle origin from those that do not. It does not provide a definitive separation of the MyoD1-positive tumors into subtypes. Thus far, all embryonal RMS types have shown loss of their constitutional heterozygosity of chromosome 11. With a greater specificity, should the gene locus prove to be 11p15.5 (SCRABLE et al. 1989) and with further technology to identify these changes short of a DNA extraction and hybridization, this would make this a practical diagnostic process.

DIAS et al. (1990) have studied MyoD1 expression in childhood solid tumors by their reactivity with anti-MyoD1 polyclonal sera on fresh or frozen normal tissue. The specificity of these antisera was demonstrated by immunoprecipitation of in vitro translated 45-kD/MyoD1 protein.

This antibody was used to stain the cells by indirect fluorescence. Each of 16 rhabdomyoblastomas was positive for MyoD1 protein, including four that did not react to anti-desmin. Two of five specimens diagnosed as STI by the IRS classification nomenclature were positive, as were two of three cases of extraosseous Ewing's sarcoma. A variety of other solid tumor types including neuroblastoma, primitive neuroectodermal tumor, non-Hodgkin's tumor, embryonal sarcoma of the liver, malignant fibrous histiocytoma, malignant rhabdoid tumor, and Ewing's sarcoma of bone did not show a positive reaction.

This technique allows this type of analysis to be done on fresh or fresh frozen tissue without using molecular probes. The importance of this study was to demonstrate the ability to identify muscle-reacting tumors which have insufficient histologic and immunochemistry features to do so. It also demonstrates that some tumors currently being diagnosed as extraosseous Ewing's sarcoma may be either heterogeneous for muscle and neural origins or of muscle histogenesis alone.

6 Classification by the Degree of Tumor Cell Differentiation

One of the many variables of the RMS group of tumors is the remarkable diversity in the degree of maturation, or differentiation of the myoblastic cells. Each of the subtypes of RMS shows a variability of maturation of these cells. The botryoid subtype characteristically contains tumor cells which appear to be miniature mature muscle firbers. This subtype enjoys a very favorable outcome. On the other hand, the alveolar tumors are most often composed of very undifferentiated cells and are more likely to have a poor outcome on current therapy. These are generalizations which need to be explored in more detail, but suggest that each classification of an RMS should indicate the degree of maturation of the average population of tumor cells.

SCHMIDT et al. (1986) studied 64 cases of embryonal RMS by light microscopy and immunohistochemistry. Three histologic subgroups were identified: primitive (<10% rhabdomyoblasts), intermediate (10%–50% rhabdomyoblasts), and well-differentiated (>50% rhabdomyoblasts). Vimentin-positive cells predominated in the primitive group, desmin- and vimentin-positive cells were common in the intermediate group of tumors, and myoglobin-positive cells were demonstrated only in the well-differentiated group. The early response to chemotherapy was best in the well-differentiated, and worst with the primitive cell tumors. Obviously this type of analysis should be applied to longer-term data to further evaluate the predictability of response to therapy by the degree of tumor cell differentiation.

MIRALLES et al. (1991) studied 100 soft tissue tumors as to their degree of differentiation. They defined five subgroups: embryonal or undifferentiated, myxoid, well-differentiated, and celomic-like. Survival of these patients was measured by the actuarial curves of Benson and Gage. Well-differentiated and myxoid lesions were associated with a longer survival (average 88 months and 94 months, respectively) than undifferentiated lesions (23 months), and embryonal (15 months), and celomic (17.3 months). This approach needs to be done on a larger scale with proper case controls.

One of the important, unanswered questions relating to maturation of RMS cells and its significance involves the issue of the degree of malignancy of relatively mature-appearing rhabdomyoblasts seen in biopsies of previously treated tumor sites. MOLENAAR et al. (1985) was the first to point out this problem, which has not yet been properly answered. A variety of analyses have been applied including flow-cytometric analysis, nuclear proliferative antigen determination, nuclear organizer region analysis, and mitotic rate determination. RAZA et al. (1992) has recommended that proliferation kinetics be determined after infusion of iododeoxyuridine (IUDR) and bromodeoxyuridine (BRDU). This has been successfully used in evaluating leukemia, as well as in hepatocellular carcinoma of adults (TARAO et al. 1991).

7 Fetal Rhabdomyoma and RMS

Mesenchymal muscle tumors are as a rule malignant. One type of skeletal muscle tumor occurring mainly in infants but occasionally in adults is an exception, namely fetal rhabdomyoma (DEHNER et al. 1972; DI SANT 'AGNESE and KNOWLES 1980). It is divided into two morphologic subgroups: myxoid and cellular. The tumor cells consist of myoblasts that are relatively mature resembling fetal skeletal muscle cells in the sixth to tenth weeks of gestation. The myxoid type needs to be differentiated from the botryoid subtype of embryonal RMS. The muscle fibers are definitely more mature in fetal rhabdomyoma, do not show the characteristic cambium layer of Micholson, do not have an increased mitotic activity, and are not infiltrative. They also occur in different areas, namely in the subcutaneous tissues of the head and neck region, particularly the posterior auricular area. A recent report was published of a patient with this type of lesion in the tongue who went on to develop an embryonal RMS in the same site (KODET et al. 1991). This would seem to be a rare exception, but suggests that the two processes could be related on occasion.

8 Should RMS of Childhood Be Graded?

Grading of a neoplasm is based on identification of general features such as amount of necrosis, number of mitotic figures per unit area, etc. Grading of a neoplasm is considered to be important in deciding therapy for adult sarcomas, often in preference to the histologic diagnosis. This is based upon the fact that there are many types of sarcomas and each type may have a wide range of degrees of biologic aggressiveness. Grading is one of the parameters required to evaluate each patient for the purpose of programming therapy for adults. This has not been the practice for deciding treatment of childhood sarcomas or, for that matter, any non-CNS childhood tumor. RMS has been considered to be a high-grade neoplasm, and therefore grading has not been a popular exercise in the evaluation of this group of tumors. Now that a number of less aggressive subtypes have been identified, perhaps this should be re-assessed as a possible parameter for determining therapy. Necrosis is a common feature of many of these tumors and is one of the more important indicators of grade (COSTA et al. 1984).

9 Electron Microscopy in Classification of RMS

Ultrastructural studies of RMS have shown that the presence of thick and thin myofilaments is required to establish the diagnosis of RMS by that means (MORALES et al. 1972; MIERAU and FAVARA 1980; GHADIALLY 1988; BALE et al. 1983). Most reports show that these features are not present in a third to a half of the cases diagnosable by light microscopy. SEIDAL and KINDBLOM (1984) were able to satisfy the requirements in all eight cases of both embryonal and alveolar RMS and considered that electron microscopy is still the cornerstone in the definition and diagnosis of RMS. MIERAU and FAVARA (1980) stated that in many tumors fewer than 1% of the cells showed myofilaments.

Most authors do not use ultrastructure to separate RMS subtypes. SEIDAL and KINDBLOOM (1984) demonstrated that the embryonal RMS lesions could be differentiated from alveolar RMS by the presence of small rounded mononuclear rhabdomyoblasts with dominating thin filaments and occasionally thick filaments. TAXY (1988) commented that:

> The yield, as in finding cells with cross striations, is small. The large component of primitive cells in both alveolar and embryonal RMS often results in tedious searches by light and by EM for cells with more abundant cytoplasm that are likely to be rhabdomyoblasts. Cells with scanty cytoplasm are usually too primitive to contain diagnostic structures.

10 Immunohistochemistry and Classification of RMS

There is no question that the addition of immunologic detection of specific antigens in tissue has both simplified and complicated the diagnosis and classification of soft tissue tumors. In the vast majority of cases of RMS, anti-desmin or anti-actin antibodies demonstrate a positive reaction, in contrast to anti-myoglobin which is usually positive only in the more differentiated tumors. This enables the surgical pathologist to establish the diagnosis of RMS more clearly than with the use of electron microscopy. Neither is needed to establish the diagnosis alone in the majority of lesions, but they are most helpful in the more primitive, less differentiated ones. These antibodies recognize that these cells are primitive or more differentiated rhabdomyoblasts, but they do not differentiate between the subtypes.

Unfortunately, many of these tumors are very undifferentiated, and in many instances only an occasional cell shows a positive reaction. This correlates well with the ultrastructural picture. Applying a battery of reagents to evaluate the possible presence of neural, epithelial, vascular, or other tissue cells presents the pathologist with the fact that a so-called skeletal muscle tumor may have positive reactions to a variety of these reagents. Is this due to the fact that these tumors are, in fact, of heterogeneous histogenesis, or is it non-specificity due to the short-comings of our present technology? My personal opinion, which is still optimistic about this added diagnostic support, is that it is probably due to both cellular heterogeneity *and* non-specificity of the immunohistochemistry. Our laboratory is currently involved in a largescale effort to study these tumors with a diverse battery of reagents on tissue fixed either with alcohol or formalin on cases entered on IRS IV, hoping to shed more light on this dilemma.

11 Heterogeneity of Soft Tissue Tumors

It has been known for some time that embryonal neoplasms occur in a variety of body sites that are composed of more than one type of neoplastic cell. Some of the more obvious ones are: malignant Triton tumor, consisting of a mixture of RMS and Schwann cells; Wilms' tumor, with a mixture of epithelial and mesodermal elements including RMS; medullomyoblastoma, a mixture of primitive neural elements and RMS; the rare hepatoblastoma that contains RMS; and others. Even a pure skeletal tumor such as RMS consists of a combination of both embryonal and alveolar subtypes in about 10% of the cases of embryonal RMS. That may not seem to be as much a contrast as the others, but with our newer understanding of the cytogenetics and molecular biology of these two elements, it is clear that they are biologically very different and thus heterogeneous. As mentioned above, as we evaluate more of the cases of RMS with a variety of immunohistochemical reagents, it is becoming increasingly clear that these tumors have subpopulations of non-muscle cells in their make-up. Further, it is clear both from the ultrastructural data as well as from immunohistochemical data that only a few of the primitive cells show specificity of their histogenesis. We assume that the rest of the cells in the tumor will in all likelihood become or have the potential to become cells of that particular origin. That may not be the case. It is reasonable to consider these primitive tumors to be formed by pleuripotential cells which are capable of forming a variety of cell types.

Extraosseous Ewing's sarcoma, which not too many years ago was diagnosed as an undifferentiated sarcoma, has now been shown to have a basically neural cell population by a variety of techniques, but it has also been shown that it can contain either obviously non-neural elements (epithelial and glial; HACHITANDA et al. 1990) to develop cytokeratin in nude mouse transplants (LLOMBART-BOSCH et al. 1990) or to demonstrate muscle antigens.

One of the tumors that has been separated out of the typical RMS group is ectomesenchymoma. This tumor type will be discussed in more detail as an example of heterogeneity.

12 Ectomesenchymoma and Its Relation to RMS

One of the first reported instances of a tumor now called ectomesen-chymoma was an instance of what appeared to be concomitant development of tumors in the middle ear and posterior fossa of a young black infant (HOLIMON and ROSENBLUM 1971). The first presentation was symptoms of a middle ear infection, followed by development of an inoperable middle ear tumor 15 months later. He lived for 6 months after diagnosis. At autopsy, in addition to pulmonary metastases, he was found to have an oval mass in the left cerebello-pontine angle which was connected by a pedicle with the rest of his tumor which had eroded through the skull and was continuous with the middle ear tumor. There were tumor cells in the subarachnoid space, but the brain was not invaded. The histology of the middle ear lesion was that of an embryonal RMS, but the mass in the cerebello-pontine angle showed many mature neurones either in masses, groups, or single cells. They suggested the name gangliorhabdomyoblastoma for this lesion, but pointed out that the logical explanation for the development was from the neural crest:

> In this region embryological studies have shown that the neural crest, an ectodermal derivative, supplies cells to the mesenchyme. Furthermore, these ectodermal cells, rather than cells from the mesoderm, produce bone, cartilage, and other tissues previously considered to be only mesodermal in origin. This portion of the mesenchyme has been termed the mesectoderm of ectomesenchyme to emphasize its derivation from the ectodermal neural crest.

This concept was credited to HORSTADIUS (1950). In retrospect, the more likely sequence of events in this case was extension of the middle ear tumor through to the CNS, as has been clearly shown in many instances of tumors arising in the parameningeal area (TEFFT et al. 1969, 1978; RANEY et al. 1987).

Malignant ectomesenchymomas are rare tumors composed of neuro-blasts and/or ganglion cells and malignant mesenchymal tissues of various types, usually RMS (KAWAMOTO et al. 1987). These tumors occur mostly in infants, but can be seen in adults. They occur in a wide variety of sites: wrist, thigh, pelvis, retroperitoneum, abdominal wall, paratesticular area, and head and neck region. This list closely mimics the soft tissue distribution of RMS. Eleven of the 13 cases summarized by KAWAMOTO et al. (1987) showed embryonal RMS as the mesenchymal component of their tumor.

HACHITANDA et al. (1992) have expanded the concept of this group of tumors by showing that in an ultrastructural examination of a group of primitive cell tumors of children (three osseous, 17 extraosseous) originally diagnosed as Ewing's sarcoma, peripheral neuroectodermal tumor (PNET), or undifferentiated sarcoma, five showed a mixture of neuronal and myoblastic elements. There were cells with neurosecretory granules and/or neuritic processes, and cells with actin-like filaments, and/or focal "Z"-disc condensations. Some tumor cells contained organelles indicating both neurogenic and myogenic differentiation in the *same* cell. The conclusion was that these tumors represented the most primitive form of ectomesenchymoma, and that their frequency would likely greatly exceed that of conventional ectomesenchymoma.

Clinical data concerning survival after modern combined therapy are very limited. Survival is usually good if the tumor is resected. One patient was treated on the IRS II protocol with the RMS type of therapy and has done well.

Those cases classified as ectomesenchymomas in the IRS studies have been lesions in which the neural component was mature ganglion cells. Often the number of ganglion cells was not high, and their recognition could have been easily misssed.

Recently reported cases of the co-existence of a malignant peripheral nerve sheath tumor and ganglioneuroma, while both are of neural origin, should probably be included in this group of tumors (GHALI et al. 1992; BANKS et al. 1989). Other elements that have been described in these tumors are: liposarcoma, melanocytes, chondroid tissue, undifferentiated sarcoma, and malignant fibrous histiocytoma (KAWAMOTO et al. 1987).

The histogenesis of these tumors is not known, but it is reasonable to suggest their origin to be from remnants of migratory neural crest cells, usually referred to as ectomesenchyme.

The possible derivation of these tumors from the neural crest was first suggested by HOLIMON and ROSENBLUM (1971), but the term ectomesenchymoma was initiated by KARCIOGLU et al. in 1977. They describe a 6-month-old with a 2-month history of an enlarging facial mass diagnosed as an embryonal RMS. A recurrence of this tumor was found to contain a mixture of RMS and ganglion cells displaying varying degrees of maturity which were intimately mixed with the RMS. A third specimen consisted mainly of mixtures of mature and immature ganglioneuroma showing Schwann cell cords arranged in interlacing fascicles, as well as groups of melanin pigment-containing cells. Only a few areas contained RMS tissue. They reviewed the concepts of the origin of the Triton tumor, as well as the previously reported instances of mixed neural and mesenchymal tumors. Their conclusions were that the concept of neural crest derivation of these lesions from ectomesenchyme was the most likely explanation.

The tumor reported by NAKA et al. (1975) arose in the retroperitoneum and consisted not only of RMS and ganglion cells, but also areas of liposarcoma, undifferentiated mesenchymatous tissue, and cartilage. Their concepts were similar to those proposed by KARCIOGLU et al. (1977) but they called their tumor ganglioneuroblastoma associated with malignant mesenchymoma. This tumor probably would also be called an ectomesenchymoma.

Another extension of this concept is illustrated in the report of the finding of alpha smooth muscle actin and desmin expression in human neuroblastoma cell lines (SUGIMOTO et al. 1991).

13 Future Considerations for Classification

It is clear that the present HORN and ENTERLINE (1958) classification scheme with modifications provides a prognostically significant way to classify RMS histologically. An international committee has reviewed this and all other currently used systems, and will be recommending an updated version of the HORN and ENTERLINE classification having tested each system utilizing histologic and clinical data from IRS II.

Obviously, when MyoD1 antibodies become available, particularly if workable on fixed tissue, this should be the standard technique to identify tumors that have a skeletal muscle origin. Immunohistochemistry may be able to enable more precise separation of other related primitive round cell and undifferentiated sarcomas. Cytogenetics has limited value since specific changes are not regularly demonstrable, but should be done routinely to capture those that show t(2,13), t(11,22) or other changes that will become established by more extensive testing.

The challenge still is to seek morphologic or biologic features which reliably identify patients that are likely to do well or poorly. This will allow future treatment programs to lessen the adverse effects of the currently necessary treatment programs, or to focus more precisely on the tumors that are failing current therapy efforts.

References

Bale PM, Parsons RE et al. (1983) Diagnosis and behavior of juvenile rhabdomyosarcoma. Hum Pathol 14: 596–611
Banks E, Yum M et al. (1989) A Malignant Peripheral Nerve Sheath Tumor in Association With a Paratesticular Ganglioneuroma. Cancer 64: 1738–1742
Berard M (1892) Tumor embryonaire du muscle strie. Lyon Med 77: 52
Burgess AM (1914) Malignant rhabdomyoma with multiple metastases. J Med Res 29: 447
Caillaud JM, Gerard-Marchant R et al. (1989) Histopathological classification of childhood rhabdomyosarcoma. Med Pediatr Oncol 17: 391–400
Cavazzana A (1992) Spindle cell tumors of the paratesticular area. Am J Surg Pathol 16: 229–235

Costa J, Wesley RA et al. (1984) The grading of soft tissue sarcomas: results of a clinico-histopathologic correlation in a series of 163 cases. Cancer 53: 530–541

Crist WM, Garnsey L et al. (1990) Prognosis in children with rhabdomyosarcoma: a report of the intergroup rhabdomyosarcoma studies I and II. J Clin Oncol 8: 443–452

Dehner LP, Enzinger FM et al. (1972) Fetal rhabdomyoma. An analysis of nine cases. Cancer 30: 160–166

Di Sant'Agnese PA, Knowles DM (4692) Extracardiac Rhabdomyoma: a Clinicopathologic Study and Review of the Literature. Cancer 1980: 780–789

Dias P, Parham D et al. (1990) Myogenic Regulatory Protein (MyoD1) Expression in childhood solid tumors. Diagnostic utility in rhabdomyosarcoma. Am J Pathol 137: 1283–1291

Gehan EA, Glover FN et al. (1981) Prognostic factors in children with rhabdomyosarcoma. Natl Cancer Inst Monogr 56: 83–92

Ghadially, FN (1988) Myofilaments in rhabdomyoma and rhabdomyosarcoma. In: Ultrastructural pathology of the cell and matrix, a text and atlas of physiological and pathological alterations in the fine structure of cellular and extracellular components. Butterworths, London, pp 854–901

Ghali VS, Gold JE et al. (1992) Malignant peripheral nerve sheath tumor arising spontaneously from retroperitoneal ganglioneuroma: a case report, review of the literature, and immunohistochemical study. Hum Pathol 23(1): 72–75

Ghavimi F, Mandell LR et al. (1989) Prognosis in childhood rhabdomyosarcoma of the extremity. Cancer 64: 2233–2237

Hachitanda Y, Tsuneyoshi M et al. (1990) Congenital primitive neuroectodermal tumor with epithelia and glial differentiation. An ultrastructural and immunohistochemical study. Arch Pathol Lab Med 114: 101–105

Hachitanda Y, Aoyama C et al. (1992) The most primitive form of ectomesenchymoma: an immunohistochemically and ultrastructurally identified entity. Pediatr Pathol 12: 5P (abstract)

Hajdu, SI (1979) Tumors of muscle. In: Hajdu SI (ed) Pathology of soft tissue tumors. Lea and Febiger, Philadelphia, pp 325–365

Hayes DM, Sutow WW, Lawrence W Jr, Moon TE (1977) Rhabdomyosarcoma: surgical therapy in extremity lesions in children. Orthop Clin North Am 8: 883–902

Holimon JL, Rosenblum WI (1971) "Ganglorhabdomyosarcoma": a tumor of ectomesenchyme. Case report. J Neurosurg 34: 417–422

Horn RC Jr, Enterline HT (1958) Rhabdomyosarcoma: a clinicopathological study and classification of 39 cases. Cancer 11: 181–199

Horstadius SO (1950) The neural crest, its properties and derivatives in the light of experimental research. Oxford University Press, London

Karcioglu Z, Someren A et al. (1977) Ectomesenchymoma a malignant tumors of migratory neural crest (ectomesenchyme) remnant showing ganglionic, schwannian, melanocytic, and rhabdomyoblastic differentiation. Cancer 39: 2486–2496

Kawamoto EH, Weidner N et al. (1987) Malignant ectomesenchymoma of soft tissue: report of two cases and review of the literature. Cancer 59: 1791–1802

Kodet R, Newton WA et al. (1991) Rhabdoid tumors of soft tissues: a clinicopathologic study of 26 cases enrolled on the intergroup rhabdomyosarcoma study. Human Pathol 22: 674–684

Kodet R, Fajstavr J et al. (1991) Is fetal cellular rhabdomyoma an entity or a differentiated rhabdomyosarcoma? A study of patients with rhabdomyoma of the tongue and sarcoma of the tongue enrolled in the intergroup rhabdomyosarcoma studies I, II, and III. Cancer 67: 2907–2913

Kodet R, Newton WA Jr et al. (1992) Childhood rhabdomyosarcoma with pleomorphic-anaplastic features. A report of Intergroup Rhabdomyosarcoma Study. Am J Surg Pathol 17: 443–453

LaQuaglia MP, Ghavimi R et al. (1990) Factors predictive of mortality in pediatric extremity rhabdomyosarcoma. J Pediatr Surg 25(2): 238–244

Lattes R, Stout AP (1982) Rhabdomyosarcoma. In: Hartmann WH (ed) Tumors of the soft tissues. Armed Forces Institute of Pathology, Washington DC, pp 169–181

Lawrence W, Gehan EA et al. (1987) Prognostic significance of staging factors of the UICC staging system in childhood rhabdomyosarcoma: a report from the Intergroup Rhabdomyosarcoma Study (IRS-II). J Clin Oncol 5: 46–54

Llombart-Bosch A, Carda C et al. (1990) Soft tissue Ewing's sarcoma: characterization in established cultures and xenografts with evidence of a neuroectodermic phenotype. Cancer 66: 2589–2601

Mierau GW, Favara BE (1980) Rhabdomyosarcoma in children. Cancer 46: 2035–2040

Miralles TG, Penn C et al. (1991) The prognostic value of tissue differentiation in soft tissue sarcomas. Pathol Res Pract 6: 187–187

Molenaar WM, Oosterhuis JW et al. (1985) Mesenchymal and muscle-specific intermediate filaments (vimentin and desmin) in relation to differentiation in childhood rhabdomyosarcomas. Hum Pathol 16: 838–843

Morales AR, Fine G et al. (1972) Rhabdomyosarcoma: an ultrastructural appraisal. Pathol Ann 7: 81–106

Naka A, Matsumoto S et al. (1975) Ganglioneurobastoma associated with malignant mesenchymoma. Cancer 36: 1050–1056

Nicholson GW (1952) Studies on tumor formation. Butterworth, London Palmer NF, Sachs NE, Foulkes M (1981) Histopathology and prognosis in rhabdomyosarcoma (abs). Int Soc Ped Oncol 9: 15–19

Peyron A (1929) Les tumeurs des muscles. Atlas du cancer, fasc 7. Alcan, Paris

Raney RB Jr, Tefft MMD et al. (1987) Improved prognosis with intensive treatment of children with cranial soft tissue sarcomas arising in nonorbital parameningeal sites. A report from the Intergroup Rhabdomyosarcoma Study. Cancer 59: 147–155

Raza A, Yousuf N et al. (1992) Contribution of in vivo proliferation/differentiation studies toward the development of a combined functional and morphologic system of classification of neoplastic diseases. Cancer 69[Suppl]: 1557–1566

Reboul-Marty J, Quintana E et al. (1001) Prognostic factors of alveolar rhabdomyosarcoma in childhood. Cancer 68: 493–498

Reilly A, Perilongo G et al. (1991) Histologic subtype determines pattern of metastases in childhood rhabdomyosarcomas (RMS). Proc ASCO 10: 316

Riopelle JL, Theriault JP (1956) Sur une forme meconnue de sarcome des parties molles: le rhabdomyosarcome alveolaire. Ann Anat Pathol 1: 88–111

Rodary C, Rey A et al. (1988) Prognostic factors in 281 children with nonmetastatic rhabdomyosarcoma (RMS) at diagnosis. Med Pediatr Oncol 16: 71–77

Schmidt D, Reimann O et al. (1986) Cellular differentiation and prognosis in embryonal rhabdomyosarcoma. Virchows Arch [Pathol Anat] 409: 183–194

Scrable H, Witte D et al. (1989) Molecular differential pathology of rhabdomyosarcoma. Genes Chrom Cancer 1: 23–35

Seidal T, Kindblom LG (1984) The ultrastructure of alveolar and embryonal rhabdomyosarcoma: a correlative light and electron microscopic study of 17 cases. Acta Pathol Microbiol Immunol Scand 92: 231–248

Shimada H, Newton WA Jr et al. (1987) Pathology of fatal rhabdomyosarcoma. Report from Intergroup Rhabdomyosarcoma Study (IRS-I and IRS-II). Cancer 59: 459–465

Shimada H, Newton WA Jr et al. (1988) Pathological features of extraosseous Ewing's sarcoma: a report from the Intergroup Rhabdomyosarcoma Study. Hum Pathol 19: 442–453

Soule EH, Newton WA Jr et al. (1978) Extraskeletal Ewing's sarcoma. A preliminary review of 26 cases encountered in the Intergroup Rhabdomyosarcoma Study. Cancer 42: 259–264

Stobbe GD, Dargeon HW (1950) Embryonal rhabdomyosarcoma of the head and neck in children and adolescents. Cancer September: 826–836

Stout A, Lattes R (1967) Rhabdomyosarcoma. In: Stout A, Lattes R (eds) Tumors of soft tissues. Armed Forces Institute of Pathology, Washington DC, pp F5/89–F5/98

Stout AP (1946) Rhabdomyosarcoma of the skeletal muscles. Ann Surg 123: 447–472

Sugimoto T, Ueyama H et al. (1991) Alpha-smooth-muscle actin and desmin expressions in human neuroblastoma cell lines. Int J Cancer 48: 277–283

Tarao K, Shimizu A et al. (1991) In vitro uptake of bromodexyuridine by human hepatocellular carcinoma and its relation of histopathologic findings and biologic behavior. Cancer 68: 1789–1794

Taxy JB (1988) Soft tissue neoplasms. In: Azar HA (ed) Pathology of human neoplasms. An atlas of diagnostic electron microscopy and immunohistochemistry. Raven, New York, pp 183–219

Tefft MMD, Vawter GFMD et al. (1969) Paravertebral "round cell" tumors in children. Radiology 92: 1501–1509

Tefft MMD, Fernandez CMD et al. (1978) Incidence of meningeal involvement by rhabdomyo-sarcoma of the head and neck in children. Cancer 42: 253–258
Tsokos M, Miser A et al. (1984) Histologic and cytologic characteristics of poor prognosis childhood rhabdomyosarcoma. Lab Invest 50: 61A–61A (abstract)
Tsokos MMD, Triche TJMD (1986) Primitive, "solid variant" rhabdomyosarcoma. Lab Invest 54: 65A
Wolbach SB (1928) A malignant rhabdomyoma of skeletal muscle. Arch Pathol 5: 775–786

Spindle Cell Rhabdomyosarcoma:
Histologic Variant of Embryonal Rhabdomyosarcoma
with Association to Favorable Prognosis

I. LEUSCHNER

1 Introduction

Rhabdomyosarcoma (RMS) is the most important malignant soft tissue tumor of childhood (ENZINGER and WEISS 1988). Following the first detailed description of an RMS of the skeletal muscles by STOUT (1946), this entity was subdivided by histologic criteria into embryonal (STOBBE and DARGEON 1950), alveolar (RIOPELLE and THERIAULT 1956), botryoid (HORN et al. 1955), and pleomorphic variants (HORN and ENTERLINE 1958). Later it could be shown that the botryoid RMS is a subtype of embryonal RMS. In clinical studies, it has been demonstrated that the distinction of these subtypes of RMS has an influence on prognosis in children (NEWTON et al. 1988). However, this classification of RMS into four subtypes does not relate to prognosis in all patients. Subsequently, the "solid alveolar RMS" was excluded from embryonal RMS (TSOKOS et al. 1984). This tumor type has the cytology of typical alveolar RMS but does not form the regressive alveolar spaces. Prognosis is similar to that of typical alveolar RMS (see chapter by D. Harms, this volume). Recently two independent studies were published concerning a subtype of embryonal RMS which is exclusively composed of spindle cells (CAVAZZANA et al. 1992; LEUSCHNER et al. 1993).

Current Topics in Pathology
Volume 89, Eds. D. Harms/D. Schmidt
© Springer-Verlag Berlin Heidelberg 1995

Prognosis of patients with such a tumor is more favorable in comparison to patients with RMS of "classical" embryonal histology.

The fact that embryonal and pleomorphic RMS can be composed of spindle cells was already described in the "conventional classification" of RMS (HORN and ENTERLINE 1958). In addition, presumably the first description of such subtype of embryonal RMS was published nearly 150 years ago (ROKITANSKY 1849). However, the prognostic relevance of this subtype was yet not realized. In the early 1980s, PALMER et al. (1981), in their systematic cytohistologic catalogue study of the Intergroup Rhabdomyosarcoma Study (IRS)-I lesions, identified a type of RMS with spindle-shaped tumor cells which they called "type A variant of rhabdomyosarcoma." This entity was included among the mixed-cell subgroup of RMS. This type A variant was associated with a favorable prognosis. Unfortunately, the PALMER classification was never used on a larger series of patients. In the newly proposed prognosis-related "international classification", the spindle cell RMS will be a subtype of RMS in the group of tumors with favorable prognosis (NEWTON et al. 1994).

2 Histology

2.1 Microscopic Findings

By conventional histology spindle cell RMS is almost entirely composed of spindle-shaped tumor cells. At low-power viewing a storiform pattern of the tumor is seen at first glance (Fig. 1). The tumor cells are arranged in whirls or tangles, sometimes in bundles, resulting in a histologic pattern of low to moderate cellularity. The tumor cells often have an elongated eosinophilic cytoplasm resembling fetal muscle cells (Fig. 2). Cross-striation can be seen in some of the tumor cells, but is not a necessary feature of the tumor. The nuclei are round to ovoid with a fine chromatin structure and sometimes with prominent nucleoli. The mitotic count ranges from zero to seven figures per ten high-power fields (CAVAZZANA et al. 1992). Periodic-acid-Schiff (PAS) staining shows a moderate to high positivity.

Two different variants of spindle cell RMS can be distinguished by the amount of collagen found in the tumor (LEUSCHNER et al. 1993). In the larger number of cases the tumor cells are surrounded by a matrix of collagen (Fig. 3) causing the low cellularity mentioned above. In other cases collagen fibers are scanty. In these tumors the spindle-shaped tumor cells are closely arranged in bundles resulting in a moderate cellularity (Fig. 4). However, it seems to be that the amount of collagen in the tumor does not have any influence on tumor growth or prognosis of patients.

Follow-up data have shown that the favorable prognosis of this tumor type is only seen if the majority of the tumor is composed of spindle cells. If

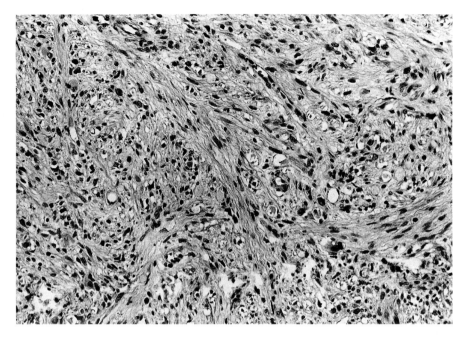

Fig. 1. Spindle cell RMS with storiform pattern and low cellularity. H&E, ×270

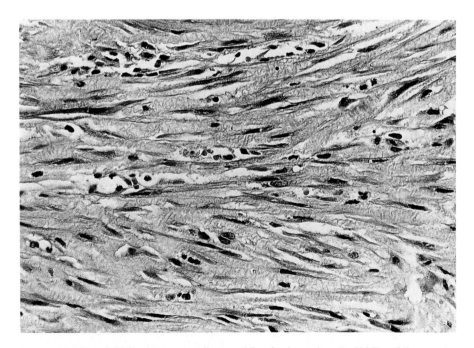

Fig. 2. Spindle cell RMS with tumor cells resembling fetal muscle cells. H&E, ×540

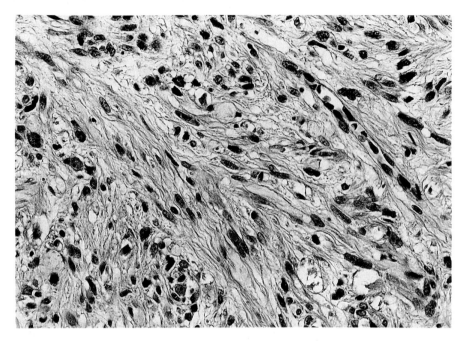

Fig. 3. Spindle cells surrounded by collagen matrix. H&E, ×540

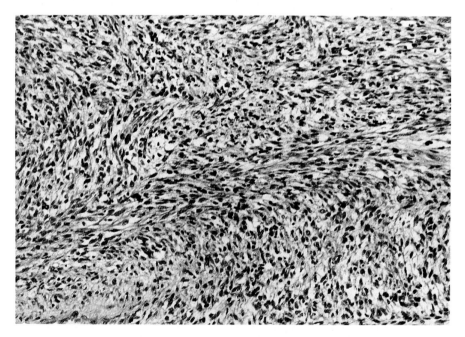

Fig. 4. Spindle cell RMS with low collagen content resulting in a moderate cellularity. H&E, ×270

the spindle cell component is less than 50%, prognosis of patients is similar to children with tumors of "classical" embryonal histology.

2.2 Invasive Growth and Lymph Node Involvement

Most spindle cell RMS are confined to a single, sometimes multilobulated nodule. In the periphery the tumor nodules are well circumscribed and in many cases a pseudocapsule is found. Aggressive tumor invasion into surrounding tissue is rarely seen. In paratesticular spindle cell RMS only one of 43 cases showed an infiltrating growth into the testicular tissue (LEUSCHNER et al. 1993). In nonparatesticular spindle cell RMS an infiltration into adjacent tissue is more frequently seen, resulting in a clinical tumor stage of extended disease. Nevertheless, a vascular invasion was never seen in the cases reviewed.

In paratesticular RMS lymph node metastases were found in lower numbers if the tumor was composed of spindle cells as compared to tumors of classical embryonal histology. Out of 43 cases of cell RMS paratesticular spindle, only seven patients had paraaortal lymph node metastases (16.3%) compared to 40 of 112 cases of paratesticular RMS with classical embryonal histology (35.7%) (LEUSCHNER et al. 1993). However, it needs to be proven in larger studies whether this low rate of lymph node involvement is only true for paratesticular lesions or whether spindle cell tumors of other sites have a similar behavior.

Distant metastases of spindle cell RMS were seen only in one (2.3%) of 43 paratesticular cases. By contrast 13 (11.6%) of 112 patients with tumors of classical embryonal histology had distant metastases at the time of diagnosis.

3 Immunohistochemistry

Many antibodies suitable for detecting myogenic antigens in paraffin-embedded tissues have been used on this tumor type (LEUSCHNER et al. 1993; CAVAZZANA et al. 1992). The results revealed a high degree of differentiation of the tumor cells. A strong expression of muscle-specific actin can be demonstrated in almost all cases (Fig. 5). Desmin expression is weaker, but also seen in all tumors investigated. In addition, myoglobin and Troponin T, both antigens expressed in later stages of skeletal muscle development, are found in a high number of cases (73% and 68.7%, respectively). Titin, a protein which is involved in organization of myofibrils, can be demonstrated in many cases (CAVAZZANA et al. 1992). The intermediate filament vimentin was expressed in 86% of cases investigated.

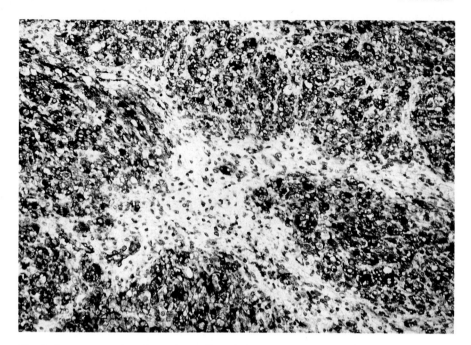

Fig. 5. Strong expression of muscle-specific actin in most tumor cells. APAAP, ×270

Taking the results of immunohistochemistry together, the degree of differentiation is comparable to a stage of normal myogenesis just before or even after fusion of myoblasts.

4 Electron Microscopy

Fifteen cases of spindle cell RMS could be studied by electron microscopy. In cases which demonstrated abundant collagen fibers by conventional histology, a rather uniform ultrastructural pattern of the tumor cells was seen in most cases. The cells were spindle shaped and surrounded by large amounts of collagen. Thick and thin filaments were seen in the cytoplasm of most tumor cells. The filaments were mainly found in large tangles, but also formed sarcomeres with Z-bands (Fig. 6). Occasionally myosin–ribosome complexes could be demonstrated. Many cells were surrounded by a basal lamina.

In cases with fewer collagen fibers seen by conventional histology the tumor cells showed a basal lamina and myosin–ribosome complexes. Thick and thin filaments and collagen fibers were also seen, forming abortive Z-bands.

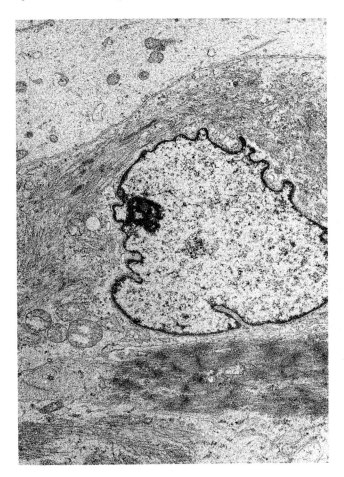

Fig. 6. High degree of ultrastrucural differentiation with Z-bands. ×19 000

5 DNA Ploidy

Ploidy analysis has proven to be of value in predicting prognosis in several different childhood tumors (SCHMIDT et al. 1986; LOOK et al. 1984). In RMS contradicting results have been published in the literature. In a study including a large number of stage III and IV cases, ploidy analysis was a reliable predictor for treatment response and clinical outcome (SHAPIRO et al. 1991). By contrast, other studies including similar number of cases revealed no correlation between ploidy and clinical outcome (KOWAL-VERN et al. 1990; LEUSCHNER et al. 1990).

We have investigated 18 cases of spindle cell RMS by flow cytometry using paraffin-embedded tissue. All but two cases showed a triploid DNA

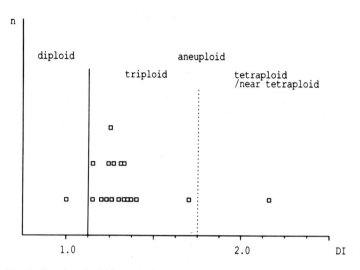

Fig. 7. Results of ploidy analysis. Each *square* represents one patient

content, the other two cases a diploid or tetraploid/near tetraploid DNA content, respectively (Fig. 7). With regard to the excellent prognosis of the spindle cell RMS the triploid DNA content seems to be associated with the low malignant potential of the tumors. A similar association of an aneuploid DNA content to a better prognosis was found by SHAPIRO et al. (1991) in stage III and IV embryonal RMS. Nevertheless, the value of ploidy analysis in RMS needs to be investigated in a larger number of cases.

6 Differential Diagnosis

Differential diagnosis can be difficult in some cases – in particular, leiomyosarcoma and fibrosarcoma should be considered. In general the pleomorphism of tumor cells and nuclei is not so prominent in spindle cell RMS as compared to the other two tumors. In addition, the nuclei of spindle cell RMS often do not have the "cigar-like" form as found in leiomyosarcoma.

Table 1. Differential diagnosis

	Spindle Cell RMS	Leiomyosarcoma	Fibrosarcoma
PAS	+/+++	−/(+)	−/(+)
Desmin	++	+	−
Muscle-specific actin	+/+++	+	−
Smooth muscle actin	−/(+)	++	−
Myoglobin	+/+++	−	−

Finally, invasion into surrounding tissue is more obvious in leiomyosarcoma and fibrosarcoma.

Using PAS stain, immunohistochemistry, and/or electron microscopy differential diagnosis will be possible to distinguish between the tumor entities (see Table 1).

7 Clinical Correlations and Prognosis

7.1 Age

A similar age distribution is found in patients with spindle cell RMS and embryonal RMS with classical histology. The mean age of patients with paratesticular spindle cell RMS was 6.6 years (median 5 years) compared to 5.9 years (median 4 years) of patients with nonparatesticular spindle cell RMS.

7.2 Tumor Size

No striking differences in tumor size at time of diagnosis could be demonstrated between the spindle cell RMS and RMS of classical embryonal histology. The mean tumor size of spindle cell RMS in the paratesticular site was 5.8 cm (2.0–18 cm, median 4.6 cm). For non-spindle cell RMS in this site a mean tumor size of 6.4 cm (1–18 cm, median 6.0) was found. In nonparatesticular sites a mean tumor size of 6.6 cm (2.0–20.0, median 5.25) for the spindle cell RMS and of 6.4 cm (0.2–27.0, median 5.0 cm) for the non-spindle cell RMS was estimated (LEUSCHNER et al. 1993).

7.3 Localization

Spindle cell RMS are predominantly found in the paratesticular site. In a study including 800 randomly selected cases of IRS-II, spindle cell RMS was seen in 57 cases: 18 cases occurred in the paratesticular site (31.6%), nine were located in the head and neck (15.8%), seven in the extremities (including shoulder and buttock) (12.3%), seven in the orbit (12.3%), five in the retroperitoneum (including the pelvis) (8.8%), six in the nonparatesticular genitourinary tract (10.5%), three in the trunk (5.3%), one in the abdomen (1.7%), and one in the buttock (1.7%) (LEUSCHNER et al. 1993).

In the paratesticular site about one quarter of the tumors show spindle cell RMS histology. Out of 173 paratesticular RMS included in the IRS studies I–III, 43 cases (24.8%) were composed almost entirely of spindle cells. Six additional cases of this study (3.5%) revealed some spindle cell areas, but these areas accounted for less than 50% of the tumor section. The major portion of these tumors was composed of a non-spindle cell pattern.

About two thirds of paratesticular RMS (112 of 173 cases, 64.7% of the study mentioned above) corresponded on the classical embryonal histology. Only three cases of the same study (1.7%) showed a purely alveolar pattern, and nine tumors (5.2%) were classified as mixed embryonal/alveolar (those with less than 50% of alveolar areas by IRS I–III definition) or as embryonal/pleomorphic type.

7.4 Clinical Stages

Almost all paratesticular embryonal RMS with spindle cell features were staged as clinical groups I and II. Thirty-two patients (74.4%) with a spindle cell type tumor had group I disease, ten patients (23.3%) group II disease, and only one patient (2.3%) group IV disease. By contrast, the non-spindle cell tumors in this site displayed a broader distribution of clinical stages. Sixty patients (53.6%) had group I disease, 29 patients (25.9%) group II disease, ten patients (8.9%) group III disease, and 13 patients (11.6%) a group IV disease.

The usually limited disease of spindle cell RMS is supported by the findings of the analysis of the 800 randomly selected cases of IRS-II. Most paratesticular tumors belonged to favorable clinical groups: out of 18 cases of spindle cell tumors 14 were group I and three group II tumors. The remaining case was a group IV tumor. With regard to all other sites 25 of 39 tumors were group III and IV tumors; seven were group I and another seven group II tumors.

7.5 Survival

Survival data of patients with paratesticular spindle cell RMS revealed an excellent prognosis. The Kaplan-Meier curves of survival showed a 95.5% survival at 5 years for the spindle cell cases in this site (Fig. 8). Only two of 43 evaluable patients with this tumor type died during this period. Patients with embryonal RMS with classical histology had a survival rate of 80% at 5 years ($p < 0.035$).

Analysis of survival of the spindle cell RMS found in the 800 randomly selected cases of IRS-II revealed a 92% 5-year survival rate for group I and II tumors of all sites except the paratesticular location (one of 15 patients died), and a 93% 5-year survival rate for group I and II tumors of the

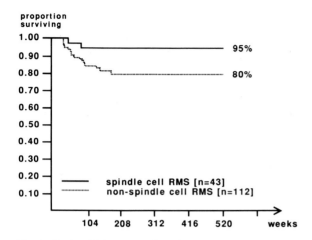

Fig. 8. Kaplan-Meier curve of survival. Paratesticular spindle cell RMS in comparision to non-spindle cell embryonal RMS. *Solid line*, spindle cell RMS ($n = 43$); *dotted line*, non-spindle cell RMS ($n = 112$). (From LEUSCHNER et al. 1993)

paratesticular site (one of 18 patients died). Survival at 5 years for spindle cell cases in all sites except the paratesticular area was 58% (15 of 39 patients died) and 88% (two of 18 patients died) for all spindle cell cases in the paratesticular site (LEUSCHNER et al. 1993).

8 Conclusion

Spindle cell RMS is a variant of embryonal RMS with special features in regard to tumor biology and prognosis of patients. This entity is easily distinguishable from other subtypes of RMS. The excellent prognosis for patients with such tumors makes it necessary to identify these tumors and separate them from RMS with classical embryonal histology. In addition, the low potential of malignancy and the site predominance in the para-testicular region make this tumor subtype an interesting object for in vitro studies with regard to differentiation, invasive growth, and metastasis.

References

Cavazzana AO, Schmidt D, Ninfo V, Harms D, Tollot M, Carli M, Treuner J, Betto R, Salviati G (1992) Spindle cell rhabdomyosarcoma. A prognostically favorable variant of rhabdomyosarcoma. Am J Surg Pathol 16: 229–235
Enzinger, FM, Weiss, SH (1988) Soft tissue tumors, 2nd edn. Mosby, St Louis, pp 448–488

Horn RC, Enterline HT (1958) Rhabdomyosarcoma: a clinicopathological study and classification of 39 cases. Cancer 11: 181–199

Horn RC Jr, Yakovac WC, Kaye R, Koop CE (1955) Rhabdomyosarcoma (sarcoma botryoides) of the common bile duct. Report of a case. Cancer 8: 468–477

Kowal-Vern A, Gonzalez-Crussi F, Turner J, Trujillo YP, Chou P, Herman C, Castelli M, Walloch J (1990) Flow and image cytometric DNA analysis in rhabdomyosarcoma. Cancer Res 50: 6023–6027

Leuschner I, Schmidt D, Möller R, Harms D (1990) Ploidy- and NOR-studies in rhabdomyosarcomas. Klin Paediatr 202: 290 (abstract)

Leuschner I, Newton WA Jr, Schmidt D, Sachs N, Asmar L, Hamoudi A, Harms D, Maurer HM (1993) Spindle cell variants of embryonal rhabdomyosarcoma of the paratesticular region: a report of the Intergroup Rhabdomyosarcoma Study. Am J Surg Pathol 17: 221–230

Look AT, Hayes FA, Nitschke R, McWilliams NB, Green AA (1984) Cellular DNA content as a predictor of response to chemotherapy in infants with unresectable neuroblastoma. N Engl J Med 311: 231–235

Newton WA Jr, Gehan EA, Webber BL, Marsden HB, van Unnik AJM, Hamoudi AB, Tsokos M, Shimada H, Harms D, Schmidt D, Ninfo V, Cavazzana A, Gonzalez-Crussi F, Parham DM, Reiman HM, Asmar L, Beltangady MS, Sachs N, Triche TJ, Maurer HM (1994) Classification of rhabdomyosarcomas and related sarcomas. Pathologic aspects and proposal for a new classification. An Intergroup Rhabdomyosarcoma Study. Cancer (in press)

Newton WA Jr, Soule EH, Hamoudi AB, Reiman HM, Shimada H, Beltangady M, Maurer H (1988) Histopathology of childhood sarcomas, Intergroup Rhabdomyosarcoma Studies I and II: clinicopathologic correlation. J Clin Oncol 6: 67–75

Palmer NF, Sachs N, Foulkes M (1981) Histopathology and prognosis in rhabdomyosarcoma. A report of the Intergroup Rhabdomyosarcoma Study (IRS). SIOP, XIIIth meeting, Marseille, 1981, 113–114 (abstract)

Riopelle JL, Theriault JP (1956) Sur une forme méconnue de sarcome des parties molles: le rhabdomyosarcome alvéolaire. Ann Anat Pathol 1: 88–111

Rokitansky (1849) Ein aus quergestreiften Muskelfasern constituiertes Aftergebilde. Z KK Ges Aerzte Wien 5: 331–333

Schmidt D, Wiedemann B, Keil W, Sprenger E, Harms D (1986) Flow cytometry analysis of nephroblastomas and related neoplasms. Cancer 58: 2494–2500

Shapiro DN, Parham DM, Douglass EC, Ashmun R, Webber BL, Newton WA, Hancock ML, Maurer HM, Look AT (1991) Relationship of tumor-cell ploidy to histologic subtype and treatment outcome in children and adolescents with unresectable rhabdomyosarcoma. J Clin Oncol 9: 159–166

Stobbe GD, Dargeon HW (1950) Embryonal rhabdomyosarcoma of head and neck in children and adolescents. Cancer 3: 826–836

Stout AP (1946) Rhabdomyosarcoma of skeletal muscles. Ann Surg 123: 447–472

Tsokos M, Miser A, Wesley R, Miser JS, Kinsella TJ, Grayson J, Pizzo PA, Glatstein E, Triche TJ (1984) Solid variant alveolar rhabdomyosarcoma: a primitive rhabdomyosarcoma with poor prognosis and distinct histology. SIOP, XVIIth meeting, Barcelona, 1984, 71–74 (abstract)

Alveolar Rhabdomyosarcoma:
A Prognostically Unfavorable Rhabdomyosarcoma Type and Its Necessary Distinction from Embryonal Rhabdomyosarcoma

D. Harms

1 Introduction

Since publication of the classic descriptions by Riopelle and Thériault (1956) and Enzinger and Shiraki (1969) the morphology of alveolar rhabdomyosarcoma (aRMS) has been well known. RMS presenting with clear and unequivocal (pseudo)alveolar spaces can be recognized at first sight as the alveolar (sub-)type of RMS. On the other hand, a diagnosis of aRMS may be difficult in cases which display neither significant evidence of rhabdomyogenesis in conventionally stained slides nor unambiguous alveolar spaces. In such cases the diagnosis of RMS must be confirmed by special staining including immunohistochemistry.

Because aRMS is associated with an unfavorable prognosis – in contrast to embryonal RMS (eRMS) which shows an intermediate prognosis under the conditions of modern multimodal therapy – it is necessary to distinguish any case of aRMS from the other RMS subtypes, above all from eRMS (Newton et al. 1989).

Applying the criterion of quantity of alveolar spaces Bale et al. (1983) considered RMS to be aRMS only if at least 70% of the tumor cut surfaces presented an alveolar pattern with alveolar spaces. By this definition, only three of 95 RMS cases could be classified as aRMS, and no prognostic difference could be found between the different RMS subtypes.

In contrast to this approach, we classified RMS exhibiting even very small foci of alveolar spaces in otherwise undifferentiated sarcomas as aRMS (Harms et al. 1985). Thus, predominantly "embryonal" RMS with

Current Topics in Pathology
Volume 89, Eds. D. Harms/D. Schmidt
© Springer-Verlag Berlin Heidelberg 1995

some alveolar foci were categorized as aRMS. Using this definition of aRMS, the difference in biological behavior and outcome between eRMS and aRMS became evident: alveolar histology means "unfavorable histology" regardless of the amount of tumor tissue with an alveolar pattern (HARMS et al. 1985).

Moreover, TSOKOS et al. (1984, 1985, 1992) clearly demonstrated that alveolar spaces are not a *conditio sine qua non* in the diagnosis of aRMS, since RMS without alveolar spaces but displaying the same cytological features as classic aRMS showed the same biological behavior as primitive aRMS. Consequently, they classified such cases in accordance with previous descriptions by RIOPELLE and THÉRIAULT (1956) and by ENZINGER and SHIRAKI (1969) as a solid variant of aRMS.

In conclusion, aRMS exhibiting a predominantly alveolar pattern and solid aRMS have to be considered the extremes of a spectrum, and at least most cases of "mixed eRMS and aRMS" within this spectrum should be categorized as aRMS.

2 Conventional Light Microscopy

Alveolar RMS is a highly proliferative, solid, mostly round-cellular tumor which may contain a variable quantity of alveolar spaces (RIOPELLE and

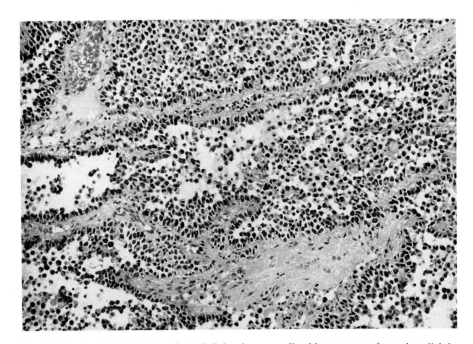

Fig. 1. Alveolar RMS displaying (pseudo-)alveolar spaces lined by one row of round to slightly elongated tumor cells attached to fibrous tissue lining the individual tumor cell aggregates; 20-year-old male. H&E, ×134

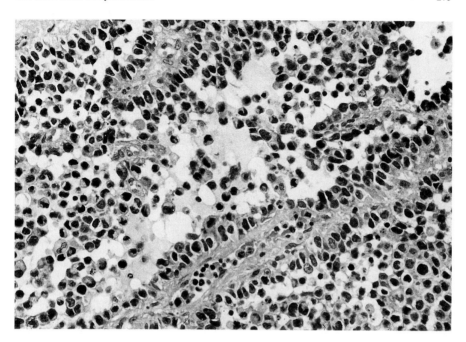

Fig. 2. Alveolar RMS at higher magnification. The slightly elongated tumor cells are arranged perpendicular to the fibrous septa. Small tumor cells containing small, but polymorphic and hyperchromatic nuclei. Poorly developed cytoplasm. Prominent loss of cell cohesion in the center of the tumor cell complexes with "free-floating" individual tumor cells. Same case as in Fig. 1; H&E, ×270

THÉRIAULT 1956; ENZINGER and SHIRAKI 1969) (Figs. 1 and 2). The individual cell complexes are surrounded by fibrous septa. These septa, which may be sclerotic and hyalinized, contain fibroblasts and myofibroblasts, collagen and reticulin fibers, in addition to blood vessels. Most important for the diagnosis of alveolar histology is the reticulin fiber stain (ENZINGER and SHIRAKI 1969): the tumor cell aggregates are surrounded by a dense framework of reticulin fibers, while the centers of the tumor cell complexes are virtually free of any fibers (Fig. 3). This is in contrast to eRMS which contains at least some reticulin fibers throughout the tumor tissue. Thus, the distinction between eRMS and aRMS in questionable cases can be achieved most easily by reticulin stain. Moreover, solid variants of aRMS show the same reticulin fiber pattern as classic aRMS.

Classic aRMS displays a "mixture" of solid areas and areas with completely or incompletely developed alveolar spaces. Solid areas (Fig. 4) are mainly located at the periphery of the tumor, while alveolar spaces tend to occur more frequently at the center of the lesion.

Typical alveolar spaces are lined by one row of round tumor cells which are attached to the fibrous septa and are arranged like a string of pearls (Figs. 1 and 2). In the center of the spaces some smaller aggregates of degenerated necrobiotic tumor cells with condensed hyperchromatic nuclei

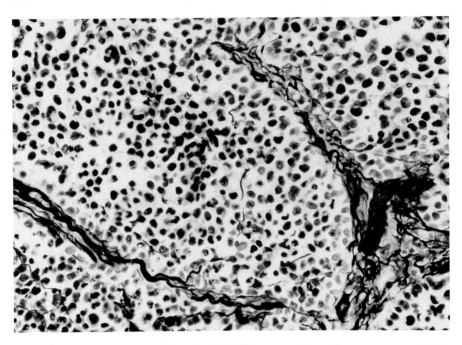

Fig. 3. Typical reticulin fiber pattern of aRMS. The tumor cell complexes are surrounded by a dense framework of reticulin fibers, while in the center of the tumor cell complexes only very few can be seen. Same case as in Fig. 1; reticulin stain, ×270

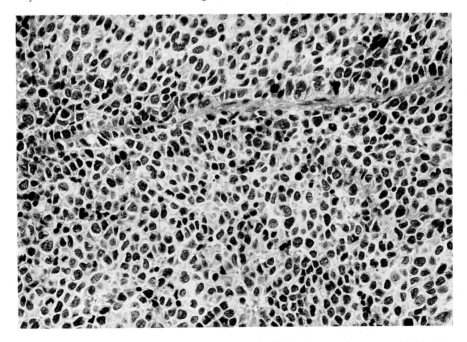

Fig. 4. Solid area of aRMS displaying the same cytologic features as other areas with alveolar pattern. Distant from the slender fibrous septum the tumor tissue is virtually devoid of vessels. Same case as in Fig. 1; H&E, ×270

are frequently seen. In addition, alveolar areas often contain large multi-nucleated tumor giant cells whose nuclei are arranged either wreath like at the cell periphery or more irregularly. Incompletely developed alveolar spaces exhibit loss of cell cohesion in varying degrees.

The formation of alveolar spaces must be considered a degenerative process which begins in the vessel-free central parts of the individual tumor cell aggregates. Loss of cell cohesion is the first morphological equivalent of cell degeneration, which is later followed by tumor cell necrobiosis and necrosis. Fully developed alveolar spaces are the final result of this degenerative process.

Cytologically, in most cases of aRMS the predominant cell types possess small to medium-sized round cells with polymorphic and hyperchromatic nuclei. The nucleoli are either small and inconspicuous or more or less prominent. The cytoplasm is generally scanty and eosinophilic. Some aRMS contain a dense population of small cells which are uniform in size and shape, and have distinct nuclear folds. Tumors composed almost entirely of such cells are classified by PALMER et al. (1983) as monomorphous RMS. De facto, monomorphous RMS are aRMS with an unfavorable prognosis. Other classic or solid aRMS consist of uniform round cells, similar to cells of Ewing's sarcoma, displaying a clear to weakly eosinophilic cytoplasm and

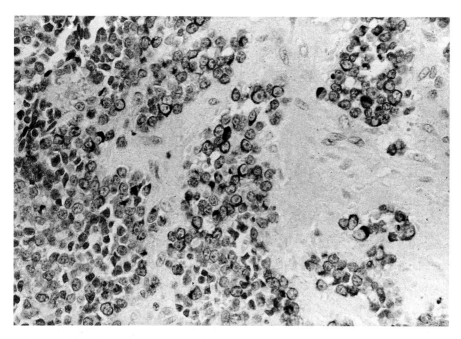

Fig. 5. Alveolar RMS reminiscent of atypical Ewing's sarcoma. Desmin-positive round tumor cells with round nuclei, moderately enlarged nucleoli, and sparse cytoplasm; 22-year-old male. Immunohisto-chemistry (PAP method), ×335

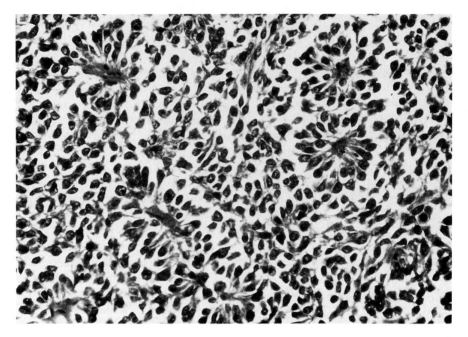

Fig. 6. Alveolar RMS displaying a rare, ependymoma-like pattern. The distinctly elongated tumor cells are arranged perpendicular to the fibrovascular structures. This tumor is desmin positive and contains other areas with typical alveolar spaces; 32-year-old male. H&E, ×270

round nuclei with ground glass-like chromatin and generally small, but usually distinct nucleoli (Fig. 5). In addition to these cell types round, cuboidal (pseudoepithelial) and club-shaped cells with distinctive rhabdomyoblastic differentiation with and without cross-striation can be seen. Generally, however, cross-striations are rare in aRMS. The same is true for strap cells which are so typical and almost diagnostic for eRMS.

Rarely, aRMS may display an ependymoma-like pattern (Fig. 6). In such cases elongated spindle cells are arranged perpendicularly to fibrovascular septa.

Another rare but important cytological feature of aRMS is the presence of round, eosinophilic cytoplasmic inclusions (Fig. 7). Such inclusions, representing (vimentin) intermediate filament accumulations at the ultrastructural level, are by no means specific for the malignant rhabdoid tumor (HAAS et al. 1981) since they can occur in a variety of other tumors (pseudo-rhabdoid pattern) (see WEEKS et al. 1986, 1989, 1991) and were described most recently in aRMS and eRMS by KODET et al. (1991).

It is notable that large pleomorphic cells with bizarre, hyperchromatic nuclei can occur in aRMS as well as in eRMS. Therefore, such RMS should be classified as aRMS or eRMS depending on the "basic" histology (KODET et al. 1993).

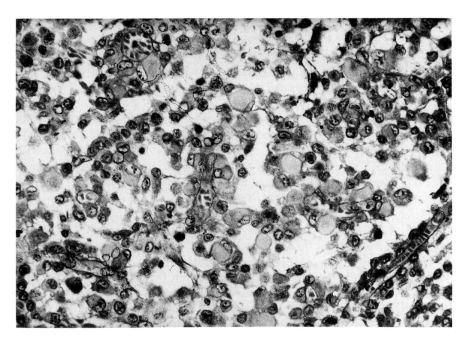

Fig. 7. Alveolar RMS presenting with so-called pseudorhabdoid pattern. Many tumor cells contain round, weakly eosinophilic, glassy cytoplasmic inclusions with nuclear displacement to the cell periphery. This case, which is indeed a RMS displaying cross-striations and strong desmin positivity, has to be distinguished from a "true" malignant renal and extrarenal rhabdoid tumor; 8-year-old male. Giemsa, ×335

Most aRMS cases are more or less (coarse, granular) PAS-positive (diastase-sensitive). Ewing's type cells of aRMS display the strongest positive PAS reaction, making it occasionally impossible to distinguish between true Ewing's sarcoma cells and Ewing's-type RMS cells by cytology and PAS reaction without additional immunohistochemistry. Nevertheless, the PAS reaction is helpful in recognizing aRMS, especially in predominantly solid tumor variants.

3 Immunohistochemistry

Immunohistochemical reactions are extremely important for confirming the diagnosis of aRMS and distinguishing aRMS from other round cell tumors. This is particularly true for poorly differentiated round-cellular aRMS devoid of detectable rhabdomyoblastic differentiation in conventional stains and even under electron-microscopic examination. With the improvement of immunohistochemical techniques most reactions can now be performed on paraffin sections after formalin fixation. Our experience has shown that the

APAAP method (CORDELL et al. 1984) is much more sensitive than the PAP method (STERNBERGER et al. 1970). Consequently, after staining with the APAAP method more cells will be positive with "muscle-specific" markers and even more undifferentiated tumor cells will react with a given antibody than after staining with the PAP method.

A large battery of muscle-specific markers has been published (for references see NINFO and CAVAZZANA 1991). In practice, desmin (ALTMANNSBERGER et al. 1982; MIETTINEN et al. 1982; HARMS et al. 1985; SEIDAL et al. 1987, 1990; DODD et al. 1989; KODET 1989), muscle-specific actin (HHF 35) (SEIDAL et al. 1990), myoglobin (BROOKS 1982; KINBDLOM et al. 1982), and vimentin are the most useful markers. Additional stains, employing antibodies against neuron-specific enolase (NSE), protein S-100, Leu 7, and cytokeratins may be useful either for detecting multidirectional, aberrant, or divergent expressions in aRMS or for differential diagnosis against other round cell tumors.

According to our experience (SCHMIDT et al. 1990) cases of aRMS react almost invariably with antibodies against desmin (41/42 = 97.6%) (Fig. 8), actin (44/45 = 97.8%), and vimentin (38/40 = 95%). It is noteworthy that desmin and actin positivity occur generally in a high percentage of tumor cells independent of the degree of the cell differentiation (Fig. 9). The

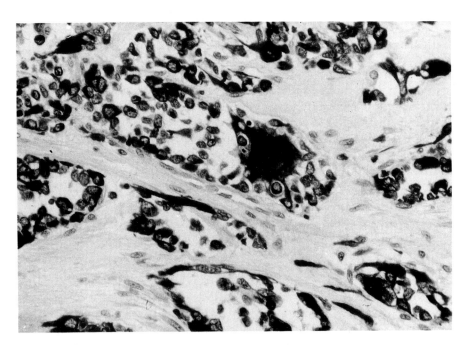

Fig. 8. Alveolar RMS with alveolar spaces lined by strongly desmin-positive tumor cells. In the center a likewise desmin-positive tumor giant cell; 12-year-old male. Immunohistochemistry (APAAP method), ×270

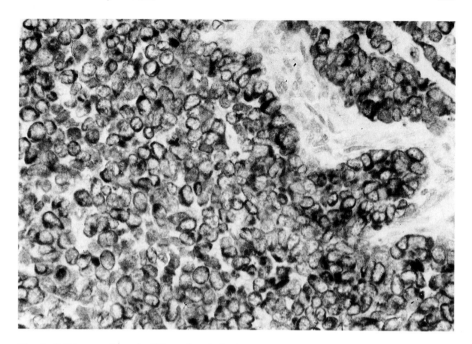

Fig. 9. Solid area of poorly differentiated aRMS with strong expression of desmin by virtually all tumor cells. This figure represents the sensitivity of immunohistochemistry; 15-year-old female. Immunohistochemistry (APAAP method), ×335

vimentin reaction, however, tends to become less positive or even negative in highly differentiated rhabdomyoblasts, but only two of our cases were completely vimentin negative. In contrast to desmin and actin, myoglobin positivity was found in 19/46 cases (41.3%), and in these cases typically the more differentiated cells expressed this skeletal-specific marker.

The myoglobin reaction is more specific for aRMS than reactions for desmin and actin (and the same is true for eRMS). However, the latter are more sensitive, supporting the diagnosis even in undifferentiated RMS, since undifferentiated RMS show desmin positivity but no myoglobin in a significant number of cases (DE JONG et al. 1984; SEIDAL et al. 1987, 1988). Thus, in practice, reactions against desmin and actin are more helpful than stainings for myoglobin, since myoglobin positivity presupposes at least some evidence of myoblastic differentiation, which in most cases can be detected either by conventional light microscopy or by additional electron microscopy.

The most frequent aberrant marker expressions in aRMS are neuron-specific enolase (NSE) (Fig. 10) and protein S-100 (Fig. 11) with 27/46 (58.7%) and 24/47 (51.1%) positive cases, respectively. The percentages of positive cells vary, but generally the amount of NSE- and protein S-100-positive cells was lower than the amount of desmin- and actin-positive cells. Furthermore, a significant number of cases expressed cytokeratins (7/47

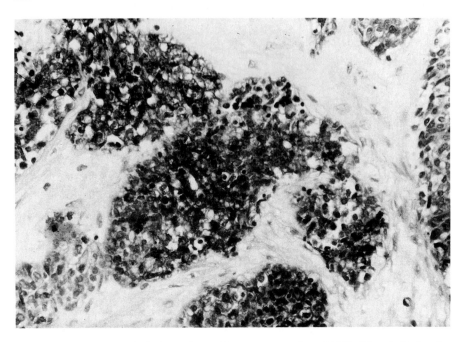

Fig. 10. Alveolar RMS displaying "aberrant" strong expression of NSE; 22-year-old female. Immunohistochemistry (APAAP method), ×270

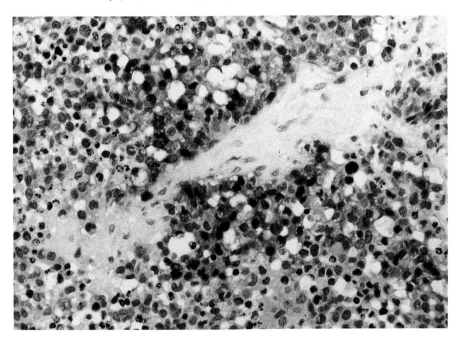

Fig. 11. Alveolar RMS expressing protein S-100 by many tumor cells (nuclear and cytoplasmic positivity); 20-year-old male. Immunohistochemistry (APAAP method), ×270

= 14.9%) after staining with the broad-spectrum anticytokeratin KL 1. Cytokeratin positivity in RMS was previously reported by COINDRE et al. (1988) and by MIETTINEN and RAPOLA (1989). In some cases cytokeratins present predominantly as globular cytoplasmic inclusions. In addition, positive reactions with the anticytokeratins AE 1 and Cam 5.2 occurred seldom (1/47 and 2/47, respectively). Finally, 26/44 (59.1%) cases were HNK 1 positive (antibody Leu 7). Such a high number of HNK 1-positive cases was observed only in aRMS, seeing that only 2/33 cases (6.1%) of eRMS expressed this antigen. The significance of HNK 1 expression in aRMS is unclear.

In summary, the immunohistochemical profile of aRMS (and eRMS) encompasses not only myogenous markers, but in fact a variety of myogenous and nonmyogenous antigens (in addition to vimentin).

4 Electron Microscopy

Electron microscopy is an unequivocally useful tool in recognizing RMS and its different subsets (MIERAU and FAVARA 1980; ERLANDSON 1987; SCHMIDT

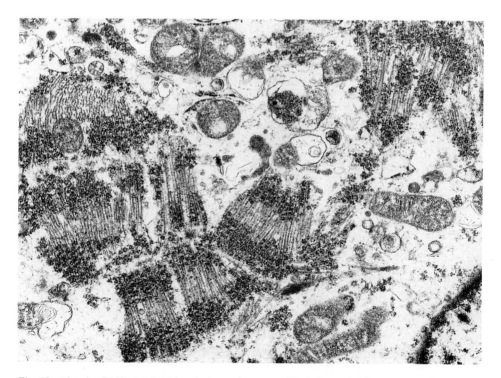

Fig. 12. Alveolar RMS examined by electron microscopy. Typical myosin/ribosome complexes as the minimal requirement for the ultrastructural diagnosis of RMS. ×19 200

et al. 1987; Mᴀᴄᴋᴀʏ 1990). Briefly, the presence of thick myosin filaments and thin actin filaments in the cytoplasm establishes the diagnosis of RMS at the ultrastructural level. In addition, ribosomes are often present and typically arranged in an indian file pattern along the thick filaments, the so-called myosin/ribosome complex (Fig. 12), which is the minimal criterion for the ultrastructural diagnosis of RMS (Eʀʟᴀɴᴅsᴏɴ 1987). In more different-iated cells Z-bands and occasional full banding can be seen.

Conversely, many RMS present as primitive, undifferentiated tumors without any diagnostic criteria. Thus, in the material of Mɪᴇʀᴀᴜ and Fᴀᴠᴀʀᴀ (1980) 17 of 31 cases were devoid of myoblastic features, and even in cases where ample block material was available for electron microscopy, only 40 of 54 RMS displayed myofilaments (Sᴄʜᴍɪᴅᴛ et al. 1987). Consequently, with their increasing sensitivity, immunohistochemical methods became the more useful tool in the diagnosis of poorly differentiated RMS (Mɪᴇᴛᴛɪɴᴇɴ et al. 1982; Sᴇɪᴅᴀʟ et al. 1988, 1990).

Independent of the "diagnostic value" of electron microscopy, ultra-structural studies have demonstrated significant differences between aRMS and eRMS (Sᴇɪᴅᴀʟ and Kɪɴᴅʙʟᴏᴍ 1984; Kᴏᴅᴇᴛ 1985). Alveolar RMS are characterized by myoblastic differentiation, while eRMS generally display both primitive fibroblast-like cells *and* myoblasts (Kᴏᴅᴇᴛ 1985). Thus, eRMS is basically a more primitive type of RMS than aRMS.

5 Cytogenetics

There is increasing evidence that the reciprocal chromosomal translocation t(2;13)(q37;q14), first described by Sᴇɪᴅᴀʟ et al. (1982), is consistent (Tᴜʀᴄ-Cᴀʀᴇʟ et al. 1986) and specific (Dᴏᴜɢʟᴀss et al. 1987) for aRMS (Eɴɢᴇʟ et al. 1988; Wᴀɴɢ-Wᴜᴜ et al. 1988; Vᴀʟᴇɴᴛɪɴᴇ et al. 1989; Nᴏᴊɪᴍᴀ and Aʙᴇ 1990). In contrast, eRMS does not display this characteristic chromosomal rearrangement. To this extent, cytogenetic analysis can discriminate aRMS from other RMS and, in addition, provides evidence that both RMS sub-types are different tumor *types* even at the chromosomal level.

6 DNA Cytometry

The concordance rate between flow and image cytometry in RMS was found to be 83% (Kᴏᴡᴀʟ-Vᴇʀɴ et al. 1990). Ploidy studies done by different investigators showed that the DNA level is variable in both RMS types. Diploidy occurs in aRMS as well as in eRMS and is prognostically an unfavorable indicator independent of histology (Sʜᴀᴘɪʀᴏ et al. 1991). Hy-perdiploid DNA levels were exclusively associated with eRMS, while near-

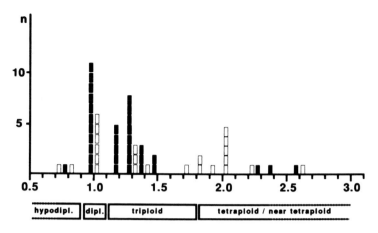

Fig. 13. Results of DNA analysis in aRMS (*open columns*) and RMS (*solid columns*). Tetraploid and near-tetraploid DNA levels occurred predominantly in aRMS, while hyperdiploid/near-triploid DNA levels were associated most often with eRMS. Diploidy can occur both in eRMS and aRMS. DNA image cytometry

tetraploidy occurred with significantly greater frequency in aRMS (SHAPIRO et al. 1991). In our own material the average DNA indices in aRMS and eRMS differed slightly (1.52 ± 0.50 and 1.31 ± 0.42, respectively) (LEUSCHNER et al. 1990). Triploid DNA levels dominated in eRMS, whereas aRMS were more often tetraploid than eRMS. Except for our finding that some aRMS were near triploid (Fig. 13), our results are similar to those presented by SHAPIRO et al. (1991).

7 Differential Diagnosis

Alveolar RMS displaying alveolar spaces and rhabdomyoblastic differentiation, at least in some cells, are easily recognizable tumors. In practice, though, aRMS may show an indistinct alveolar pattern and, more frequently particularly in small biopsy specimens, present as undifferentiated so-called round- and blue-cell tumors at the cytological level. Generally speaking, in conventionally stained slides unequivocal rhabdomyoblastic differentiation is more rare in aRMS than in the embryonal counterpart. This is especially true for cross-striations, which occur only in a small percentage of aRMS cases. Thus, in a significant number of cases the diagnosis of RMS remains uncertain by conventional hemotoxylin and eosin stain, therefore requiring special stains and immunohistochemical reactions. Of course, the application of electron microscopy in conjunction may be useful, too. However, many RMS lack any evidence of rhabdomyoblastic differentiation (MIERAU and FAVARA 1980). Thus, due to the increased sensitivity, modern immuno-

Table 1. Differential diagnosis between predominantly round-cell rhabdomyosarcoma and other round-cell tumors of childhood and adolescence by immunohistochemistry and by the PAS reaction. Note that none of the single criteria is axiomatic (diagnostic or exclusive) and that aberrant marker expressions occur frequently. Thus, only the main and most characteristic immunohistochemical profiles of the different tumor entities are mentioned in this table

	PAS	Cyto-keratins	Vimentin	Desmin	Myoglobin	Neuro-filaments	Muscle-specific actin	S-100	NSE	Panleukocytic antigen	Chromogranin A	Placental alkaline phosphatase	HBA71
Rhabdomyosarcoma	+	0	+	+	+/0	0	+	0	0	0	0	0	0
Malignant rhabdoid tumor	+	+	+	0	0	0	0	+	+	0	0	0	0
Ewing's sarcoma	+	0	+	0	0	0	0	0	0	0	0	0	+
Malignant peripheral neuroectodermal tumor	+	0	+	0	0	0	0	+	+	0	0	0	+
Neuroblastoma, undifferentiated	0	0	0	0	0	+	0	+/0	+	0	+	0	0
Nephroblastoma, blastemic	0	+	+	0	0	0	0	0	0	0	0	0	0
Medulloblastoma	0	0	0	0	0	+	0	0	+	0	0	0	0
Malignant non-Hodgkin's lymphomas, leukemias	0	0	+	0	0	0	0	0	0	+[b]	0	0	0
Germinomas[a]	+	0	0	0	0	0	0	0	0	0	0	+	0

[a] Including dysgerminoma.
[b] In large-cell anaplastic, CD30-positive lymphoma (so-called Ki-1-lymphoma) the reaction against panleukocytic antigen is negative in approximately 50% of cases.

histochemistry seems to be more effective in identifying RMS (SEIDAL et al. 1988).

In differential diagnosis the following list of somewhat common round-cell tumors of childhood and adolescence mimicking aRMS has to be taken into account in a given case of probable aRMS (this list is not complete, but includes most tumors which must be distinguished from aRMS in practice): malignant rhabdoid tumor, neuroblastomas including ganglioneuroblastoma, blastemic variants of nephroblastoma, Ewing's sarcoma and peripheral neuroepithelioma (malignant peripheral neuroectodermal tumor), germinomas including dysgerminoma and seminoma, malignant non-Hodgkin's lymphomas, tumorous leukemic infiltrates and medulloblastomas.

Usually, the distinction between these histogenetically different tumors is possible using a comparably small panel of immunohistochemical reactions in addition to the PAS reaction (in questionable cases with and without diastase digestion). Of course, the composition of such panels is variable from one laboratory to another, but most markers listed in Table 2 are commonly used (SWANSON and DEHNER 1991). Additional immunohistochemical reactions may be necessary in uncertain cases exhibiting no characteristic immunohistochemical profiles in the "standard panel." In practice, even "undifferentiated" RMS can be distinguished from other round-cell malignancies by strong expression of desmin and muscle-specific actin in a significant number of tumor cells, this in addition to a positive (diastase-sensitive) PAS reaction.

Although the alveolar pattern is highly characteristic for aRMS, a variety of other round-cell tumors may also display alveolar structures. These include alveolar soft part sarcoma (diagnostic diastase-resistant PAS-positive crystals), malignant rhabdoid tumor, malignant peripheral neuroectodermal tumor (Fig. 14), malignant melanoma, malignant extranodal non-Hodgkin's lymphomas and, of practical importance, tumors of the germinoma group with or without multinucleated syncytial trophoblastic cells, which can

Table 2. Differential diagnosis of aRMS and other round-cell tumors which can present with alveolar pattern

Tumor type	Main criteria for distinction[a]
Alveolar RMS	Desmin+, actin+, myoglobin+/0
Malignant rhabdoid tumor	Nuclear morphology, intracytoplasmic inclusions, cytokeratin+, S-100+, NSE+
Malignant peripheral neuroectodermal tumor	"Ewing's" cytology, NSE+, S-100+, desmin 0, HBA71+
Malignant melanoma	Nuclear morphology, melanin+/0, S-100+, melanoma antibody (HMB45)+, PAS 0
Malignant (extranodal) non-Hodgkin's lymphomas	PAS 0, panleukocytic antigen+
Germinomas (including dysgerminoma and seminoma)	Placental alkaline phosphatase+ (syncytial giant cells β-HCG+)

[a] Further immunohistochemical criteria – cf. Table 1.

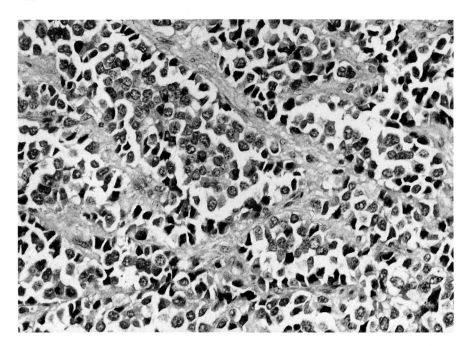

Fig. 14. Alveolar pattern in malignant peripheral neuroectodermal tumor (malignant peripheral neuroectodermal tumor; peripheral neuroepithelioma). This case could be distinguished from aRMS only by immunohistochemistry (negative desmin reaction!); 8-year-old male. H&E, ×270

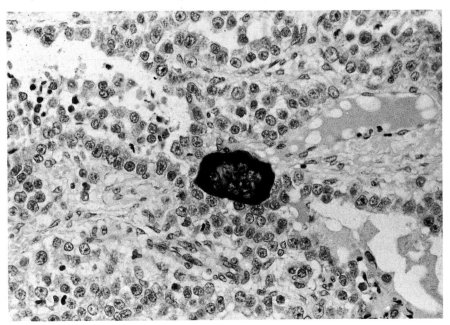

Fig. 15. Alveolar pattern in a dysgerminoma of the ovary. Lining of alveolar spaces by tumor cells. In the center a multinucleated giant cell which reacted strongly with an antibody against β-HCG; 9-year-old female. Immunohistochemistry (PAP method), ×270

mimic multinucleated giant cells in aRMS (Fig. 15). Thus, an alveolar pattern compels to the exclusion of several tumor types in the histopathologic differential diagnosis of aRMS.

In conclusion, the distinction between aRMS and other soft tissue malignancies will be possible in most cases by conventional histology and immunohistochemistry (provided that adequate tumor material is available). Other diagnostic techniques, e.g., electron microscopy, will be necessary only in a comparably small number of cases.

8 Important Clinicopathologic Data

Alveolar RMS can occur at any age, even in the newborn and during infancy (RAGAB et al. 1986; KOSCIELNIAK et al. 1989; HARMS 1990; PAIS and RAGAB 1991). In our own material comprising 215 cases of aRMS, 21.4% developed in the first quinquennium of life, 27.0% in the second, 26.0% in the third, and 25.6% of the patients were older than 15 years. Thus, with the exception of a slightly lower percentage of cases in the first quinquennium, cases of aRMS are distributed almost equally among the age groups of childhood and adolescence. Similar data have been reported previously by HAYS et al. (1982).

In contrast, most cases of eRMS (75.0% of 541 cases) occurred in the first two quinquennia of life. Only 25.0% of eRMS presented in children and adolescents older than 10 years. The proportion of eRMS to aRMS in the different age groups is 7:1 in children less than 10 years of age, but only 1.2:1 in children older than 10 years and in adolescents. Thus, the decrease in the proportion of eRMS to aRMS with increasing age is mainly due to the decreased incidence of eRMS and is attributable only to a minor degree to an increase of the alveolar tumor type (cf. HAYS et al. 1982; RUYMANN and GRUFFERMAN 1991).

Overall, the percentage of aRMS is considerably lower than that of eRMS. According to the data of the Kiel Pediatric Tumor Registry, 28.1% of all RMS display alveolar histology, while 70.6% are eRMS. By contrast, pleomorphic RMS is so rare (1.3%) that it can be neglected in statistical evaluations. Compared with these percentages, data from the Intergroup Rhabdomyosarcoma Study (IRS) show an almost identical percentage distribution of alveolar, embryonal, and pleomorphic RMS: 26.0%, 73.2%, and 0.8%, respectively (NEWTON et al. 1988).

Unlike eRMS, which occurs mainly in the head and neck region (including the orbit) and in the genitourinary tract, aRMS predominantly develops at the extremities. According to the Cooperative Soft Tissue Sarcoma Study (CWS) 45 of 115 cases of aRMS (39.1%) were located at the extremities, whereas only 23/363 eRMS (6.3%) occurred in this location (data from CWS 81/86, protocol patients). In the IRS-II material 94/208

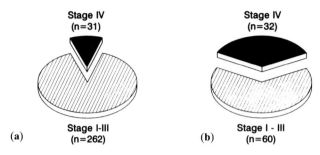

Fig. 16a,b. Relative incidence and stage distribution (I–III versus IV) of eRMS (**a**) and aRMS (**b**). Patients with aRMS present significantly more often with stage IV (metastatic disease) than patients with eRMS. Data from the CWS Study (Chairman: Prof. Dr. J. Treuner) (CWS 81/86, 8/90; protocol and non-protocol patients)

cases of aRMS (45.2%) and only 39/565 cases of eRMS (6.9%) manifested at the extremities (RUYMANN and GRUFFERMAN 1991). Thus, despite the low total number of cases aRMS is absolutely more frequent at the extremities than eRMS.

However, it would be incorrect to consider aRMS a sarcoma restricted only to the extremities, since 60.9% of the CWS cases and 54.8% of the IRS-II cases (RUYMANN and GRUFFERMAN 1991) were observed in non-extremity sites. In absolute numbers eRMS is generally much more frequent in these regions than aRMS. With regard to the main RMS locations both the lowest frequency and the lowest percentages of aRMS were seen in the genitourinary region: seven cases (6.1%) and five cases (2.4%) in the CWS and the IRS-II (RUYMANN and GRUFFERMAN 1991), respectively.

In conclusion, aRMS and eRMS differ in age distribution, relative and absolute frequency, and main tumor locations. These facts are by no means only of academic and statistical interest, since both RMS types display important differences concerning biological behavior and prognosis.

Data from the IRS show that a higher percentage of aRMS than eRMS present with metastatic disease at the time of diagnosis (GEHAN et al. 1981; RANEY et al. 1988). In the combined CWS 81/86 material (Fig. 16), 34.8% of the patients with aRMS had distant metastases at the time of presentation (stage IV, corresponding to group IV in the IRS staging system), while only 10.6% of eRMS were stage IV cases (protocol *and* non-protocol patients evaluated, since stage IV patients generally are considered to be non-protocol patients in the German CWS). This important difference between aRMS and eRMS is highly significant.

In contrast, most eRMS (89.4%) presented with stages I–III, hence as local or locoregional disease, whereas this was true for only 65.2% of aRMS cases. Similar data were gathered recently in a European multicenter analysis (KOSCIELNIAK et al. 1992).

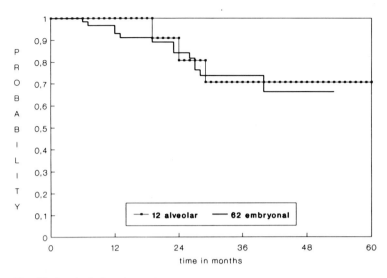

Fig. 17. Survival of patients with stage III RMS according to histology (protocol patients). No difference exists between aRMS and eRMS. Data from the CWS Study (CWS 88, 8/90)

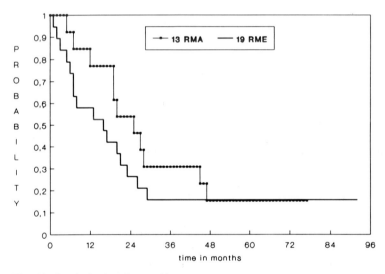

Fig. 18. Survival of patients with stage IV RMS according to histology (protocol and non-protocol patients). No difference exists between alveolar and embryonal RMS. Data from the Cooperative Soft Tissue Sarcoma Study (CWS 81, 8/90)

Thus, eRMS is basically a locoregional disease at the time of diagnosis, while aRMS tends to be a disseminated (metastatic) disease. The latter statement is supported by several reports of leukemia- or lymphoma-like bone marrow involvement at the time of presentation (Toch 1972; Nunez et

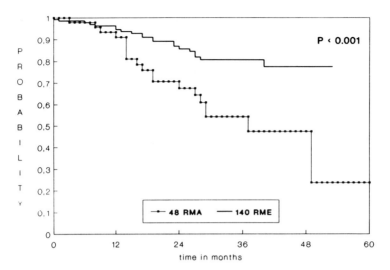

Fig. 19. Overall survival of patients with RMS according to histology (all stages, protocol and non-protocol patients): a highly significantly worse prognosis for patients with aRMS. Data from the CWS Study (CWS 88, 8/90)

al. 1983; RUYMANN et al. 1984; ENGEL et al. 1988; MECHTERSHEIMER et al. 1989) and the observation that in IRS-group I RMS alveolar histology was the factor with the worst prognosis. It was the only patient characteristic consistently related to survival (CRIST et al. 1990). Furthermore, patients with extremity RMS and hence a high proportion of alveolar histology present with metastatic disease in a higher percentage of cases than RMS of all other sites (27% versus 18%) (HAYS et al. 1982; WIENER and HAYS 1991). Overall, the mortality of aRMS is higher than that of eRMS. This can be clearly demonstrated with data from the IRS (HAYS et al. 1982; SHIMADA et al. 1987).

According to CWS data the *stage*-related survival of RMS is independent of histologic RMS type (alveolar vs. embryonal) (see Figs. 17 and 18). At first glance this finding is unexpected; however, patients suffering from aRMS had a significantly worse prognosis (probability of survival) than patients with eRMS (Fig. 19, data from CWS 86). Thus, it can be concluded that stage determines prognosis in RMS, but stage is related to histology! In summary, histology has proven to be a major prognostic factor in RMS.

9 Conclusions

Alveolar RMS (including the solid variant) is a distinct tumor entity which differs from eRMS (including botryoid and spindle-cell variant) in many respects:

1. Histologically, the tumor cell complexes are arranged in solid aggregates, lacking capillaries and reticulin fibers. These aggregates are surrounded by fibrous tissue. The formation of alveolar spaces is due to the loss of cell cohesion with consecutive cell degeneration in the center of the individual cell aggregates. Thus, the amount of alveolar pattern is variable both from tumor to tumor and in individual tumors. Moreover, the alveolar space is not an essential criterion for the diagnosis of aRMS if other histologic and cytologic criteria of aRMS are realized (solid variant of aRMS).

2. By conventional histology, the tumor cells in aRMS are often less well-differentiated than in eRMS. Thus, modern techniques like immunohistochemistry (± electron microscopy) are necessary for the identification of aRMS in a considerable number of cases. Desmin intermediate filaments and muscle-specific actin are the most sensitive and useful markers of poorly differentiated aRMS (as well as for eRMS) in addition to a positive, diastase-sensitive PAS reaction.

3. Electron microscopically, aRMS shows myoblastic differentiation, while in eRMS a primitive, fibroblast-like cell predominates. Thus, at the ultrastructural level eRMS is a more primitive form of RMS than aRMS.

4. Cytogenetically, aRMS display a specific chromosomal translocation t(2;13) (q37;q14), this in sharp contrast to eRMS.

5. Alveolar RMS are more often near tetraploid than eRMS, as demonstrated by DNA cytometry. Hyperdiploidy is associated predominantly with eRMS, while diploidy can occur in both RMS types (indicating an unfavorable outcome).

6. Clinicopathologic data display further important differences between aRMS and eRMS: (a) the age distribution of aRMS is almost constant in childhood and adolescence, while most eRMS occur in the first 10 years of life; (b) overall, eRMS are more frequent than aRMS – in two large series (IRS and CWS) the relative frequency of aRMS is 26% and 28.1%, respectively; (c) most RMS of the extremities are aRMS, whereas eRMS dominates in the head and neck region (including the orbit) and in the genitourinary tract; (d) a higher percentage of aRMS cases presents with metastatic disease at the time of diagnosis (aRMS: 34.8%; eRMS: 10.6%). Thus, the tendency to hematogeneous tumor dissemination is much more pronounced in aRMS than in eRMS; (e) overall, the prognosis of aRMS is significantly more unfavorable than the prognosis of eRMS.

In summary, aRMS is a well-defined RMS type with characteristic morphology and biologic behavior. It is necessary to distinguish aRMS from all other RMS types, especially eRMS.

References

Almannsberger M, Osborn M, Treuner J, Hölscher A, Weber K, Schauer A (1982) Diagnosis of human childhood rhabdomyosarcoma by antibodies to desmin, the structural protein of muscle specific intermediate filaments. Virchows Arch [B] 39: 203–215

Bale PM, Parsons RE, Stevens MM (1983) Diagnosis and behavior of juvenile rhabdomyosarcoma. Hum Pathol 14: 596–611

Brooks JJ (1982) Immunohistochemistry of soft tissue tumors. Myoglobin as a tumor marker for rhabdomyosarcoma. Cancer 50: 1757–1763

Coindre JM, de Mascarel A, Trojani M, de Mascarel J, Pages A (1988) Immunohistochemical study of rhabdomyosarcoma. Unexpected staining with S 100 protein and cytokeratin. J Pathol 155: 127–132

Cordell JL, Falini B, Erber WN, Ghosh AK, Zainalabideen A, MacDonald S, Pulford KAF, Stein H, Mason DY (1984) Immunoenzymatic labeling of monoclonal antibodies using immune complexes of alkaline phosphatase and monoclonal anti-alkaline phosphatase (APAAP complexes). J Histochem Cytochem 32: 219–229

Crist WM, Garnsey L, Beltangady MS, Gehan E, Ruymann F, Webber B, Hays DM, Wharam M, Maurer HM (1990) Prognosis in children with rhabdomyosarcoma: a report of the Intergroup Rhabdomyosarcoma Studies I and II. J Clin Oncol 8: 443–452

de Jong ASH, van Vark M, Albus-Lutter CE, van Raamsdonk W, Voûte PA (1984) Myosin and myoglobin as tumor markers in the diagnosis of rhabdomyosarcoma. A comparative study. Am J Surg Pathol 8: 521–528

Dodd S, Malone M, McCulloch W (1989) Rhabdomyosarcoma in children: a histological and immunohistochemical study of 59 cases. J Pathol 158: 13–18

Donglass EC, Valentine M, Etcubanas E et al. (1987) A specific chromosomal abnormality in rhabdomyosarcoma. Cytogenet Cell Genet 45: 148–155

Engel R, Ritterbach J, Schwabe D, Lampert F (1988) Chromosome translocation (2;13)(q37; q14) in a disseminated alveolar rhabdomyosarcoma. Eur J Pediatr 148: 69–71

Enzinger FM, Shiraki M (1969) Alveolar rhabdomyosarcoma. An analysis of 110 cases. Cancer 24: 18–31

Erlandson RA (1987) The ultrastructural distinction between rhabdomyosarcoma and other undifferentiated "sarcomas". Ultrastruct Pathol 11: 83–101

Gehan EA, Glover FN, Maurer HM, Sutow WW, Hays DM, Lawrence W Jr, Newton WA Jr, Soule EH (1981) Prognostic factors in children with rhabdomyosarcoma. Natl Cancer Inst Monogr 56: 83–92

Haas JE, Palmer NF, Weinberg AG, Beckwith JB (1981) Ultrastructure of malignant rhabdoid tumor of the kidney. A distinctive renal tumor of children. Hum Pathol 12: 646–657

Harms D (1990) Cancer in the first year of life – pathology. Report from the Kiel Pediatric Tumor Registry. Gaslini 22: 115–121

Harms D, Schmidt D, Treuner J (1985) Soft-tissue sarcomas in childhood. A study of 262 cases including 169 cases of rhabdomyosarcoma. Z Kinderchir 40: 140–145

Hays DM, Soule EH, Lawrence W Jr, Gehan EA, Maurer HM, Donaldson M, Raney RB, Tefft M (1982) Extremity lesions in the Intergroup Rhabdomyosarcoma Study (IRS-I): a preliminary report. Cancer 48: 1–8

Hays DM, Newton W Jr, Soule EH, Foulkes MA, Raney RB, Tefft M, Ragab A, Maurer HM (1983) Mortality among children with rhabdomyosarcomas of the alveolar histologic subtype. J Pediatr Surg 18: 412–417

Kindblom LG, Seidal T, Karlsson K (1982) Immuno-histochemical localization of myoglobin in human muscle tissue and embryonal and alveolar rhabdomyosarcoma. Acta Pathol Microbiol Immunol Scand [A] 90: 167–174

Kodet R (1985) Rabdomyosarkom v detskem veku. II. Ultrastruktura (Rhabdomyosarcoma in childhood. II. Ultrastructure). Cesk Patol 21: 201–208

Kodet R (1989) Rhabdomyosarcoma in childhood. An immunohistochemical analysis with myoglobin, desmin and vimentin. Pathol Res Pract 185: 207–213

Kodet R, Newton WA Jr, Hamoudi AB, Asmar L (1991) Rhabdomyosarcomas with intermediate-filament inclusions and features of rhabdoid tumors. Light microscopic and immunohistochemical study. Am J Surg Pathol 15: 257–267

Kodet R, Newton WA Jr, Hamoudi AB, Asmar L, Jacobs DL, Maurer HM (1993) Childhood rhabdomyosarcoma with anaplastic (pleomorphic) features. A report of the Intergroup Rhabdomyosarcoma Study. Am J Surg Pathol 17: 443–453

Koscielniak E, Harms D, Schmidt D, Ritter J, Keim M, Riehm H, Treuner J (1989) Soft tissue sarcomas in infants younger than 1 year of age: a report of the German Soft Tissue Sarcoma Study Group (CWS-81). Med Pediatr Oncol 17: 105–110

Koscielniak E, Rodary C, Flamant F, Carli M, Treuner J, Pinkerton R, Grotto P (1992) Metastatic rhabdomyosarcoma and histologically similar tumors in childhood: a retrospective European multi-center analysis. Med Pediatr Oncol 20: 209–214

Kowal-Vern A, Gonzalez-Crussi F, Turner J, Trujillo Y, Chou P, Herman C, Castelli M, Walloch J (1990) Flow and image cytometric DNA analysis in rhabdomyosarcoma. Cancer Res 50: 6023–6027

Leuschner I, Schmidt D, Möller R, Harms D (1990) DNA-Ploidie und "nuclear organizer regions" bei Rhabdomyosarkomen. Ein Vergleich mit den klinischen Stadien und dem Verlauf. Verh Dtsch Ges Pathol 74: 589

Mackay B (1990) Electron microscopy of soft tissue tumours. In: Fletcher CDM, McKee PH (eds) Pathobiology of soft tissue tumours. Churchill Livingstone, Edinburgh, pp 199–220

Mechtersheimer G, Haas R, Katus HA, Möller P (1989) Leukämieverdächtige Panzytopenie als Initialsymptom eines alveolären Rhabdomyosarkoms des Hodens. Pathologe 10: 252–256

Mierau GM, Favara BE (1980) Rhabdomyosarcoma in children: Ultrastructural study of 31 cases. Cancer 46: 2035–2040

Miettinen M, Rapola J (1989) Immunohistochemical spectrum of rhabdomyosarcoma and rhabdomyosarcoma-like tumors. Expression of cytokeratin and the 68-kD neurofilament protein. Am J Surg Pathol 13: 120–132

Miettinen M, Lehto VP, Badley RA, Virtanen I (1982) Alveolar rhabdomyosarcoma. Demonstration of the muscle type of intermediate filament protein, desmin, as a diagnostic aid. Am J Pathol 108: 246–251

Newton WA Jr, Soule EH, Hamoudi AB, Reiman HM, Shimada H, Beltangady M, Maurer H (1988) Histopathology of childhood sarcomas, Intergroup Rhabdomyosarcoma Studies I and II: clinicopathologic correlation. J Clin Oncol 6: 67–75

Newton W, Triche T, Marsden H, Ninfo V, Harms D, Gehan E, Maurer H (1989) International Childhood Soft Tissue Sarcoma Pathology Classification Study: design and implementation utilizing Intergroup Rhabdomyosarcoma Study II clinical and pathology data. Med Pediatr Oncol 17: 308 (abstract)

Ninfo V, Cavazzana AO (1991) Tumors of muscle tissue. In: Ninfo V, Chung EB, Cavazzana AD (eds) Tumors and tumorlike lesions of soft tissue. Churchill Livingstone, New York, pp 91–121

Nojima T, Abe S (1990) A case of alveolar rhabdomyosarcoma with a chromosomal translocation, t(2;13) (q37;q14). Virchows Arch [A] 417: 357–359

Nunez C, Abboud SL, Lemon NC, Kemp JA (1983) Ovarian rhabdomyosarcoma presenting as leukemia. Case report. Cancer 52: 297–300

Pais RC, Ragab AH (1991) Rhabdomyosarcoma in infancy. In: Maurer HM, Ruymann FB, Pochedly C (eds) Rhabdomyosarcoma and related tumors in children and adolescents. CRC Press, Boca Raton, pp 373–384

Palmer NF, Foulkes MA, Sachs N, Newton WA (1983) Rhabdomyosarcoma: a cytological classification of prognostic significance. Proc Am Soc Clin Oncol 2: 229

Ragab AH, Heyn R, Tefft M, Hays DN, Newton WA Jr, Beltangady M (1986) Infants younger than 1 year of age with rhabdomyosarcoma. Cancer 58: 2606–2610

Raney RB Jr, Tefft M, Maurer HM, Ragab AH, Hays DM, Soule EH, Foulkes MA, Gehan EA (1988) Disease patterns and survival rate in children with metastatic soft-tissue sarcoma. A report from the Intergroup Rhabdomyosarcoma Study (IRS)-I. Cancer 62: 1257–1266

Riopelle JL, Thériault JP (1956) Sur une forme méconnue de sarcome des parties molles: Le rhabdomyosarcome alvéolaire. Ann Anat Pathol 1: 88–111

Ruymann FB, Grufferman S (1991) Introduction and epidemiology of soft tissue sarcomas. In: Maurer HM, Ruymann FB, Pochedly C (eds) Rhabdomyosarcoma and related tumors in children and adolescents. CRC Press, Boca Raton, pp 3–18

Ruymann FB, Newton WA Jr, Ragab AH, Donaldson MH, Foulkes M (1984) Bone marrow metastases at diagnosis in children and adolescents with rhabdomyosarcoma. Cancer 53: 368–373

Schmidt D, Harms D, Pilon VA (1987) Small-cell pediatric tumors: histology, immunohistochemistry, and electron microscopy. Clin Lab Med 7: 63–89

Schmidt D, Leuschner I, Moeller R, Harms D (1990) Immunhistochemische Befunde bei Rhabdomyosarkomen. Pathologe 11: 283–289

Seidal T, Kindblom LG (1984) The ultrastructure of alveolar and embryonal rhabdomyosarcoma. A correlative light and electron microscopic study of 17 cases. Acta Pathol Microbiol Immunol Scand [A] 92: 231–248
Seidal T, Mark J, Haymar B, Angervall L (1982) Alveolar rhabdomyosarcoma: a cytogenetic
and correlated cytological and histological study. Acta Pathol Microbiol Immunol Scand [A]
90: 345–354
Seidal T, Kindblom LG, Angervall L (1987) Myoglobin, desmin and vimentin in ultrastructurally proven rhabdomyomas and rhabdomyosarcomas. An immunohistochemical study
utilizing a series of monoclonal and polyclonal antibodies. Appl Pathol 5: 201–219
Seidal T, Kindblom LG, Angervall L (1988) Alveolar and poorly differentiated rhabdomyosarcoma. A clinicopathologic, light-microscopic, ultrastructural and immunohistochemical
analysis. Acta Pathol Microbiol Immunol Scand [A] 96: 825–838
Seidal T, Angervall L, Kindblom LG (1990) Expression of muscle-specific actins and myosin in
light microscopically undifferentiated small and dark cell malignancies of soft tissues. Acta
Pathol Microbiol Immunol Scand [A] 98: 1105–1112
Shapiro DN, Parham DM, Douglass EC, Ashmun R, Webber BL, Newton WA Jr, Hancock
ML, Maurer HM, Look AT (1991) Relationship of tumor-cell ploidy to histologic subtype
and treatment outcome in children and adolescents with unresectable rhabdomyosarcoma. J
Clin Oncol 9: 159–166
Shimada H, Newton WA Jr, Soule EH, Beltangady MS, Maurer HM (1987) Pathology of fatal
rhabdomyosarcoma. Report from Intergroup Rhabdomyosarcoma Study (IRS-I and IRS-II).
Cancer 59: 459–465
Sternberger LA, Hardy PH Jr, Cuculis JJ, Meyer HG (1970) The unlabeled antibody enzyme
method of immunohistochemistry. Preparation and properties of soluble antigen-antibody
complex (horseradish peroxidase-antihorseradish peroxidase) and its use in identification of
spirochetes. J Histochem Cytochem 18: 315–333
Swanson PE, Dehner LP (1991) Pathology of soft tissue sarcomas in children and adolescents.
In: Maurer HM, Ruymann FB, Pochedly C (eds) Rhabdomyosarcoma and related tumors in
children and adolescents. CRC Press, Boca Raton, pp 385–420
Toch R (1972) Case records of the Massachusetts General Hospital. Case 4 – 1972. N Engl J
Med 286: 205–212
Tsokos M, Miser A, Pizzo P, Triche T (1984) Histologic and cytologic characteristics of poor
prognosis childhood rhabdomyosarcoma. Lab Invest 50: 61A
Tsokos M, Miser A, Wesley R, Miser JS, Kinsella TJ, Grayson J, Pizzo PA, Glatstein E,
Triche TJ (1985) Solid variant alveolar rhabdomyosarcoma: a primitive rhabdomyosarcoma
with poor prognosis and distinct histology. Interational Society of Paediatric Oncology,
XVIIth meeting, Venice (abstract-volume), pp 71–74
Tsokos M, Webber BL, Parham DM, Wesley RA, Miser A, Miser JS, Etcubanas E, Kinsella
T, Grayson J, Glatstein E, Pizzo PA, Triche TJ (1992) Rhabdomyosarcoma. A new class-
ification scheme related to prognosis. Arch Pathol Lab Med 116: 847–855
Turc-Carel C, Lizard-Nacol S, Justrabo E, Favrot M, Philip T, Tabone E (1986) Consistent
chromosomal translocation in alveolar rhabdomyosarcoma. Cancer Genet Cytogenet 19:
361–362
Valentine M, Douglass EC, Look AT (1989) Closely linked loci on the long arm of chromosome
13 flank a specific 2; 13 translocation breakpoint in childhood rhabdomyosarcoma. Cytogenet
Cell Genet 52: 128–132
Wang-Wuu S, Soukup S, Ballard E, Gotwals B, Lampkin B (1988) Chromosomal analysis of
sixteen human rhabdomyosarcomas. Cancer Res 48: 983–987
Weeks DA, Beckwith JB, Mierau GW (1986) "Pseudo-rhabdoid" tumors of the kidney. Lab
Invest 54: 10P
Weeks DA, Beckwith JB, Mierau GW, Luckey DW (1989) Rhabdoid tumor of kidney. A
report of 111 cases from the National Wilms' Tumor Study Pathology Center. Am J Surg
Pathol 13: 439–458
Weeks DA, Beckwith JB, Mierau GW, Zuppan CW (1991) Renal neoplasms mimicking
rhabdoid tumor of kidney. A report from the National Wilms' Tumor Study Pathology
Center. Am J Surg Pathol 15: 1042–1054
Wiener ES, Hays DM (1991) Rhabdomyosarcoma in extremity and trunk sites. In: Maurer
HM, Ruymann FB, Pochedly C (eds) Rhabdomyosarcoma and related tumors in children
and adolescents. CRC Press, Boca Raton, pp 363–372

Malignant Peripheral Neuroectodermal Tumor

D. Schmidt

1 Definition

Primitive neuroectodermal tumors (PNETs) constitute a diverse group of small cell neoplasms which may occur in the central nervous system and in peripheral sites including the soft tissues and bone. Accordingly, they have been subdivided into central and peripheral PNETs. The revised classification system of the World Health Organization (WHO) on pediatric brain tumors by Rorke et al. (1985) provoked a continuous discussion on the former group of tumors with some principal investigators deeming it a too simplistic scheme and favoring the retention of the conventional classification system (Rubinstein 1987).

No such controversy surrounds the peripheral PNETs which have been well characterized during recent years by modern techniques including cytogenetics, molecular genetics, and molecular biology (Dehner 1986, 1993; Thiele 1991). The group of peripheral PNETs comprises the different forms of neuroblastoma (NB), Ewing's sarcoma (ES), malignant peripheral neuroectodermal tumor (MPNT), pigmented neuroectodermal tumor (retinal anlage tumor or progonoma), ectomesenchymoma, and the very rare peripheral medulloepithelioma (Table 1). Olfactory neuroblastoma (esthesioneuroblastoma) used to be considered by most investigators as belonging to the group of central PNETs, together with retinoblastoma. However, this concept is probably no longer tenable in view of the finding that olfactory neuroblastoma reveals the same reciprocal translocation t(11;22)(q24;q12)

Current Topics in Pathology
Volume 89, Eds. D. Harms/D. Schmidt
© Springer-Verlag Berlin Heidelberg 1995

Table 1. Peripheral primitive neuroectodermal tumors (PPNETs)

Neuroblastoma
Ewing's sarcoma
Malignant peripheral neuroectodermal tumor (of soft tissue and bone)
Olfactory neuroblastoma
Pigmented neuroectodermal tumor
Ectomesenchymoma
Peripheral medulloepithelioma

as ES and MPNT (WHANG-PENG et al. 1987). The same holds true for the malignant small cell tumor of the thoracopulmonary region (ASKIN et al. 1979) which is now widely accepted as a clinical and topographic variant of MPNT. Several synonyms have been proposed for MPNT including neuro-epithelioma (BAILEY and CUSHING 1926), peripheral neuroepithelioma (PN) (STOUT 1918), primitive neuroectodermal tumor (neuroblastoma) (NESBITT and VIDONE 1976), primitive neuroectodermal tumor (LIEBERMANN 1979), malignant neuroepithelioma (peripheral neuroblastoma) (HASHIMOTO et al. 1983), primitive neuroectodermal (neuroepithelial) tumor of soft tissue (SHUANGSHOTI 1986), and peripheral neuroectodermal sarcoma of soft tissue (LLOMBART-BOSCH et al. 1989). Very often, no clear distinction is made between primitive peripheral neuroectodermal tumors (PPNETs) and the central counterparts (PNETs in the more common clinical sense), which may cause considerable confusion in diagnosis and treatment. Therefore, we continue to call primitive peripheral neuroectodermal tumors MPNT and this term is also used throughout in this chapter.

2 Histogenesis

Among the clinicopathologic features of MPNT extensively studied during recent years, none has attracted as much interest as the question of its origin. A definite answer to this question would help in delineating MPNT from classical neuroblastoma, and also from the other entities in this group of tumors. This, in turn, would provide new insights into the different clinical and prognostic features. The suspicion of a neuroepithelial origin of MPNT dates back to as early as 1918 when A.P. STOUT described a tumor of the ulnar nerve which consisted of small, round cells arranged in masses and strands and separated by trabeculae of connective tissue. Further evidence for the capacity of neural differentiation in these tumors was provided over the years following through many studies applying electron microscopy (SCHMIDT et al. 1982), immunohistochemistry (LLOMBART-BOSCH et al. 1988), cell culture (CAVAZZANA et al. 1988), and molecular biology (YEGER et al. 1990). Besides demonstrating a neural phenotype in MPNT, these investigations also yielded convincing evidence that MPNT is histogenetically related to ES (MCKEON et al. 1988; USHIGOME et al. 1989; AMBROS et al. 1991; FELLINGER et al. 1991; FRIEDMAN et al. 1992), but not to classical neuroblastoma. In contrast to neuroblastoma, which may show N-myc amplification and/or N-myc overexpression, both ES and PNET express high levels of c-myc, but not of N-myc. This thesis was further supported by cytogenetic investigations which demonstrated a reciprocal translocation t(11;22)(q24; q12) in both MPNT (WHANG-PENG et al. 1984; LADANYI et al. 1990; GORMAN et al. 1991) and ES (AURIAS et al. 1984; DOUGLASS et al. 1986; SPELEMAN et al. 1992). The breakpoints have recently been defined (ZHANG et al. 1990; SELLERI et al. 1991) and cloned (DELATTRE et al. 1992). The same type of chromosomal anomaly was also found in the malignant small cell tumor of the thoracopulmonary region (SEEMAYER et al. 1985; WHANG-PENG et al. 1986), which is commonly referred to as an Askin tumor. A neural origin of this type of neoplasm was originally suggested by the finding of neurosecretory granules in three cases studied (ASKIN et al. 1979). Eventually, a unifying concept was proposed suggesting that ES and MPNT are related tumors representing a broad spectrum of tumors with different grades of neural differentiation (USHIGOME et al. 1989). According to this concept typical ES would represent the most immature form of peripheral neuroectodermal tumor, and MPNT with rosettes the most differentiated variant. Although this concept is no longer debated, the question as to the origin of ES and MPNT is still open. Most authors have proposed a derivation from neural crest cells, analogous to the concept which has been established for neuroblastoma. The rare demonstration of an elevated VMA excretion in urine has been used as an argument to support this view (VOSS et al. 1984). In neuroblastoma, the origin has been traced to neural crest cells which migrate to the developing sympathetic nervous system during embryogenesis. One questions, however, whether this concept applies to ES and MPNT, since no normal cellular correlate has ever been demonstrated for these tumors. Therefore, a strong point could be made in favor of a derivation from an uncommitted pluripotential cell, which may express a "neural" phenotype under certain circumstances, as was suggested by FUJII et al. (1989) and DEHNER (1990). Moreover, this cell could express combined neural (glial) and non-neural phenotypes including epithelial (MOLL et al. 1987; ALBA GRECO et al. 1988; HACHITANDA et al. 1990) and myogenic differentiation (PARHAM et al. 1992) as evidenced by intermediate filament typing and electron microscopy. If one accepted this hypothesis it would no longer be necessary to exhaust the neural crest theory as an explanation of a "neural" tumor in an unusual location.

3 Clinical Features

3.1 Age, Sex, and Location

Among the clinical findings routinely evaluated in the diagnosis and differential diagnosis of MPNT serum catecholamine levels and the excretion of VMA and HVA in 24-hour urine are of great importance. With a few exceptions, the levels of these compounds have been reported to be within normal limits, in contrast to most cases of NB, in which at least one of the compounds of the catecholamine metabolic pathway is elevated.

In contrast to NB, which usually affects infants and young children, MPNT occurs in all age groups including adults (MACKAY et al. 1976; VERWEY et al. 1985) with a peak age incidence in adolescence and young adulthood. Variations in mean age are often influenced by the case material which is received. Thus, the mean age of the patients in the files of the Kiel Pediatric Tumor Registry is 15.2 years (SCHMIDT et al. 1991), compared to 21 years in the series of HASHIMOTO et al. (1983). KUSHNER et al. (1991) studied 54 cases from the Memorial Sloan-Kettering Cancer Center and found a median age of 17 years. In our study, patients with MPNT were older than those with ES. This was one of the clinical findings which emerged using a new classification system for ES and MPNT.

In accordance with previous findings we found that male patients were more often affected than females including cases of MPNT in the chest wall. Another interesting finding was the different tumor locations. Cases of MPNT were mostly found in the thoracopulmonary region (Fig. 1), whereas ES predominated in the pelvis and the lower extremities. Thus, our data support the earlier findings of ASKIN et al. (1979) that MPNT is a tumor with preferential localization in the chest wall. Most of the cases in our study were soft tissue tumors with secondary involvement of adjacent bones. However, MPNTs are by no means restricted to the soft tissues, since they have been found in bone (JAFFE et al. 1984; USHIGOME et al. 1984; YUNIS 1986; LLOMBART-BOSCH et al. 1988; MACKAY and ORDONEZ 1988; STEINER et

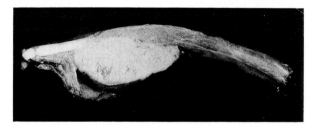

Fig. 1. Gross appearance of a thoracopulmonary MPNT demonstrating a destructive growth into a rib

al. 1988; LLORETA et al. 1990) and other sites including the testis (NISTAL and PANIAGUA 1985). Demonstration of a relationship to a peripheral nerve is no longer a prerequisite to establish the diagnosis (HARKIN and REED 1969; NESBITT and VIDONE 1976; BOLEN and THORNING 1980).

3.2 Prognosis

Contradictory findings have been reported on the prognosis of MPNT, although in most investigations the survival rates in cases of MPNT were lower than those of ES (HASHIMOTO et al. 1983; LLOMBART-BOSCH et al. 1988). In a previous investigation from this institution using the case material of the Cooperative Ewing's Sarcoma Study (CESS) of the German Society of Pediatric Oncology (GPO), we could not support these data (JÜRGENS et al. 1988). However, when we reinvestigated this material using a larger collection of cases and a different approach to the diagnosis of ES and MPNT, a significant difference in overall and disease-free survival between both types of tumors was evident (SCHMIDT et al. 1991). Only 37.5% of the patients with MPNT were living without evidence of disease compared to 54.4% of patients with ES. From these data we concluded that it is necessary to continue to distinguish between ES and MPNT despite a likely common origin. An additional finding in this study was that Leu 7 positivity apparently conferred a more unfavorable prognosis, whereas it was more favorable in cases with protein S-100 positivity. Apart from this study, only DAUGAARD et al. (1989) have investigated the influence of the immunohistochemical properties on the prognosis in Ewing's sarcoma, and they could find no relationship.

4 Histopathology

Malignant peripheral neuroectodermal tumor is usually described as a small-cell neoplasm with lobular or diffuse arrangement of the uniformly appearing neoplastic cells (Fig. 2). These cells have round or oval nuclei with marginated chromatin, distinct nuclear membranes, small but clearly discernible nucleoli, and a sparse cytoplasm. The latter contains varying amounts of glycogen in most cases, although cases of MPNT without detectable glycogen may occur. It was probably the glycogen-containing tumors with neural differentiation that were called glycogen-positive NB in the past (TRICHE and ROSS 1978; YUNIS et al. 1979). Mitotic activity varies, but is usually high. Despite a rich vascular network the tumors may present extensive areas of necrosis, which are sometimes geographic (Fig. 3). Reticulin fibrils are scarce and are mostly present around blood vessels, whereas the cellular

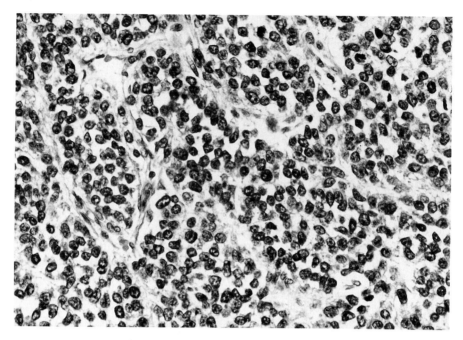

Fig. 2. Malignant peripheral neuroectodermal tumor with typical lobular arrangement of the cells. H&E, ×335

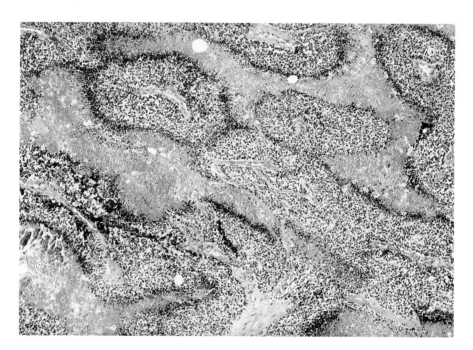

Fig. 3. Malignant peripheral neuroectodermal tumor with geographic necroses. H&E, ×53

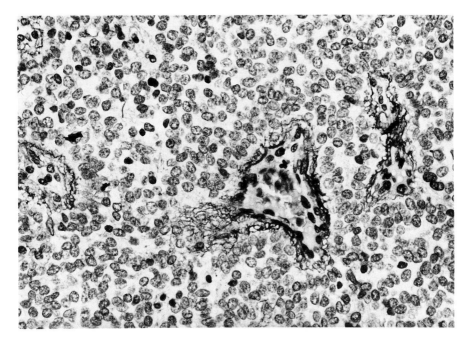

Fig. 4. Malignant peripheral neuroectodermal tumor. No reticulin fibrils are visible between the cells. Silver impregnation, ×335

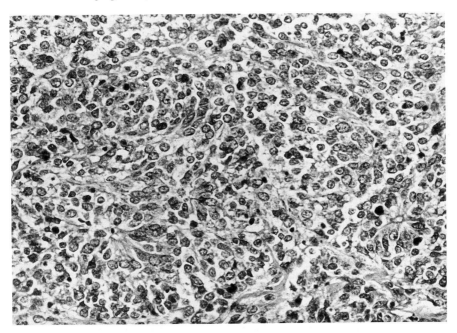

Fig. 5. Malignant peripheral neuroectodermal tumor with formation of true rosettes. H&E, ×335

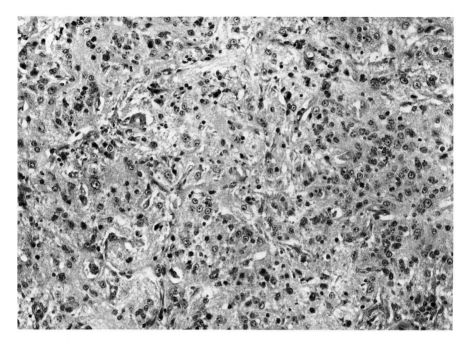

Fig. 6. Malignant peripheral neuroectodermal tumor containing immature ganglion cells with prominent nucleoli. H&E, ×135

aggregates are usually devoid of reticulin fibrils (Fig. 4). Variations of this common histopathological appearance are not infrequent and are essentially related to the grade of neural differentiation (SCHMIDT et al. 1989). Thus, the histopathological features of the most primitive form of MPNT (alternatively, this tumor could be called atypical ES) fit with those described above for the most common form of MPNT. However, cases with overt neural differentiation contain Homer–Wright or Flexner-type rosettes (Fig. 5), and even immature (Fig. 6) or, very rarely, mature ganglion cells may be present. In one case, which we studied several years ago, neural tube-like structures could be demonstrated (SCHMIDT et al. 1985). In terms of differential diagnosis from other small-cell tumors the possible occurrence of some rare growth patterns must be kept in mind. These include cases with a histological appearance suggestive of malignant non-Hodgkin's lymphoma, Burkitt-type, or tumors which present with a pseudoalveolar pattern and which must therefore be distinguished from alveolar rhabdomyosarcoma. Either the presence of areas of typical MPNT or additional investigations, notably immunohistochemistry, will usually solve the diagnostic problems. No diagnostic difficulties should be encountered in cases with a focal hemangio-pericytoma-like pattern, since this pattern is a well-known feature of malignant soft tissue tumors. Moreover, in other portions of the tumor the overall histological appearance is that of MPNT.

5 Electron Microscopy

Electron microscopy provided the first evidence of neural differentiation in MPNT. A neural phenotype was suspected in the thoracopulmonary tumor described by Askin et al. (1979), and it was strongly suggested in four cases which we described under the term "Ewing's sarcoma with neuroblastoma-like features" (Schmidt et al. 1982). This term was not intended to confuse readers, but was derived from the observation that tumors indistinguishable from ES by conventional light microscopy and clinical presentation revealed some ultrastructural findings which had only been observed in NB. These included cells with long cytoplasmic projections containing dense-core, neurosecretory-type granules associated with microtubules and intermediate filaments, supposedly neurofilaments. In contrast to NB, however, the cells contained ample amounts of glycogen similar to cells in typical ES. Several studies (Nesland et al. 1985; Llombart-Bosch et al. 1988) confirmed that dense-core granules with a size of about 150–250 nm, microtubules, and intermediate filaments are regular features in MPNT but, in contrast to NB cytoplasmic processes, usually do not interdigitate in a neuropil-like manner. Nevertheless, they can be long and slender. Except for the membrane-bound dense-core granules, the other cytoplasmic organelles are noncharacteristic. They include some rough endoplasmatic reticulum, abundant ribosomes and polyribosomes, some mitochondria, and a Golgi complex. Between the cells small desmosomes can be found.

6 Immunohistochemistry

For the definition of MPNT and the distinction from the other small-, round-, blue-cell tumors, immunohistochemistry has been equally important as electron microscopy, although some of the first findings must be interpreted differently today. Many poly- and monoclonal antibodies have been successfully employed including antibodies against intermediate filaments (vimentin, cytokeratins, neurofilaments, glial fibrillary acidic protein) and different so-called neural markers (neuron-specific enolase, protein S-100, chromogranin A, Leu 7). A comparison of the immunophenotype of MPNT with that of other small-, round-, blue-cell tumors to be considered in differential diagnosis is provided in Table 2. The most important antibody today is that against the $p30/32^{MIC2}$ protein (Fig. 7). In the past, neuron-specific enolase (γ/γ enolase, NSE) was regarded as the most useful marker to detect a neural differentiation and to distinguish MPNT from ES and non-neural tumors. Thus, it was common practice to classify a tumor with Ewing's cytology and NSE positivity as MPNT. Several years of experience, however, have shown that this procedure is no longer justified, because this

Table 2. Immunoreactivity of different antibodies in the differential diagnosis of small-, round-cell tumors retrieved from paraffin material

Antibody	NBL	RMS	ES	MPNT
Vimentin	Mostly negative	Always strongly positive	Positive	Faintly positive
Desmin	Negative	Always positive	Negative	Negative
Cytokeratin	Negative	Occasionally positive	Occasionally positive	Occasionally positive
Neurofilaments	Mostly positive	Occasionally positive	Negative	Occasionally positive
GFAP	Negative	Negative	Negative	Occasionally positive
NSE	Positive	Positive	Negative/positive	Positive/negative
Protein S-100	Often positive	Often positive	Negative/positive	Positive/negative
Leu 7	Occasionally positive	Occasionally positive	Negative/positive	Positive/negative
Chromogranin	Mostly positive	Negative	Negative	Occasionally positive
HBA 71	Negative	Negative	Positive	Positive

NBL, undifferentiated neuroblastoma; RMS, rhabdomyosarcoma; ES, Ewing's sarcoma; MPNT, malignant peripheral neuroectodermal tumor; GFAP, glial fibrillary acidic protein; NSE, neuron-specific enolase; HBA 71, antibody against MIC2 gene product.

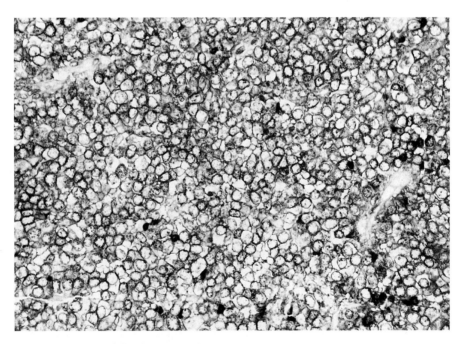

Fig. 7. Malignant peripheral neuroectodermal tumor demonstrating strong reactivity for HBA 71. ×535

enzyme does not only occur in cells of neural origin. Moreover, not all antibodies currently available are specific for the γ/γ form, so that cross-reactions with other dimers may occur. Therefore, the immunohistochemical reaction for NSE is now viewed with much skepticism both in the diagnosis and the definition of histogenesis of a given tumor. Nevertheless, it can still be useful provided it is used in conjunction with other markers.

In a previous study (SCHMIDT et al. 1991) we were able to demonstrate different grades of neural differentiation in cases of ES and MPNT using a monoclonal antibody against NSE, as well as the two markers protein S-100 and Leu 7. In accordance with findings from previous studies (HASHIMOTO et al. 1983; TSOKOS et al. 1984; KAWAGUCHI and KOIKE 1986; LLOMBART-BOSCH et al. 1989; LIZARD-NACOL et al. 1989; LADANYI et al. 1990) we found that most cases of MPNT were NSE positive (Fig. 8), whereas 55.5% expressed protein S-100 (Fig. 9), and 30.5% reacted positively for Leu 7. Interestingly, and most importantly, the prognosis of the protein S-100 positive cases proved to be more favorable, whereas it was worse in the cases with Leu 7 positivity. No similar clinical relevance could be shown for the other markers including the different types of intermediate filaments. Their expression did not differ significantly between ES and MPNT. Specifically, both tumor types revealed a coexpression of vimentin and cytokeratins in some cases (ES: 3.4%, MPNT: 8.3%). This is not surprising, since the expression of

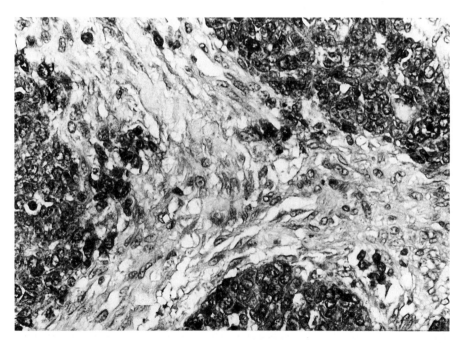

Fig. 8. Malignant peripheral neuroectodermal tumor with strong positivity for neuron specific enolase. ×335

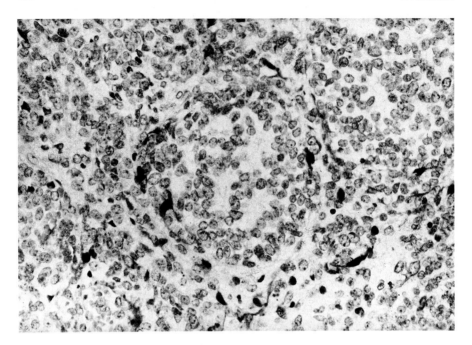

Fig. 9. Malignant peripheral neuroectodermal tumor with several protein S-100 positive spindle cells. These cells probably represent early schwannian differentiation. ×335

cytokeratins in these tumors has been repeatedly reported, both in tumor tissue and in cell lines derived therefrom (DELLAGI et al. 1987; MOLL et al. 1987).

7 DNA Ploidy

The evaluation of DNA ploidy has become an important tool in the diagnostic work-up of a tumor, since for many tumor types ploidy has been identified as an independent prognostic factor. Ploidy can be determined by either DNA flow or image cytometry, and it can be used successfully not only on fresh tumor specimens but also on archival paraffin material (HEDLEY et al. 1983). Thus, large retrospective studies are potentially feasible. However, data on DNA ploidy in cases of ES and MPNT are still limited, especially with regard to the relationship between ploidy and prognosis. The latter issue was addressed in a most recent study by KOWAL-VERN et al. (1992) who studied 21 cases of Ewing's sarcoma by both flow and image cytometry. No correlation between DNA ploidy and probability of survival was found. This is surprising in view of the fact that both diploid and aneuploid tumors were encountered, albeit diploid cases were more frequent. A predominance of diploid cases was also found by KISS et al. (1991) who investigated 32 cases of ES and by SWANSON et al. (1992) on a series of 16 cases of PPNET. In a preliminary series of 11 cases of ES and MPNT which we investigated by image cytometry we only observed diploid tumors. More detailed information on DNA ploidy is given in the chapter by MELLIN et al. (this volume). Conclusive data are also lacking on the relationship between cellular proliferation and biological behavior in ES and MPNT. In ploidy investigations the proliferative activity is usually assessed by the proliferation index or the percentage of S phase cells. From the number of mitoses in conventionally stained slides of ES or MPNT it would appear that the proliferative activity is moderately high. However, we found that proliferation indices ranged from 6% to 41%. Similarly, the percentage of cells in S phase varied between 2.5% and 40.2%. Thus, the proliferative activity in ES and MPNT varies to a large degree. Future studies will show whether these differences will account for differences in the biological behavior.

References

Alba Greco A, Steiner GC, Fazzini E (1988) Ewing's sarcoma with epithelial differentiation: fine structural and immunocytochemical study. Ultrastruct Pathol 12: 317–325

Ambros IM, Ambros PF, Strehl S, Kovar H, Gadner H, Salzer-Kuntschik M (1991) MIC2 is a specific marker for Ewing's sarcoma and peripheral primitive neuroectodermal tumors. Evidence for a common histogenesis of Ewing's sarcoma and peripheral neuroectodermal tumors from MIC2 expression and specific chromosome aberration. Cancer 67: 1886–1893

Askin FB, Rosai J, Sibley RK, Dehner LP, McAlister B (1979) Malignant small cell tumor of the thoracopulmonary region in childhood. A distinctive clinicopathologic entity of uncertain histogenesis. Cancer 43: 2438–2451

Aurias A, Rimbaut C, Buffe D, Zucker J-M, Mazabraud A (1984) Translocation involving chromosome 22 in Ewing's sarcoma. A cytogenetic study of four fresh tumors. Cancer Genet Cytogenet 12: 21–25

Bailey P, Cushing H (1926) A classification of the tumors of the glioma group on a histogenetic basis with a correlated study of prognosis. Lippincott, Philadelphia

Bolen JW, Thorning D (1980) Peripheral neuroepithelioma: a light and electron microscopic study. Cancer 46: 2456–2462

Cavazzana AO, Miser JS, Jefferson J, Triche TJ (1987) Experimental evidence for a neural origin of Ewing's sarcoma of bone. Am J Pathol 27: 507–518

Daugaard S, Kamby C, Sunde LM, Myrhe-Jense O, Schiodt T (1989) Ewing's sarcoma. A retrospective study of histological and immunohistochemical factors and their relation to prognosis. Virchows Arch [Pathol Anat] 414: 243–251

Dehner LP (1986) Peripheral and central primitive neuroectodermal tumors. A nosologic concept seeking a consensus. Arch Pathol Lab Med 110: 997–1005

Dehner LP (1990) Whence the primitive neuroectodermal tumor? Arch Pathol Lab Med 114: 16–17

Dehner LP (1993) Primitive neuroectodermal tumor and Ewing's sarcoma. Am J Surg Pathol 17: 1–13

Delattre O, Zucman J, Plougastel B, Desmaze C, Melot T, Peter M, Kovar H, Joubert I, de Jong P, Roulot G, Aurias A, Thomas G (1992) Cloning of the recurrent t(11;22) translocation of Ewing's sarcoma and peripheral neuroepithelioma. Proc Am Assoc Cancer Res 33: 604–605

Dellagi K, Lipinski M, Paulin D, Portier MM, Lenoir GM, Brouet JC (1987) Characterization of intermediate filaments expressed by Ewing's sarcoma tumor cell lines. Cancer Res 47: 1170–1173

Douglass EC, Valentine M, Green AA, Hayes FA, Thompson EI (1986) t(11;22) and other chromosomal rearrangements in Ewing's sarcoma. J Natl Cancer Inst 77: 1211–1215

Fellinger EJ, Garin-Chesa P, Triche TJ, Huvos AG, Rettig W (1991) Immunohistochemical analysis of Ewing's sarcoma cell surface antigen p30/32^{MIC2}. Am J Pathol 139: 317–325

Friedman JM, Vitale M, Maimon J, Israel MA, Horowitz ME, Schneider BS (1992) Expression of the cholecystokinin gene in pediatric tumors. Proc Natl Acad Sci USA 89: 5819–5823

Fujii Y, Hongo T, Nakagawa Y, Nasuda K, Mizuno Y, Igarashi Y, Naito Y, Maeda M (1989) Cell culture of small round cell tumor originating in the thoracopulmonary region. Evidence for derivation from a primitive pluripotent cell. Cancer 64: 43–51

Gormann PA, Malone M, Pritchard J, Sheer D (1991) Cytogenetic analysis of primitive neuroectodermal tumors. Cancer Genet Cytogenet 51: 13–22

Hachitanda Y, Tsuneyoshi M, Enjoji M, Nakagawara A, Ikeda K (1990) Congenital primitive neuroectodermal tumor with epithelial and glial differentiation. Arch Pathol Lab Med 114: 101–105

Harkin JC, Reed RJ (1969) Tumors of the peripheral nervous system. Atlas of tumor pathology, 2nd series, fasc 3. Armed Force Institute of Pathology, Washington, DC.

Hartmann K, Triche TJ, Kinsella TJ, Miser JS (1991) Prognostic value of histopathology in Ewing's sarcoma: long-term follow-up of distal extremity primary tumors. Cancer 67: 163–171

Hashimoto H, Kiryu H, Enjoji M, Daimaru Y, Nakajima T (1983) Malignant neuroepithelioma (peripheral neuroblastoma). A clinicopathologic study of 15 cases. Hum Pathol 7: 309–318

Jaffe R, Agostini RM Jr, Santamaria M, Medina J, Yunis E, Goodman M, Hrinya Tannery N (1984) The neuroectodermal tumor of bone. Am J Surg Pathol 8: 885–898

Jürgens H, Bier V, Harms D, Beck J, Brandeis W, Etspüler G, Gadner H, Schmidt D, Treuner J, Winkler K, Göbel U (1988) Malignant peripheral neuroectodermal tumors. A retrospective analysis of 42 patients. Cancer 61: 349–357

Kawaguchi K, Koike M (1986) Neuron-specific enolase and Leu 7 immunoreactive small round cell neoplasm. The relationship to Ewing's sarcoma in bone and soft tissue. Am J Clin Pathol 86: 79–83

Kiss R, Larsimont D, Huvos AG (1991) Digital image analysis of Ewing's sarcoma. Anal Quant Cytol Histol 13: 356–362

Kowal-Vern A, Walloch J, Chou P, Gonzalez-Crussi F, Price J, Potocki D, Herman C (1992) Flow and image cytometric DNA analysis in Ewing's sarcoma. Mod Pathol 5: 56–60

Ladanyi M, Heinemann FS, Huvos A, Rao PH, Chen Q, Jhanwar SC (1990) Neural differentiation in small round cell tumors of bone and soft tissue with the translocation t(11;22) (q24;q12): an immunohistochemical study of 11 cases. Hum Pathol 21: 1245–1251

Liebermann PH (1979) Case twenty-one. In: Lieberman PH, Good RA (eds) Diseases of the hematopoietic system. Am Soc Clin Pathol, Chicago, pp 100–105

Lizard-Nacol S, Lizard G, Justrabo E, Turc-Carel C (1989) Immunologic characterization of Ewing's sarcoma using mesenchymal and neural markers. Am J Pathol 135: 847–855

Llombart-Bosch A, Lacombe MJ, Peydro-Olaya P, Perez-Bacete M, Contesso G (1988) Malignant peripheral neuroectodermal tumours of bone other than Askin's neoplasm: characterization of 14 new cases with immunohistochemistry and electron microscopy. Virchows Arch [Pathol Anat] 412: 421–430

Llombart-Bosch A, Terrier-Lacombe MJ, Peydro-Olaya A, Contesso G (1989) Peripheral neuroectodermal sarcoma of soft tissue (peripheral neuroepithelioma). Hum Pathol 20: 273–280

Lloreta J, Tusquets I, Prieto V, Serrano S, Prat J (1990) Primary neuroectodermal tumor of bone. Report of a case in an adult. Surg Pathol 3: 325–331

Mackay B, Ordóñez NG (1988) Adult neuroblastoma of bone: A case report. Ultrastruct Pathol 11: 455–464

Mackay B, Luna MA, Butler JJ (1976) Adult neuroblastoma. Electron microscopic observations in nine cases. Cancer 37: 1334–1351

McKeon C, Thiele CJ, Ross RA, Kwan M, Triche TJ, Miser JS, Israel MA (1988) Indistinguishable patterns of protooncogene expression in two distinct but closely related tumors: Ewing's sarcoma and neuroepithelioma. Cancer Res 48: 4307–4311

Moll R, Lee I, Gould VE, Berndt R, Roessner A, Franke WW (1987) Immunohistochemical analysis of Ewing's tumors. Patterns of expression of intermediate filaments and desmosomal protein indicate cell type heterogeneity and pluripotential differentiation. Am J Pathol 127: 288–304

Nesbitt KA, Vidone RA (1976) Primitive neuroectodermal tumor (neuroblastoma) arising in sciatic nerve of a child. Cancer 37: 1562–1570

Nesland JM, Sobrinho-Simoes MA, Holm R, Johannessen JV (1985) Primitive neuroectodermal tumor (peripheral neuroblastoma). Ultrastruct Pathol 9: 59–64

Nistal M, Paniagua (1985) Primary neuroectodermal tumour of the testis. Histopathology 9: 1351–1359

Parham DM, Dias P, Kelly DR, Rutledge JC, Houghton P (1992) Desmin positivity in primitive neuroectodermal tumors of childhood. Am J Surg Pathol 16: 483–492

Rorke LB, Gilles FH, Davis RL, Becker LE (1985) Revision of the World Health Organization classification of brain tumors for childhood brain tumors. Cancer 56: 1869–1886

Rubinstein LJ (1987) Letter to the editor: "Primitive neuroectodermal tumors". Arch Pathol Lab Med 111: 310

Schmidt D, Mackay B, Ayala AG (1982) Ewing's sarcoma with neuroblastoma-like features. Ultrastruct Pathol 3: 143–151

Schmidt D, Harms D, Jürgens H (1989) Maligne periphere neuroektodermale Tumoren. Histologische und immunhistochemische Befunde an 41 Fällen. Zentralbl Allg Pathol Anat 135: 257–267

Schmidt D, Herrmann C, Jürgens H, Harms D (1991) Malignant peripheral neuroectodermal tumor and its necessary distinction from Ewing's sarcoma. Cancer 68: 2251–2259

Seemayer TA, Vekemans M, de Chadarévian J-P (1985) Histological and cytogenetic findings in a malignant tumor of the chest wall and lung (Askin tumor). Virchows Arch [Pathol Anat] 408: 289–296

Selleri L, Hermanson GG, Eubanks JH, Lewis KA, Evans GA (1991) Molecular localization of the t(11;22)(q24;q12) translocation of Ewing sarcoma by chromosomal *in situ* suppression hybridization. Proc Natl Acad Sci USA 88: 887–891

Shuangshoti S (1986) Primitive neuroectodermal (neuroepithelial) tumour of soft tissue of the neck in a child: demonstration of neuronal and neuroglial differentiation. Histopathology 10: 651–658

Speleman F, Van Roy N, Wiegant J, Dierick A, Uyttendaele D, Leroy JG (1992) Molecular cytogenetic analysis of a complete (10;22;11) translocation in Ewing's sarcoma. Genes Chrom Cancer 4: 188–191

Steiner GC, Graham S, Lewis MM (1988) Malignant round cell tumor of bone with neural differentiation (neuroectodermal tumor). Ultrastruct Pathol 12: 505–512

Stout AP (1918) A tumor of the ulnar nerve. Proc NY Pathol Soc 18: 2–12

Swanson PE, Jaszcz W, Nakhleh RE, Kelly DR, Dehner LP (1992) Peripheral primitive neuroectodermal tumors. A flow cytometric analysis with immunohistochemical and ultrastructural observations. Arch Pathol Lab Med 116: 1202–1208

Thiele CJ (1991) Biology of pediatric peripheral neuroectodermal tumors. Cancer Met Rev 10: 311–319

Triche TJ, Ross WE (1978) Glycogen-containing neuroblastoma with clinical and histopathologic features of Ewing's sarcoma. Cancer 41: 1425–1432

Tsokos M, Linnoila RI, Chandra RS, Triche TJ (1984) Neuron-specific enolase in the diagnosis of neuroblastoma and other small-, round-cell tumors in children. Hum Pathol 15: 575–584

Ushigome S, Shimoda T, Takai K, Nikaido T, Takakuwa T, Ishikawa E, Spjut HJ (1989) Immunocytochemical and ultrastructural studies of the histogenesis of Ewing's sarcoma and putatively related tumors. Cancer 64: 52–62

Verwey J, Slater R, Kamphorst W, Pinedo HM (1985) Neuroepithelioma (neuroblastoma) arising in an adult. A case report. J Cancer Res Clin Oncol 110: 165–169

Voss BL, Pysher TJ, Humphrey GB (1984) Peripheral neuroepithelioma in childhood. Cancer 54: 3059–3064

Whang-Peng J, Triche TJ, Knutsen T, Miser JS, Douglass EC, Israel MA (1984) Chromosome translocation in peripheral neuroepithelioma. N Engl J Med 311: 584–585

Whang-Peng J, Triche TJ, Knutsen T, Miser J, Kao-Shan S, Tsai S, Israel MA (1986) Cytogenetic characterization of selected small round cell tumors of childhood. Cancer Genet Cytogenet 21: 185–208

Whang-Peng J, Freter CE, Knutsen T, Nanfro JJ, Gazdar A (1987) Translocation t(11;22) in esthesioneuroblastoma. Cancer Genet Cytogenet 29: 155–157

Yeger H, Mor O, Pawlin G, Kaplinsky C, Shiloh Y (1990) Importance of phenotypic and molecular characterization for identification of a neuroepithelioma tumor cell line, NUB-20. Cancer Res 50: 2794–2802

Yunis EJ (1986) Ewing's sarcoma and related small cell neoplasms in children. Am J Surg Pathol 10[Suppl 1]: 54–62

Yunis EJ, Walpusk JA, Agostini RM, Hubbard JD (1979) Glycogen in neuroblastomas. Am J Surg Pathol 3: 313–323

Zhang FR, Aurias, Delattre O, Stern MH, Benitez J, Rouleau G, Thomas G (1990) Mapping of human chromosome 22 by in situ hybridization. Genomics 7: 319–324

Leiomyosarcoma

A.O. Cavazzana, V. Ninfo, R. Tirabosco,
A. Montaldi, and R. Frunzio

1 Introduction

1.1 Frequency, Incidence, Distribution, Age

Malignant tumors of smooth muscle origin are one of the more frequent sarcomas; their relative frequency has been estimated from 2% (Myhre-Jensen et al. 1983; Trojani et al. 1984) to 8.8% (Enjoji and Hashimoto 1984) – 9.3% (Markhede et al. 1982) of all soft tissue sarcomas. The annual incidence of leiomyosarcoma (LMS) is calculated to be 1.136 per million for whites and 1.984 per million for blacks regardless of the sites of origin (Polednak 1986). According to the same source, LMS also represents the most frequent sarcoma with a frequency of 30% in whites and 39% in blacks.

Owing to the ubiquitous distribution of smooth muscle cells, LMS can virtually arise anywhere in the body and consequently have been subdivided into three major groups: superficial and deep soft tissue, and visceral LMS. The uterus and gastrointestinal tract are the most commonly involved visceral sites, while the retroperitoneum and external soft tissues are the preferred extravisceral sites; LMS arising from major blood vessels (Verela-

DURAN et al. 1979), heart (BEARMAN 1974), and bones (MYERS et al. 1991) have also been reported.

A clear sexual distribution is lacking; while some authors have reported female prepoderance (HASHIMOTO et al. 1986) for external soft tissue LMS, others deny it (WILE et al. 1981). No sex difference has been noticed for gastrointestinal tumors (EVANS 1985), and a female preponderance has been noted in retroperitoneal LMS (WILE et al. 1981; SMOOKLER and LAUER 1983). Leiomyosarcomas are almost exclusively tumors of adulthood, with a peak incidence around the fifth and sixth decades (HASHIMOTO et al. 1986; WILE et al. 1981; NEUGUT and SORDILLO 1989); they are found more rarely in childhood (STOUT and HILL 1958; YANNOPOULOS and STOUT 1962; SWANSON et al. 1991).

2 Diagnosis

2.1 Histology

The diagnosis of smooth muscle tumors may be an easy or an exceedingly difficult task because these lesions display a broader spectrum of morphologic features than commonly thought. Nevertheless, the diagnosis of LMS can be

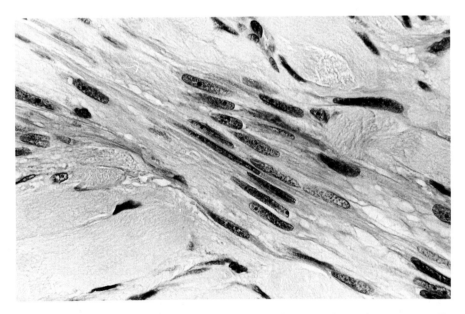

Fig. 1. The characteristic elongated, cigar-shaped nuclei of smooth muscle cells are easily recognized under high power. H&E; ×420

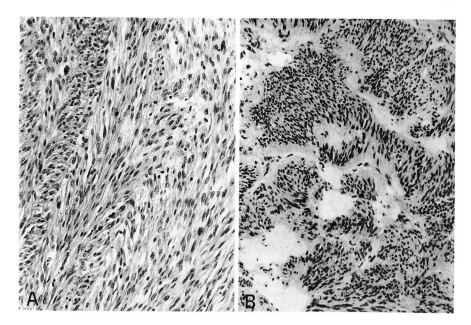

Fig. 2A,B. Long fascicles intersecting at right angles (**A**) and palisades (**B**) are the two most frequently observed patterns in LMS. H&E; **A** ×280, **B** ×88

confidently achieved in most cases on the basis of typical cytologic and architectural features.

Smooth muscle cells are characterized cytologically by an elongated, fusiform appearance with centrally placed nuclei and a fibrillary eosinophilic cytoplasm. The nuclei have blunt edges with a distinctive cigar-shaped appearance (Fig. 1) and characteristically show an artifactual clear para-nuclear halo in formalin-fixed paraffin-embedded sections (HAYASHI et al. 1990). The cells show a tendency to align regularly in bundles that intersect at right angles (Fig. 2A) or in rhythmic palisades, similar to those observed in nerve sheath tumors (Fig. 2B).

Depending on the degree of tumor differentiation, these familiar features may at times not be apparent. In fact, LMS may have a bland benign-looking appearance with highly fibrillary cytoplasms or a more primitive, fibroblast-like, uncommitted aspect (Fig. 3). The myogenic nature of the tumor may thus become more manifest after short-term tissue culture in vitro (Fig. 4), or at relapse (Fig. 5). In the myxoid variants, the smooth muscle cells may display a multivacuolated cytoplasm closely mimicking immature fat cells; at times the fasciculated pattern is substituted by a trabecular, lace-like pattern that confers a microcystic appearance to the tumor (Fig. 6A,B). Pale, epithelioid-like cells with bland round nuclei and arranged in a pseudoglandular or trabecular pattern are characteristically observed in leiomyoblastoma (Fig. 7). Superficially located LMS may present

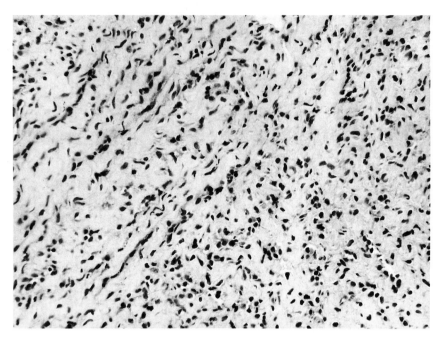

Fig. 3. A loose proliferation of oval and uncommitted spindle cells may be encountered in undifferentiated forms of LMS. H&E; ×250

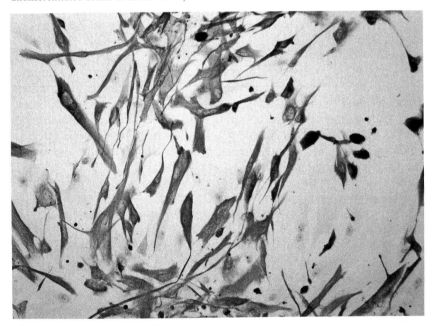

Fig. 4. Same case as Fig. 3: after 6 days in culture (RPMI 1640 supplemented with 10% fetal bovine serum), tumor cells displayed an elongated fusiform shape and an intense positivity to anti-desmin antibody. ABC; ×400

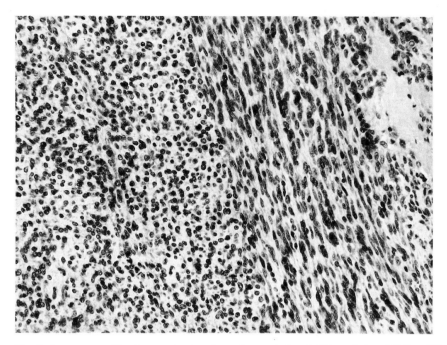

Fig. 5. Same case as Fig. 3: preoperative chemotherapy-induced differentiation. H&E; ×125

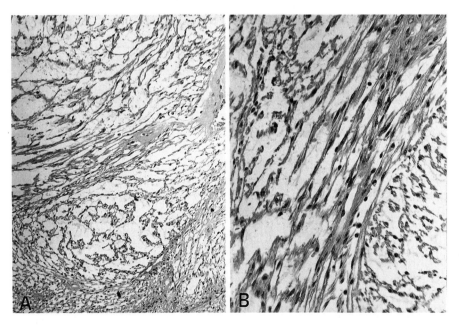

Fig. 6A,B. Retroperitoneal and visceral LMS may occasionally display a microcystic pattern due to intercellular edema (**A**); at higher magnification, empty spaces are surrounded by elongated, strongly eosinophilic cells (**B**). H&E; **A** ×105, **B**×420

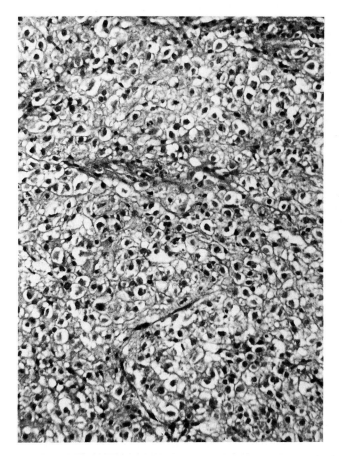

Fig. 7. Sheets of polygonal clear cells characterize epithelioid LMS. H&E; ×400

a granular cytoplasm (NISTAL et al. 1980; LEBOIT et al. 1991) which makes the cytologic distinction from other granular cell neoplasms difficult. Furthermore, bizarre, highly anaplastic, mono- or multinucleated giant cells are often observed in recurrent and in dedifferentiated LMS (Fig. 8). In the latter case, the morphologic diagnosis is based mainly on the recognition of typical, more differentiated areas.

This high morphologic variability may partially explain the discrepancies in the relative frequencies reported in the literature and justifies the application of ancillary techniques for the diagnosis of difficult cases.

2.2 Ultrastructure

The use of the transmission electron microscope has considerably improved the pathologist's capacity to resolve difficult cases of soft tissue tumors

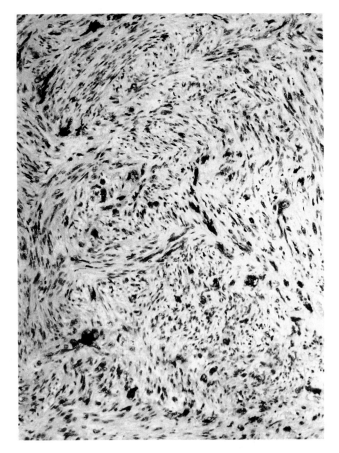

Fig. 8. Pleomorphic LMS: the presence of bizarre mono-, or multinucleated giant cells may induce the misinterpretation of this lesion as an MFH

(FISCHER 1990). Although LMS show the same variability of features at the electron microscope as at the light microscope in relation to the degree of tumor differentiation, some aspects are constant and thus enable a correct diagnosis in the majority of cases.

The cytoplasm is characterized by profiles of rough endoplasmic reticulum, a variable number of mitochondria, and generally numerous subplasmalemal micropinocytotic vescicles and dense bodies. Cells are coated by profiles of an external lamina that often incompletely surrounds the plasma membrane (Fig. 9).

The nucleus has an oval or spindle shape with blunt edges, an irregularly crenated surface (Fig. 9), and an evident nucleolus. However, the ultrastructural hallmark of smooth muscle differentiation is the presence of bundles of filaments with dense bodies along their course (Fig. 10). This finding probably represents the single most important ultrastructural criterion in diagnosing a smooth muscle tumor, with the exception of the epithelioid

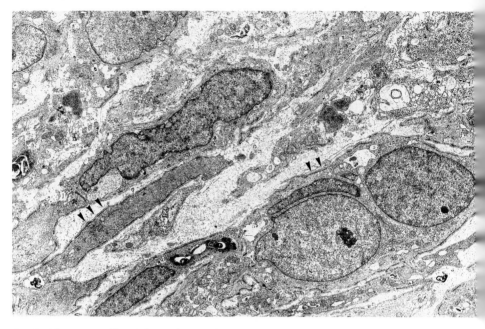

Fig. 9. Ultrastructurally, LMS are characterized by spindle cells with typically crenated nuclear profiles. The plasma membrane profiles are outlined by numerous subplasmalemal densities (*arrowhead*) and coated by an evident external lamina. Uranyl acetate and lead citrate; ×2250

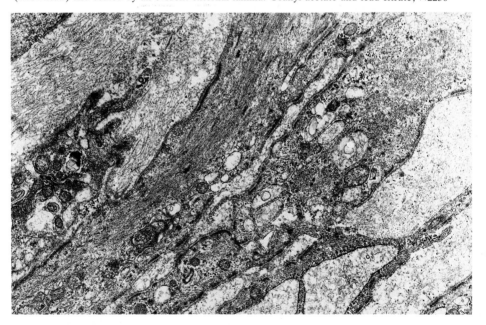

Fig. 10. At higher magnification, the recognition of broad bundles of intermediate filaments is of utmost importance in the ultrastructural diagnosis of smooth muscle tumors. Uranyl acetate and lead citrate; ×9000

cells of leiomyoblastoma where filaments are scarce and the typical arrangement with focal densities is barely appreciable, if at all present (FISCHER
1990; WEISS and MACKAY 1981; KNAPP et al. 1984).

2.3 Immunocytochemistry

A number of monoclonal antibodies have been successfully employed in
diagnosing smooth muscle tumors. While most studies have focused their
attention on the expression of some specific muscle markers, such as vimentin, actins, and desmin, other nonspecific markers, such as laminin, and
collagen IV, have also been investigated (MIETTINEN et al. 1983; OGAWA et
al. 1986). A detailed discussion of these latter markers is beyond our scope,
but actins and desmin deserve a brief comment.
   Actin has at least six different tissue-specific and developmentally regulated isoforms that differ from each other due to the diversity of the
tryptic digestion products of their N terminal region (VANDEKERCKHOVE and
WEBER 1978). Beta and gamma non-muscle actins are common to most
mammalian cells (VANDEKERCKHOVE and WEBER 1981), whereas smooth
and striated (skeletal and cardiac) muscles have specific isoforms, namely
alpha and gamma smooth muscle actins, and alpha sarcomeric (cardiac and
skeletal) actins. Alpha smooth muscle actin is found mainly in the vessel
walls (GABBIANI et al. 1981), while alpha and gamma isoforms constitute the
main filaments in parenchymal smooth muscles (SCHURCH et al. 1987).
   Monoclonal antibodies raised against some of these different actin forms
are now commercially available and seem to offer more reliable and reproducible results in identifying the smooth muscle nature of a tumor compared
to desmin (UEYAMA et al. 1992; TSUKADA et al. 1987; JONES et al. 1990).
The excellence of these antibodies seems to be partially limited by the
susceptibility of the actin filaments to aldehyde-based fixatives, such as
formalin, which greatly impair protein antigenicity; the preventive use of
ethylenediaminetetra-acetic acid (EDTA) seems to overcome this problem
(TSUKADA et al. 1987).
   Desmin is considered the best single marker of myogenic differentiation;
it is a muscle-specific intermediate filament (LAZARIDES 1980), with a molecular weight of approximately 50 kD, that forms a complex network linking
cytoplasmic dense bodies to dense plaques (RICCI et al. 1987). Its positivity
in smooth muscle tumors (Fig. 11) varies greatly according to different
authors, ranging from about 100% to 30%–40% of cases (FISCHER 1990;
UEYAMA et al. 1992; RANGDAENG and TRUONG 1991; MIETTINEN 1988a;
OLIVER et al. 1991). Nevertheless, it is now apparent that negative results
are also not uncommon in otherwise morphologically evident tumors with
special regard to visceral tumors (UEYAMA et al. 1992; SAUL et al. 1987).
With this caveat in mind, it seems reasonable not to exclude a diagnosis of

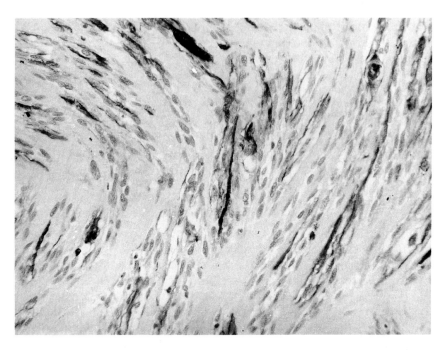

Fig. 11. While desmin expression in a spindle cell tumor is highly variable, it represents a "certain" marker of muscle differentiation. ABC; ×600

LMS in the face of a lesion that fulfills the morphologic criteria but not the immunocytochemical profile of LMS. Indeed, we recently found that immunocytochemistry techniques may fail to recognize muscular antigens, in particular the gamma actin, in both paraffin-embedded and frozen material; in these cases the smooth muscle origin of a desmin and S-100 protein-negative tumor may be demonstrated through a Western blot analysis of the cytoskeleton proteins (TIRABOSCO et al., submitted).

Keratin was long considered a highly specific marker for epithelial differentiation, and its expression in smooth muscle-derived tumors represents a biologic enigma. An immunocytochemical reactivity to simple epithelium keratins (such as keratins 18 and 8) has been reported by several authors (BROWN et al. 1987; MIETTINEN 1988b, 1991). The biochemical demonstration of a class of intermediate filaments of approximately 50 kD molecular weight reacting with anti-keratin 8 antibody (Fig. 12), ruled out the possibility of a cross-reactivity among intermediate filaments as previously supposed (MIETTINEN 1988b), and thus confirmed the immunocytochemical findings. On the other hand, keratins 8 and 18 are transiently expressed by nonepithelial cells during mammalian embryogenesis (FRANKE et al. 1982; KURUC and FRANKE 1988), and a loss of regulatory genetic controls might explain this aberrant expression in transformed mesenchymal phenotypes (KNAPP and FRANKE 1989).

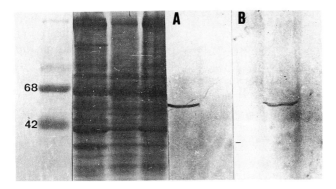

Fig. 12A,B. The coexpression of different classes of intermediate filaments such as desmin (**A**) and cytokeratin 8 (**B**) is confirmed in LMS by Western blot analysis of whole protein extract

3 Differential Diagnosis

The differential diagnosis includes a wide spectrum of spindle cell neoplasms, encompassing both mesenchymal and nonmesenchymal tumors; among the mesenchymal lesions, nerve sheath tumors, synovial sarcoma, fibrosarcoma, malignant fibrous histiocytoma, and Kaposi sarcoma are the most important pitfalls.

Nerve sheath-derived tumors are probably the most challenging, since they share many histologic features with LMS. Smooth muscle tumors in the gastrointestinal tract may closely mimic nerve sheath tumors by virtue of the presence of evident nuclear palisades similar to those observed in schwannomas (Fig. 3). The distinction between these two different tumor classes relies on histochemical and immunocytochemical findings. Smooth muscle tumors show histochemically detectable amounts of cytoplasmic glycogen in formalin-fixed, paraffin-embedded specimens, while a distinct fibrillary cytoplasm is highlighted by the trichrome stain; moreover, they show a positive reaction with muscle markers, such as smooth muscle actins and desmin.

Adult-type fibrosarcoma may occasionally enter the differential diagnosis, especially in poorly differentiated LMS; fibrosarcoma-like areas are also commonly observed in dedifferentiated LMS. The search for more differentiated areas will generally clarify the diagnosis.

There is a growing body of evidence that many of the so-called malignant fibrous histiocytomas (MFH) diagnosed in the past could represent a pleomorphic variant of other phenotypically distinct sarcomas, including LMS. This conclusion is based mainly on immunocytochemical findings, since these tumors reacted positively with anti-desmin and/or muscle actin antibodies (FLETCHER 1992; ROHOLL et al. 1990). Nevertheless, it is known that LMS, like liposarcomas and malignant nerve sheath tumors, may display dedifferentiated features both in primary and recurrent lesions more often than other soft tissue sarcomas (BROOKS 1986). Thus, from a practical point of view, when diagnosing a pleomorphic sarcoma, it is safe to confirm the morphologic impression with immunohistochemical and/or ultrastructural studies; a positive reaction with muscle markers or ultrastructural evidence of smooth muscle differentiation will rule out the diagnosis of pleomorphic MFH. Kaposi sarcoma in the nodular stage may also mimic an LMS; the presence of vascular slits, intratumoral red blood cells extravasation, and a nodular lymphocytic infiltration favor the diagnosis of Kaposi sarcoma over LMS.

The positivity to keratins may suggest the differential with a monophasic synovial sarcoma. Synovial sarcoma is characterized by shorter fascicles of spindle cells, often arranged in a curl-like pattern, with interspered small nests of clear round cells.

Among the nonmesenchymal tumors, the main differential includes melanoma, spindle cell carcinoma, and carcinoid. Nodular melanoma may present as a fascicular tumor, composed of spindle cells with abundant eosinophilic cytoplasm closely resembling smooth muscle cells. An ulceration of the overlying epidermis, and the presence of prominent nucleoli, as well as a diffuse lymphocytic infiltrate in a nodular neoplasm of the upper dermis, should always alert the pathologist to look for evidence of junctional activity.

Epidermoid carcinoma, arising in sun-exposed skin or in hollow organs, such as the esophagus, larynx, and urinary bladder, may present as a spindle cell neoplasm. The presence of dysplastic changes in the adjacent epithelium and diffuse positivity to keratins enable a correct diagnosis.

Epithelioid leiomyosarcoma in the gastrointestinal tract may be misdiagnosed as a carcinoid due to the presence of small nests of pale round to oval cells with bland, central nuclei. The negativity to neuroendocrine markers and the presence of more classic spindle cell areas will assist in making the correct diagnosis.

4 Prognosis

Leiomyosarcomas are fully malignant neoplasms regardless of their site of origin and, although some major differences have been noted among different anatomic sites, they often show a capricious and unpredictable behavior.

4.1 Gastrointestinal Tract

The mitotic count, tumor size, histologic grade, and immunophenotypic differentiation have been reported to be major factors in influencing the final outcome for gastrointestinal tumors. A mitotic rate of ten mitoses per ten high power fields (hpf) has been recommended as the cut-off point between low- and high-grade tumors (EVANS 1985). For small bowel tumors, the histologic tumor grade, based on assessment of mitoses, cellularity, cellular differentiation, necrosis, and atypia, was found to be a more reliable parameter than the mitotic count alone in predicting disease behavior; 5-year survival rates of 50%, 33%, and 0% were reported for grades I, II, and III, respectively (RICCI et al. 1987).

For gastric lesions, tumor size seems to play a more important role than other prognostic factors; in their study, ROY and SOMMERS (1989) found that only 20% of the gastric tumors with an average diameter of 1.5–6 cm metastasized, while larger tumors showed significantly higher percentages. Gastric tumors were reported to behave in a less aggressive fashion than intestinal tumors, with 10-year survival rates of 74% and 17%, respectively (UEYAMA et al. 1992). It is worth noting that small tumors with a low mitotic count may also metastasize and lead to death (EVANS 1985).

There is universal consensus that retroperitoneal tumors have the most unfavorable prognosis of all (WILE et al. 1981; SMOOKLER and LAUER 1983), with a reported 2-year survival rate of 16% (RANCHOD and KEMPSON 1974).

4.2 Somatic Soft Tissues

The category of somatic soft tissues encompasses all dermal, subcutaneous, and deeper (intramuscular) tumors. Tumor size is the most important parameter in predicting outcome because it is strongly influenced by the anatomic location of the tumor. Dermal tumors are usually smaller than deeper tumors, such as subcutaneous and intramuscularly located lesions, and pursue a more indolent clinical course (ENJOJI and HASHIMOTO 1984; HASHIMOTO et al. 1986; WILE et al. 1981; NEUGUT and SORDILLO 1989; STOUT and HILL 1958; DAHL and ANGERVALL 1974).

4.3 Uterus

The most important prognostic factors for uterine LMS are cellularity, anaplasia, and mitotic count. A benign clinical course is expected for bland-looking, paucicellular tumors that display even up to ten mitoses per 10 hpf; on the other hand, for epithelioid and symplastic smooth muscle tumors, a mitotic rate greater than five mitoses per 10 hpf is indicative of malignancy. An excellent review of the literature on uterine sarcomas was reported by HENDRICKSON and KEMPSON (1991).

4.4 DNA Index

Flow cytometric measurement of the DNA content has been extensively used as an adjunctive parameter in evaluating the malignant potential of solid tumors; DNA aneuploidy is, in fact, commonly associated with aggressive behavior (ATKIN and KAY 1979). Ploidy findings in soft tissue tumors, however, are contradictory. It is now clear that DNA content does not distinguish between benign and malignant soft tissue tumors (AGARWAL et al. 1991; KROESE et al. 1990; KIYABU et al. 1988), nevertheless in malignant tumors, ploidy may constitute an additional parameter to predict the clinical course. Aneuploid leiomyosarcomas in fact seem to behave in a more aggressive fashion than diploid forms (OLIVER et al. 1991; KIYABU et al. 1988; TSUSHIMA et al. 1988).

5 Genetics

5.1 Cytogenetics

A characteristic t(12;14)(q14–15;q23–24) reciprocal chromosomal translocation was recently associated with at least one group of benign uterine leiomyomas (HEIM et al. 1988). Other abnormalities consistently identified thus far in benign leiomyomas include del(7)(q21.2q31.2) and trisomy 12 (NILBERT et al. 1988, 1990a).

To date, no specific and unique chromosomal abnormality has been detected in malignant smooth muscle tumors, even though a certain number of different karyotypic anomalies have been described.

The most frequently associated structural changes include partial monosomy of chromosome 1 [del (1)(p12–13)], and monosomy of chromosomes 18 and 22 (SALT et al. 1988). NILBERT et al. (1990b) reported the rearrangement of the same chromosomal regions involved in leiomyoma – 12q and 14q – in two malignant smooth muscle tumors.

BOGHOSIAN et al. (1989) recently proposed the subdivision of LMS into three distinct cytogenetic groups based on their chromosome mode and structural abnormalities. The first group is characterized by a hypodiploid chromosome number, with a highly characteristic pattern of monosomies involving chromosomes 1, 18, and 22. A second group of pseudodiploid tumors is associated with simple chromosomal translocations, while the third is a heterogeneous group with different numerical and structural changes.

In four cases observed at Padua University, we could not find any recurrent abnormality even though numerous clonal abnormalities were identified. Beside the numerical changes, the structural changes involved chromosomes 2, 3, 6, 10, 12, 13, and 16. A trisomy 8 was observed in two

Table 1. Cytogenetic data in four cases of leiomyosarcoma

Case no.	Site	DNA index	Karyotype
1	Forearm	1.0	48,XY,−2,−20,+der(2)t(2;20)(p33;p11),del(3)(p14),
2	Thigh	1.0	+8,+11,+17,del(10)(p13)
3[a]	Kidney	1.33/1.55	46,XX,t(13;16)(q14;q24)
4[a]	Liver[b]	2.0	46,XX,inv9(p11;q13),+8
			46,XY,t(6;12)(p21.2;p13)
			46,XY,del(12)(p13),13q+,−19,+der(19)t(19;?)(p11;?)

[a] The karyotype of these two tumors is not representative of the lesion due to the discrepancies between the DNA content values and chromosome mode; this finding reflects a high tumor heterogeneity.
[b] Metastatic LMS from small bowel.

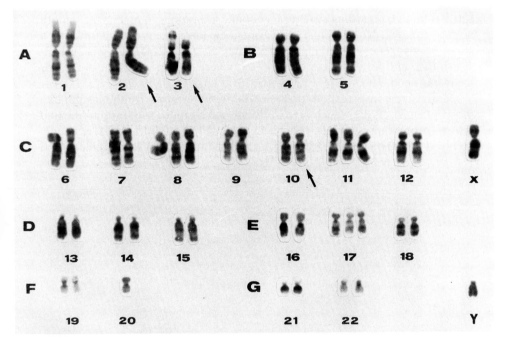

Fig. 13A–G. Cytogenetic findings in the case shown in Fig. 3. Despite an apparently diploid DNA content, the tumor showed numerous chromosomal abnormalities (see Table 1, case no. 1). The patient died 18 months after surgery with metastatic disease to lungs and liver

cases. The complete karyotypes are reported in Table 1. In two cases (case nos. 1 and 2), the cytofluorometric measurements revealed a DNA index of 1, with a corresponding chromosome mode of 48 and 46, respectively. In the first case, there was a massive structural genomic rearrangement (Fig. 13), while in the second case the only observed abnormality was a balanced chromosomal translocation t(13;16)(q14;q24). These findings further stress the high genomic variability of LMS also in the absence of significant quantitative differences in DNA content; the utility of flow cytometric studies as a tool to predict the clinical behavior of a given neoplasm is thus limited.

The grading system proposed by FLETCHER et al. (1990) seems more interesting. Unlike their benign counterparts, malignant smooth muscle tumors are in fact characterized by a higher genomic instability. This genomic instability is reflected by the presence of different cellular clones showing different nonrandom chromosomal abnormalities in addition to the stemline changes.

5.2 Molecular Genetics

Little is known regarding structural genomic alterations in malignant smooth muscle tumors. No structural abnormalities have been found utilizing a panel of oncogenes, including N- and H-ras, N- and c-myc, yes, mos, erb-B-1, erb-B-2, and fos (MAILLET et al. 1992), whereas rearrangement of the RB locus has been detected in a few cases (STRATTON et al. 1989).

Extensively investigated for their role in myogenesis are the insulin-like growth factors (IGF), which are two small polypeptides with insulin-like and growth-promoting activities (FROESCH et al. 1985). While IGF-I is mainly involved in postnatal life, IGF-II is important in fetal development and

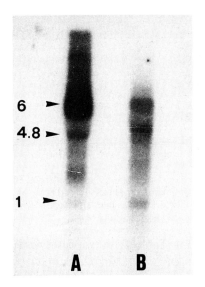

Fig. 14A,B. Northern blot analysis of IGF-II fetal mRNAs. **A** hepatoma cell line used as positive control; **B** 6.0-, 4.8-, and 1.0-Kb mRNAs are expressed by a gastric leiomyosarcoma

differentiation (TOLLEFSEN et al. 1989). High levels of IGF-II mRNAs are commonly detected in fetal smooth, cardiac, and skeletal muscles (SCOTT et al. 1985); IGF-II is presumed to act as an autocrine growth and differentiating agent in muscles since the level of IGF-II mRNAs expression declines rapidly after birth and is undetectable in adult muscle (BROWN et al. 1986; GRAY et al. 1987).

The re-expression of fetal forms of IGF-II mRNAs in malignant hepatic tumors has suggested a possible role for this gene in tumorigenesis (SCHIRMACHER et al. 1992). Reactivation of the IGF-II gene was further documented in some mesenchymal tumors, such as smooth and skeletal muscle-derived tumors (Fig. 14) (HOPPENER et al. 1988; MINNITI et al. 1992) and liposarcomas (TRICOLI et al. 1986).

In smooth muscle tumors, enhanced levels of IGF-II expression have been found in malignant lesions, thus suggesting a possible role for this factor in malignant smooth muscle tumor progression (HOPPENER et al. 1988; GLOUDEMANS et al. 1990).

Although its role as a progression factor needs further investigation, we documented high levels of fetal mRNAs expression in three out of seven LMS (CAVAZZANA et al. 1992). Interestingly, the three IGF-II-positive tumors were located in the gastrointestinal tract and showed a low degree of muscle differentiation; in fact, all displayed only muscle-specific actin expression, but failed to express desmin. This finding further supports the role of IGF-II in the early stages of myoblast differentiation.

Acknowledgement. We wish to thank A. Leorin and L. Rinaldi for technical assistance and P. Segato for help in preparing the manuscript.

References

Agarwal V, Greenebaum E, Wersto R, Koss LG (1991) DNA plody of spindle cell soft-tissue tumors and its relationship to histology and clinical outcome. Arch Pathol Lab Med 6: 558–562

Atkin NB, Kay R (1979) Prognostic significance of modal DNA value and other factors in malignant tumors, based on 1.465 cases. Br J Cancer 40: 210–220

Bearman RM (1974) Primary leiomyosarcoma of the hearth. Report of a case and review of the literature. Arch Pathol 98: 62–65

Boghosian L, dal Cin P, Turc-Carel C, Rao U, Karakousis C, Sait SJ, Sandberg AA (1989) Three possible cytogenetic subgroups of leiomyosarcoma. Cancer Genet Cytogenet 43: 39–49

Brooks JJ (1986) The significance of double phenotypic patterns and markers in human sarcomas. A novel model of mesemchymal differentiation. Am J Pathol 125: 113–123

Brown AL, Graham DE, Nissley SP, Hill DJ, Strain AJ, Rechler MM (1986) Developmental regulation of insulin-like growth factor II mRNA in different rat tissues. J Biol Chem 261: 13144–13150

Brown DC, Theaker JM, Banks PM, Gatter KC, Mason DY (1987) Cytokeratin expression in smooth muscle and smooth muscle tumours. Histopathology 11: 477–486

Cavazzaha AO, Tirabosco R, Frunzio R, Scalerta R, Panozzo M, Schiaroli S, Rossi R, Lise M, Ninfo V, Spagnoli LG (1992) IGF-II correlates with tumor differentiation and not with tumor progression in malignant smooth muscle tumors. Patologia 25: 3(8A)

Dahl I, Angervall L (1974) Cutaneous and subcutaneous leiomyosarcoma: a clinicopathologic study of 47 patients. Pathol Eur 9: 307–315

Enjoji M, Hashimoto H (1984) Diagnosis of soft tissue sarcomas. Pathol Res Pract 178: 215–226

Evans HL (1985) Smooth muscle tumors of the gastrointestinal tract. A study of 56 cases followed for a minumum of 10 years. Cancer 56: 2242–2250

Fisher C (1990) The value of electronmicroscopy and immunohistochemistry in the diagnosis of soft tissue sarcomas: a study of 200 cases. Histopathology 16: 441–454

Fletcher C (1992) Pleomorphic malignant fibrous histiocytoma: fact or fiction?: a critical reappraisal based on 159 tumors diagnosed as pleomorphic sarcoma. Am J Surg Pathol 16: 213–228

Fletcher JA, Morton CC, Pavelka K, Lage JM (1990) Chromosome aberrations in uterine smooth muscle tumors: potential diagnostic relevance of cytogenetic instability. Cancer Res 50: 4092–4097

Franke WW, Grund C, Kuhn C, Jackson BW, Illmensee K (1982) Formation of cytoskeleton of elements during mouse embryogenesis. III. Prymary mesenchymal cells and the first appearance of vimentin filaments. Differentiation 23: 4349

Froesch ER, Schmid C, Schwander J, Zapf J (1985) Actions of insulin-like growth factors. Annu Rev Physiol 47: 443–467

Gabbiani G, Schmid E, Winter S, Chaponier C, de Chastonay C, Vandekerckhove J, Weber K, Franke WW (1981) Vascular smooth muscle cells differ from other smooth muscle cells: predominance of vimentin filaments and a specific alpha-typeactin. Proc Natl Acad Sci USA 78: 298–302

Gloudemans T, Prinsen I, van Unnik JA, Lips CJ, den Otter W, Sussenbach JS (1990) Insulin-like growth factor gene expression in human smooth muscle tumors. Cancer Res 50: 6689–6695

Gray A, Tam AW, Dull TJ, Hayflick J, Pintar J, Cavanee WK, Koufos A, Ullrich A (1987) Tissue-specific and developmentally regulated transcription of the insulin-like growth factor 2 gene. DNA 6: 283–295

Hashimoto H, Daimaru Y, Tsuneyoshi M, Enjoji M (1986) Leiomyosarcoma of the external soft tissues. A clinicopathologic, immunohistochemical, and electron microscopic study. Cancer 57: 2077–2088

Hayashi T, Shimada O, Anami M, Karasuyama M, Sato N, Muraoka N, Tsuda N (1990) Histogenesis of the clear cytoplasm in the tumor cells of the smooth muscle origin. Rinsho Byori 3: 317–322

Heim S, Nilbert M, Vanni R, Floderus U-M et al. (1988) A specific translocation, t(12;14) (q14–15;q23–24), characterizes a subgroup of uterine leiomyomas. Cancer Genet Cytogenet 32: 13–17

Hendrickson MR, Kempson RL (1991) The uterine corpus. In: Sternberg SS, Mills SE (eds) Surgical pathology of the female reproductive system and peritoneum. Raven, New York

Hoppener JWM, Mosselman S, Roholl PJM, Lambrechts C, Slebos RJC, de Pagter-Holthuizen P, Lips CJM, Jansz HS, Sussenbach JS (1988) Expression of insulin-like growth factor-I and -II genes in human smooth muscle tumors. EMBO J 7: 1379–1385

Jones H, Steart PV, du Bolay CEH, Roche WR (1990) Alpha-smooth muscle actin as marker for soft tissue tumours: a comparison with desmin. J Pathol 126: 29–33

Kiyabu MT, Bishop PC, Parker JW, Turner RR, Fitzgibbons PL (1988) Smooth muscle tumors of the gastrointestinal. Flow cytometric quantification of DNA and nuclear antigen content and correlation with histologic grade. Am J Surg Pathol 12: 954–960

Knapp AC, Franke WW (1989) Spontaneous losses of control of cytokeratin gene expression in transformed, non-epithelial human cells occurring at different levels of regulation. Cell 59: 67–79

Knapp RH, Wick MR, Goeller JR (1984) Leiomyoblastoma and their relationship to other smooth-muscle tumors of the gastrointestinal tract. Am J Surg Pathol 8: 449–461

Kroese MC, Rutgers DH, Wils IS, van Unnik JA, Roholl PJ (1990) The relevance of the DNA index and proliferation rate in the grading of the benign and malignant soft tissue tumors. Cancer 8: 1782–1788

Kuruc N, Franke WW (1988) Transient coexpression of desmin and cytokeratin 8 and 18 in developing myocardial cells of some vertebrate species. Differentiation 38: 177–193

Lazarides E (1980) Intermediate filaments as mechanical integrators of cellular space. Nature 283: 249–256

LeBoit PE, Barr RJ, Burall S, Metcalf JS, Yen TS, Wick MR (1991) Primitive polypoid granular-cell tumor and other cutaneous granular-cell neoplasms of apparent nonneural origin. Am J Surg Pathol 1: 48–58

Maillet MW, Robinson RA, Burgart LJ (1992) Genomic alterations in sarcomas: a histologic correlative study with use of oncogene panels. Mod Pathol 5: 410–414

Markhede G, Angervall L, Stener B (1982) A multivariate analysis of the prognosis after surgical treatment of malignant of malignant soft-tissue tumors. Cancer 49: 1721–1733

Miettinen M (1988a) Antibody specific to muscle actins in the diagnosis and classification of soft tissue tumors. Am J Pathol 130: 205–215

Miettinen M (1988b) Immunoreactivity for cytokeratin and epithelial membrane antigen in leiomyosarcoma. Arch Pathol Lab Med 112: 637–640

Miettinen M (1991) Keratin subsets in spindle cell sarcomas. Keratins are widespread but synovial sarcoma contains a distinctive keratin polypeptide pattern and desmoplakins. Am J Pathol 138: 505–513

Miettinen M, Foidart J, Ekblom P (1983) Immunohistochemical demonstration of laminin, the major glycoprotein ofbasement membranes, as an aid in the diagnosis of soft tissue tumors. Am J Clin Pathol 79: 306–311

Minniti CP, Kohn EC, Grubb JH, Sly WS, Oh Y, Muller HL, Rosenfeld RG, Helman LJ (1992) The insulin-like growth factor II (IGF-II)/mannose 6-phosphate receptor mediates IGF-II-induced motility in human rhabdomyosarcoma cells. J Biol Chem 267: 9000–9004

Myers JL, Arocho J, Bernreuter W, Dunham W, Mazur MT (1991) Leiomyosarcoma of bone. A clinicopathologic, immunohistochemical, and ultrastructural study of five cases. Cancer 67: 1051–1056

Myhre-Jensen O, Kaae S, Hjollund Madsen E, Sneppen O (1983) Histopathological grading in soft-tissue tumours. Acta Pathol Microbiol Immunol Scand [A] 91: 145–150

Neugut AI, Sordillo PP (1989) Leiomyosarcomas of the extremities. J Surg Oncol 40: 65–67

Nilbert M, Heim S, Mandhal N, Flodérus UM, Willén H, Mitelman F (1988) Karyotypic rearrangements in 20 uterine leiomyomas. Cytogenet Cell Genet 49: 300–304

Nilbert M, Heims S, Mandhal N, Flodérus UM, Willén H, Mitelman F (1990a) Trisomy 12 in uterine leiomyoma – a new cytogenetic subgroup. Cancer Genet Cytogenet 45: 63–66

Nilbert M, Mandhal N, Heim S, Rydholm A, Helm G, Willen H, Baldetorp B, Mitelman F (1990b) Complex karyotypic changes, including rearrangements of 12q13 and 14q24, in two leiomyosarcomas. Cancer Genet Cytogenet 48: 217–223

Nistal M, Paniagua R, Picazo ML et al. (1980) Granular changes of leiomyosarcoma. Virchow Arch [A] 386: 239–248

Ogawa K, Oguchi M, Yamabe H, Nakashima Y, Hamashima Y (1986) Distribution of collagen IV in soft tissue tumors. An immunohistochemical study. Cancer 58: 269–277

Oliver GF, Reiman HM, Gonchoroff NJ, Muller SA, Umbert IJ (1991) Cutaneous and subcutaneous leiomyosarcoma: a clinicopathologic review of 14 cases with reference to antidesmin staining and nuclear DNA patterns studied by flow cytometry. Br J Dermatol 124: 252–257

Polednak AP (1986) Incidence of soft-tissue cancers in blacks and whites in New York State. Int Cancer 38: 21–26

Ranchod M, Kempson RL (1977) Smooth muscle tumors of the gastrointestinal tract and retroperitoneum. A pathologic analysis of 100 cases. Cancer 39: 266–262

Rangdaeng S, Truong LD (1991) Comparative immunohistochemical staining for desmin and muscle-specific actin. A study of 576 cases. Am J Clin Pathol 96: 32–45

Ricci A, Ciccarelli O, Cartun RW, Newcomb P (1987) A clinicopathologic and immunohistochemical study of 16 patients with small intestinal leiomyosarcoma. Limited utility of immunophenotyping. Cancer 60: 1790–1799

Roholl PJ, Elbers HR, Prinsen I, Claessens JA, van Unnik JA (1990) Distribution of actin isoforms in sarcomas: an immunohistochemical study. Hum Pathol 21: 1269–1274

Roy M, Sommers SC (1989) Metastatic potential of gastric leiomyosarcoma. Pathol Res Pract 185: 874–877

Sait SN, dal Cin P, Sandberg AA (1988) Consistent chromosome changes in leiomyosarcoma. Cancer Genet Cytogenet 35: 47–50

Saul SH, Rast ML, Brooks JJ (1987) The immunohistochemistry of gastrointestinal stromal tumors. Evidence supporting an origin from smooth muscle. Am J Surg Pathol 11: 464–473

Schirmacher P, Held WA Yang D, Chisari FV, Rustum Y, Rogler CE (1992) Reactivation of insulin-like growth factor II during hepatocarcinogenesis in transgenic mice suggests a role in malignant growth. Cancer Res 52: 2549–2556

Schurch W, Skalli O, Seemayer TA, Gabbiani G (1987) Intermediate filaments proteins and actin isoforms as markers for soft tissue tumor differentiation and origin. I. Smooth muscle tumors. Am J Pathol 128: 91–103

Scott J, Cowell J, Robertson ME, Priestly LM et al. (1985) Insulin-like growth factor-II gene expression in Wilms' tumour and embryonic tissues. Nature 317: 260–262

Smookler BM, Lauer DH (1983) Retroperitoneal leiomyosarcoma. A clinicopathologic analysis of 36 cases. Am J Surg Pathol 7: 269–280

Stout AP, Hill WT (1958) Leiomyosarcoma of the superficial soft tissues. Cancer 11: 844–854

Stratton Mr, Williams S, Fisher C, Ball A, Westbury G, Gusterson BA et al. (1989) Structural alterations of the RB1 gene in human soft tissue tumours. Br J Cancer 60: 201–205

Swanson PE, Wick MR, Dehner LP (1991) Leiomyosarcoma of somatic soft tissues in childhood: an immunohistochemical analysis of six cases with ultrastructural correlation. Hum Pathol 6: 569–577

Tirabosco R, Cavazzana AO, Santeusanio G, Spagnoli LG Gastrointestinal stromal tumor: evidence for a smooth muscle origin. Mod Pathol (submitted)

Tollefsen SE, Sadow JL, Rotwein P (1989) Coordinate expression of insulin-like growth factor II and its receptor during muscle differentiation. Proc Natl Acad Sci USA 86: 1543–1547

Tricoli JV, Rall LB, Karakousis CP, Herrera L, Petrelli NJ, Bell GI, Shows TB (1986) Enhanced levels of insulin-like growth factor messenger RNA in human colon carcinomas and liposarcomas. Cancer Res 46: 6169–6173

Trojani M, Contesso G, Coindre JM et al. (1984) Soft-tissue sarcomas of adults: study of pathological prognostic variables and definition of a histopathologic grading system. Int J Cancer 33: 37–42

Tsukada T, Mc Nutt MA, Ross R, Gown AM (1987) HHF-35, a muscle actin-specific monoclonal antibody. II. Reactivity in normal, reactive, and neoplastiic human tissues. Am J Pathol 127: 389–403

Tsushima K, Stanhope CR, Gaffey TA, Lieber MM (1988) Uterine leiomyosarcomas and benign smooth muscle tumors: usefulness of nuclear DNA patterns studied by flow cytometry. Mayo Clin Proc 61: 248–255

Ueyama T, Guo KJ, Hashimoto H, Daimaru Y, Enjoji M (1992) A clinicopathologic and immunohistochemical study of gastrointestinal stromal tumors. Cancer 4: 947–955

Verela-Duran J, Oliva H, Rosai J (1979) Vascular leiomyosarcoma: the malignant counterpart of vascular leiomyoma. Cancer 44: 1684–1691

Vandekerckhove J, Weber K (1978) At least six different actins are expressed in a higher mammal: an analysis based on the amino acid sequence of the amino-terminal tryptic peptide. J Mol Biol 126: 783–802

Vandekerckhove J, Weber K (1981) Actin typing on total cellular extracts: a highly sensitive protein-chemical procedure able to distinguish different actins. Eur J Biochem 113: 595–603

Weiss RA, Mackay B (1981) Malignant smooth muscle tumors of the gastrointestinal tract: an ultrastructural study of 20 cases. Ultrastruct Pathol 12: 231–240

Wile AG, Evans HL, Romsdahl MM (1981) Leiomyosarcoma od soft tissue: a clinicopathologic study. Cancer 48: 1022–1032

Yannopoulos K, Stout AP (1962) Smooth muscle tumors in children. Cancer 15: 958

Malignant Peripheral Nerve Sheath Tumours

C.D.M. Fletcher

1 Introduction

Malignant peripheral nerve sheath tumour (MPNST) is the term presently preferred to either malignant schwannoma or neurofibrosarcoma because many sarcomas of nerve sheath bear no reproducible morphological relationship to conventional benign schwannomas or neurofibromas and their constituent cells are typically heterogeneous: in other words, tumour cells in these lesions usually show variable degrees of Schwann cell, perineural and fibroblastic differentiation and hence it is generally impossible to impute a single cell of origin. Therefore the term MPNST more accurately reflects the cellular composition of these neoplasms.

In our experience and that of others (Enzinger and Weiss 1988), MPNST accounts for about 10% of all soft tissue sarcomas, although other authors have suggested a much lower figure (Storm et al. 1980; Enjoji and Hashimoto 1984). This probably reflects differences in the criteria used for making this diagnosis. This somewhat controversial topic is discussed below.

Current Topics in Pathology
Volume 89, Eds. D. Harms/D. Schmidt
© Springer-Verlag Berlin Heidelberg 1995

2 Diagnostic Criteria

2.1 Conventional (Spindle Cell) MPNST

It has long been suggested that MPNST has such a variable and non-reproducible, or at least non-distinctive, range of morphological patterns that very strict non-histological criteria must be set for this diagnosis. In my view, this is not entirely true and largely reflects outdated attitudes, generated during the era prior to electron microscopy or immunohisto-chemistry: quite rightly, it is now being recognised more widely that the majority of MPNSTs have distinctive histological features.

Originally it was believed that, to make a diagnosis of MPNST, one must demonstrate convincing origin from either a nerve (D'AGOSTINO et al. 1963a) or a pre-existing benign nerve sheath tumour. Subsequently the definition was broadened somewhat to include tumours with appropriate spindle cell morphology arising in the context of von Recklinghausen's disease (neurofibromatosis type 1) and tumours showing ultrastructural evidence of Schwann cell differentiation – particularly, cells with long interdigitating convoluted cytoplasmic processes and well-formed, often reduplicated external lamina (TAXY et al. 1981).

With the passage of time and with the ever improving recognition of other sarcoma types which might mimic MPNST (e.g. monophasic synovial sarcoma), it has become apparent that the majority of cases that fulfil the above criteria also show reproducible morphological patterns – which can then be recognised even in the absence of the original criteria (TSUNEYOSHI and ENJOJI 1979). These distinctive features are described later in this chapter.

Our ability to recognise these patterns has been aided, but only partially, by the advent of immunohistochemistry. It was realised in the early 1980s that the calcium-binding protein S-100 is expressed by Schwann cells and antibodies to S-100 were then used with considerable enthusiasm in the diagnosis of nerve sheath neoplasms (STEFANSSON et al. 1982; WEISS et al. 1983). While such antibodies remain of considerable value today, their use must always be interpreted with caution and in the light of a specific context since it was soon clear (KAHN et al. 1983) that S-100 positivity is also a feature of many other neural crest cells (e.g., melanocytes and neuro-endocrine cells), chondrocytes, adipocytes, myoepithelial cells, a small proportion of carcinomas and, with many polyclonal antibodies, skeletal muscle cells. Whether this widespread distribution of S-100 protein can be narrowed down by the use of antibodies specific to the alpha and beta isoforms (TAKAHASHI et al. 1984) has yet to be widely substantiated.

However, in the context of diagnostic criteria, it is clear that only around 50% of MPNSTs are S-100 positive; therefore, while a positive result might be useful, in the context of a fascicular spindle cell sarcoma, in confirming the diagnosis of MPNST, negativity means nothing. Furthermore, other conventional morphological parameters will still always need to be carefully assessed, since a small proportion of synovial sarcomas are also S-100 positive (ORDONEZ et al. 1990; FISHER and SCHOFIELD 1991).

Taking all these data together, the current criteria we personally use for the recognition of most cases of MPNST are as follows:

1. A spindle cell malignant neoplasm arising from (and within) an identifiable nerve, or
2. A spindle cell malignant neoplasm arising from (or within) a pre-existing tumour with the typical features of a benign neurofibroma, schwannoma or rarely ganglioneuroma, or
3. A malignant neoplasm showing clear ultrastructural evidence of Schwann cell differentiation, or
4. A spindle cell malignant neoplasm with typical morphological features of MPNST (see below) arising in the context of neurofibromatosis, or
5. A spindle cell malignant neoplasm with typical morphological features of MPNST (see below) showing at least focal S-100 positivity, or
6. A tumour with the usual features of a neurofibroma but showing mitotic activity (usually accompanied by at least some degree of nuclear hyperchromasia or pleomorphism)

Having presented these six options, it should be pointed out (a) that sarcomas with typical morphology but negative or unavailable electron microscopy, negative immuno histochemistry and no neurofibromatosis we classify as "spindle cell sarcoma, probably MPNST"; and (b) that patients with neurofibromatosis are at increased risk of sarcoma generally (not only MPNST) and that not all sarcomas arising from a nerve are examples of MPNST (CHAUDHURI et al. 1980): because of the plasticity of neural crest differentiation, one may very rarely encounter pure sarcomas of theoretically almost any type.

2.2 Epithelioid MPNST

The accurate recognition of the epithelioid variant of MPNST, the typical features of which are described later in this chapter, requires somewhat different (or at least modified) criteria because of its very close resemblance to amelanotic malignant melanoma, at least in some parts of the tumour. This problem is particularly acute in pure epithelioid neoplasms. The criteria we employ are as follows:

1. A tumour fulfilling the criteria for MPNST as described above, which is composed in part of large, rounded cells arranged in nests or cords, or
2. A purely epithelioid malignant neoplasm, resembling amelanotic melanoma, which either clearly originates in a nerve or shows Schwann cell

features ultrastructurally and is S-100 positive but negative for melanoma antigens (such as HMB-45).

In real day-to-day practice, the diagnosis of pure epithelioid MPNST can be exceedingly difficult, a point well made in the original description by DiCarlo et al. (1986).

3 Clinical Features

The clinical features of MPNST vary somewhat, depending upon whether the tumour is sporadic or arises in the context of neurofibromatosis. Up to 50% of MPNSTs are associated with stigmata or a family history of NF-1 (Sordillo et al. 1981; Ducatman et al. 1986; Hruban et al. 1990), although this proportion depends heavily on the diagnostic criteria used and also on the clinical rigour with which this possibility is pursued. It seems probable that this proportion will fall as morphological recognition of MPNST improves, irrespective of NF-1 status. Among all patients with NF-1, the ultimate risk of developing an MPNST is estimated to be 2% (Sorensen et al. 1986).

3.1 Sporadic MPNST

The absolute age range in sporadic MPNST is wide but the majority of cases arise in adulthood with a mean of around 40 years. The sex incidence is approximately equal in our material, although some authors have shown a female predominance (Ducatman et al. 1986). Sporadic cases arise most often in the limbs, followed by the trunk (including retroperitoneum) and then the head/neck region. In our experience demonstrable origin from a nerve is less common than in NF-1 patients, but limb tumours arising from a major nerve in either group invariably require amputation. Patients usually present with a mass, sometimes associated with pain and less commonly with neurological symptoms. With the exception of small or histologically low-grade lesions, the overall prognosis is generally not good with a reported 5-year survival of 50% or often less (Ghosh et al. 1973; Ducatman et al. 1986): many patients eventually develop pulmonary metastases. Nodal metastases are extremely rare.

3.2 MPNST Associated with NF-1

This group of patients differs from the sporadic group in that they typically present at a younger age (mean around 30 years) and show a male predominance; the tumours more often originate from an identifiable nerve or pre-existing benign neoplasm and, most importantly, in most studies, tend to have a much poorer prognosis with a 5-year survival of around 20% or less (D'AGOSTINO et al. 1963b; GHOSH et al. 1973; GUCCION and ENZINGER 1979; SORDILLO et al. 1981; DUCATMAN et al. 1986). However, this latter point has been disputed in a recent study (HRUBAN et al. 1990).

3.3 Post-irradiation MPNST

Up to 10% of cases of MPNST arise in previously irradiated tissues, most often following treatment of lymphoma or carcinoma (FOLEY et al. 1980; DUCATMAN and SCHEITHAUER 1983). Such tumours are inevitably more common in adults, have a variable post-treatment latency period which generally exceeds 10 years, affect patients with or without NF-1 and, like all post-irradiation sarcomas (LASKIN et al. 1988), are believed to carry a rather poor prognosis with a mortality of 80% or more.

3.4 Epithelioid MPNST

The epithelioid variant accounts for about 5% of MPNSTs and is most often a deep-seated lesion with no particular clinically distinctive features (LODDING et al. 1986; LASKIN et al. 1991; WOODRUFF 1991), other than a tendency for lymph node metastasis. Worthy of note, however, is the significant group of cases which arise in superficial (subcutaneous) tissues, since these tumours appear remarkably indolent with a good prognosis (LASKIN et al. 1991).

3.5 MPNST in Children

It has generally been believed that MPNST in young patients is very uncommon and most series recognise only about 5%–10% of cases in this age group, very often associated with NF-1 (DUCATMAN et al. 1984). However, a recent large study of 78 cases from the Armed Forces Institute of Pathology (AFIP) (MEIS et al. 1992) suggests that this incidence has been underestimated, albeit the clinical and prognostic features of such childhood cases are very similar to those seen in adults. Interpretation of this data depends heavily on diagnostic criteria since there is particular potential for overlap with primitive neuroectodermal tumours, monophasic synovial sarcoma and infantile fibrosarcoma in this age category.

3.6 Melanotic (Pigmented) MPNST

The majority of melanotic schwannomas are benign lesions which arise from spinal nerve roots (MENNEMEYER et al. 1979; KILLEEN et al. 1988). However, the group of pigmented nerve sheath tumours which arise in the limbs or from the sympathetic chain often pursue a malignant clinical course (KRAUSZ et al. 1984; ROWLANDS et al. 1987; ENZINGER and WEISS 1988). Anatomical location appears to provide the principal clue to aggressive behaviour, since histological distinction of benign from malignant melanotic PNST is generally impossible.

3.7 MPNST Arising in a Schwannoma or Ganglioneuroma

Malignant peripheral nerve sheath tumours quite often originate in a pre-existent neurofibroma, particularly if large, deep-seated and/or plexiform, and this may provide the key to diagnosis in up to 25% or more of cases (see Sect. 2.1). It is not so widely appreciated that rare cases may also arise in a pre-existing benign schwannoma (RASBRIDGE et al. 1989) or in a ganglioneuroma, either de novo or following irradiation-induced maturation of a neuroblastic tumour (FLETCHER et al. 1988; GHALI et al. 1992). Those arising in a ganglioneuroma tend, as expected, to be deep-seated thoracic or retroperitoneal neoplasms but, other than this, these rare subgroups are not clinically distinctive.

4 Pathological Features

4.1 Macroscopic Features

Other than those tumours arising from an identifiable nerve, MPNST is not macroscopically distinctive. Most cases appear as a circumscribed, pale mass with a variably firm, myxoid or necrotic cut surface, just like other sarcomas. Size is very variable, often depending upon presenting symptoms: those causing dysaesthesiae tend to be smaller when found, but in most cases the maximum diameter exceeds 10 cm. Those arising from a nerve typically show adjacent fusiform swelling of the affected nerve, which tapers proximally; passage of the nerve (or its remnants) through the tumour is often hard to identify. Tumours arising in a pre-existing benign PNST may be hard to recognise by the naked eye, unless there happens to be a dramatically "zoned" difference in appearance or if the pre-existing tumour was overtly plexiform.

4.2 Histological Features

4.2.1 Conventional (Spindle Cell) MPNST

The majority of MPNSTs, whether arising sporadically or in association with NF-1, have a predominantly fascicular spindle-celled morphology. Although much has been previously made of neural-type nuclear features, these are a less consistent finding than some of the architectural pointers evident at low to medium magnification. In addition to the presence of long interlacing fascicles, two frequent and useful features are the abrupt alternation between cellular and more myxoid areas, which gives a rather banded appearance (Fig. 1), and the apparent perivascular accentuation or piling-up of tumour

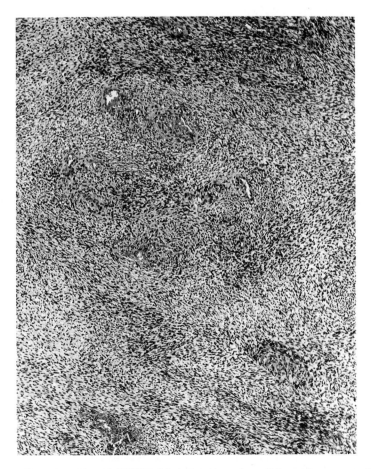

Fig. 1. Conventional MPNST. Note the alternating cellular and more myxoid fascicles. H&E; ×63

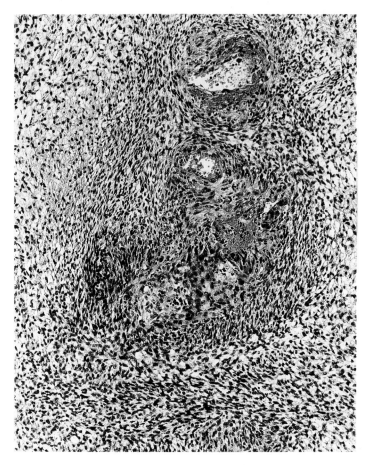

Fig. 2. Conventional MPNST. Note the striking perivascular accentuation (or whorling) and apparent subendothelial spread of tumour cells. H&E; ×100

cells both around and within vessel walls, which sometimes lead to luminal occlusion or thrombosis (Fig. 2).

The other particularly common pattern is less distinctive and is essentially very similar to monophasic synovial sarcoma or the rare fibrosarcoma, consisting of densely cellular closely packed fascicles, in which the cells have only small amounts of ill-defined cytoplasm (Fig. 3). In lesions with this pattern, it may be of help to analyse nuclear features, but synovial sarcoma is more reliably excluded by immunohistochemistry (especially EMA positivity) and by checking for features such as calcification, wiry stromal hyalinisation and an haemangiopericytoma-like vasculature. It should also be noted that stromal mast cells are a prominent feature of many synovial sarcomas, whereas they are generally absent in MPNST – despite the age-

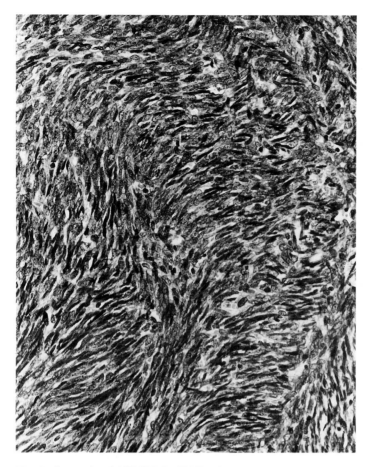

Fig. 3. Conventional MPNST. In H&E-stained sections, distinction of fascicular cases from monophasic synovial sarcoma or fibrosarcoma is often impossible. H&E; ×250

old, somewhat simplistic teaching about the association between mast cells and neural tumours!

The nuclear features which may be a useful clue to the diagnosis of MPNST are a narrow, tapering outline, often shorter than in a smooth muscle tumour, with a wavy or buckled configuration in some areas (Fig. 4). However, the latter well-known feature is not present in quite a proportion of cases. The nuclei usually tend to be dense and hyperchromatic with inconspicuous nucleoli and show at least focal pleomorphism. Mitoses are generally easy to find. Nuclear palisading is evident in fewer than 10% of cases and is no more frequent than in leiomyosarcoma. Other recognised features such as Meissnerian differentiation and hyaline stromal nodules are rare and therefore of no great diagnostic value.

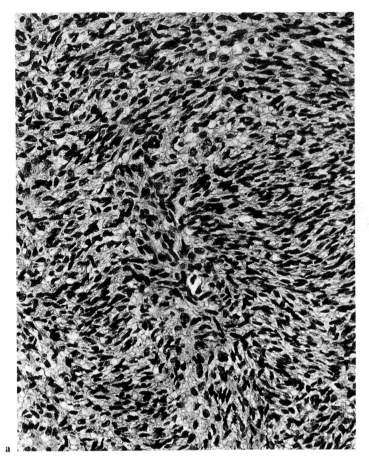
a

Fig. 4a,b. Conventional MPNST. Note the hyperchromatic, tapering nuclei with rather wavy or buckled outlines in these two cases. H&E; **a** ×250; **b** ×400

4.2.2 Myxoid MPNST

Around 10% of cases have a diffusely (rather than focally) myxoid stroma, causing possible confusion with other types of myxoid sarcoma. These lesions, which are most often low grade, show more widely dispersed cells, with the same nuclear characteristics as described above but with virtually indiscernible cytoplasm. Perivascular whorling or subendothelial proliferation often appears especially conspicuous due to the adjacent hypocellularity (Fig. 5). Delicate branching vessels and mucin pooling are not usual features.

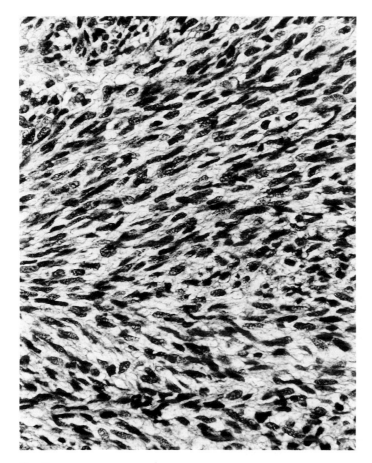

Fig. 4b

4.2.3 Malignant Change in a Neurofibroma

The development of an MPNST within a neurofibroma generally takes one of two forms. There may either be a fairly abrupt transition from bland benign neurofibroma to MPNST, showing the features described above, in which case the diagnosis is usually easy (Fig. 6). Less often, and probably reflecting an earlier stage of the same process, malignant change is evidenced simply by the presence of mitotic activity in a neurofibroma (usually deep-seated). Such mitoses are almost invariably accompanied by a mild increase in cellularity and at least focal nuclear hyperchromasia or pleomorphism (Fig. 7): in fact, these latter features, in any neurofibroma, should prompt a careful search for mitoses. We prefer to regard the presence of *any* mitoses at all in a neurofibroma as evidence of at least low-grade malignancy. This

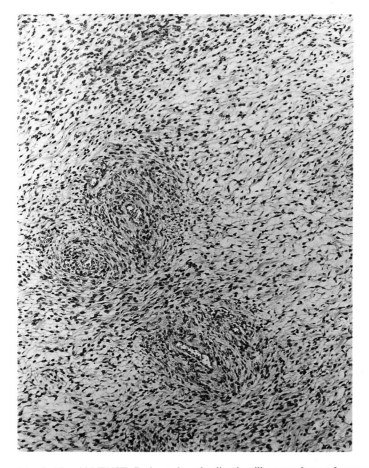

Fig. 5. Myxoid MPNST. Perivascular whorling is still a conspicuous feature. H&E; ×100

type of malignant change is seen most often in patients with NF-1. Clearly the same rule does not apply in benign schwannoma, in which scattered mitoses are quite frequent.

4.2.4 Heterologous Differentiation in MPNST

A distinctive feature seen in around 10% of MPNSTs is the presence of heterologous elements (Ducatman and Scheithauer 1984): this is usually regarded as a reflection of the plasticity of neural crest differentiation and the role of the neural crest in programming ectomesenchymal differentiation in utero. In any event, such elements are seen most often in NF-1 patients and may be a useful clue to the diagnosis of MPNST in some cases. The most common line of differentiation seen is rhabdomyoblastic, the so-called

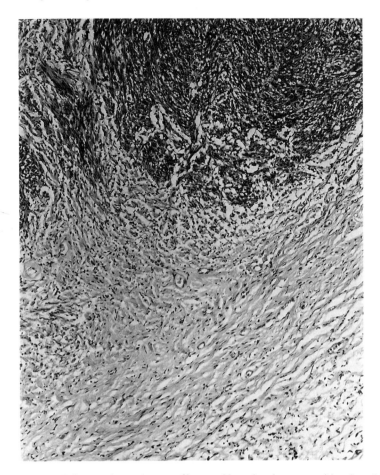

Fig. 6. Malignant change in neurofibroma. Note the abrupt transition from bland collagenous neurofibroma to spindle cell sarcoma. H&E; ×100

malignant Triton tumour (DAIMARU et al. 1984; BROOKS et al. 1985) (Fig. 8), and such tumours are generally believed to carry an especially poor prognosis. The proportion and degree of rhabdomyoblastic differentiation is extremely variable. The next most common line of additional mesenchymal differentiation is chondroblastic or osteoblastic and, while sometimes this appears cytologically banal, in some cases it has malignant features. Traditionally, however, the term malignant mesenchymoma is not used for these lesions (NEWMAN and FLETCHER 1991).

The other main form of heterologous differentiation is epithelial and takes the form of glandular structures lined by cuboidal, columnar or goblet cells with mucin secretion (WOODRUFF 1976). Less often there is squamous differentiation (DUCATMAN and SCHEITHAUER 1984; CROSS and CLARK 1988).

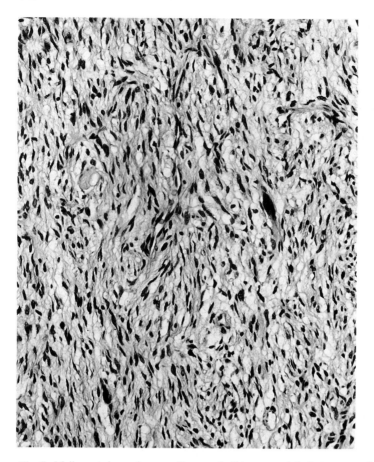

Fig. 7. Malignant change in neurofibroma. In this more subtle lesion, note the hypercellularity and focal nuclear pleomorphism. Scattered mitoses were quite easily found in other fields at higher power. H&E; ×250

Glandular MPNST needs to be distinguished from biphasic synovial sarcoma and this is achieved by the presence of goblet cells in MPNST and the fact that glandular epithelium in MPNST is CEA positive and also shows immunohistochemical evidence of neuroendocrine differentiation (WARNER et al. 1983; CHRISTENSEN et al. 1988).

4.2.5 Epithelioid MPNST

As mentioned in Sect. 2, epithelioid differentiation in MPNST may be focal or diffuse. The epithelioid component is typically arranged in cords, nests or

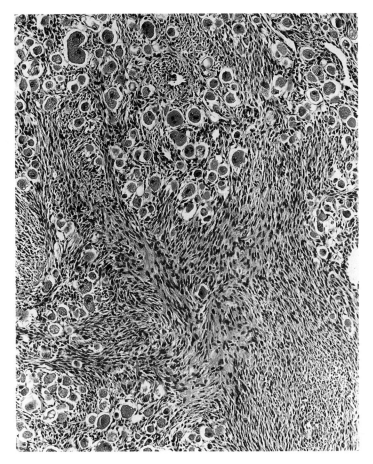

Fig. 8. Malignant Triton tumour. In this example, rhabdomyoblasts were both numerous and large and therefore easy to recognise. H&E; ×100

even small lobules, and cytologically often resembles amelanotic melanoma. The tumour cells are generally rounded with variable amounts of eosinophilic or amphophilic cytoplasm (Fig. 9). Nuclei are ovoid and vesicular, usually with a single prominent nucleolus. Personal experience suggests that the cells in superficial (subcutaneous) epithelioid MPNST are somewhat smaller and more naevoid than in deeper lesions. Distinction from metastatic melanoma, the commonest problem in differential diagnosis, is afforded by the identification of more typical spindle cell areas or by immunohisto-chemistry and electron microscopy (see below). Carcinomas, whether primary or metastatic, are readily distinguished by their immunoprofile and also are usually rather more pleomorphic than epithelioid MPNST.

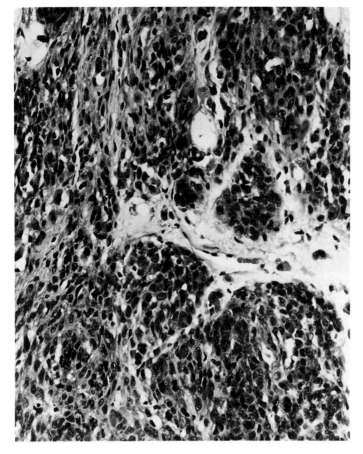

Fig. 9. Epithelioid MPNST. Note the lobulation and the similarity of the nuclei to those seen in melanoma. H&E; ×250

4.2.6 Other Histological Patterns in MPNST

A detailed discussion of pigmented (melanotic) MPNST is beyond the scope of this chapter since, as mentioned earlier, the histological features are often indistinguishable from benign melanotic schwannoma (KILLEEN et al. 1988; CARNEY 1990), which is generally regarded as a quite separate clinically distinctive lesion, arising mainly from spinal nerve roots or the sympathetic chain, and sometimes having major syndromic associations. Quite separately, however, it is important to note that very rare conventional MPNSTs, showing otherwise typical features, may also show focal melanin pigmentation: we have two such cases on file and others have been reported (JANZER and MAKEK 1983; OOI et al. 1992). Reliable distinction from a malignant melanoma is of paramount importance in such cases.

It should also be mentioned that a small percentage of MPNSTs are indistinguishable, in haemotoxylin and eosin-stained sections, from so-called pleomorphic malignant fibrous histiocytoma – i.e., high-grade poorly differentiated sarcoma (FLETCHER 1992). Such cases are very uncommon and generally require electron microscopy for accurate diagnosis (HERRERA et al. 1982; GOODLAD and FLETCHER 1991).

5 Immunohistochemistry

As mentioned earlier, immunohistochemistry, particularly using antibodies to S-100 protein, has some role in the diagnosis of MPNST, more often in a confirmatory context or else in the differential from monophasic synovial

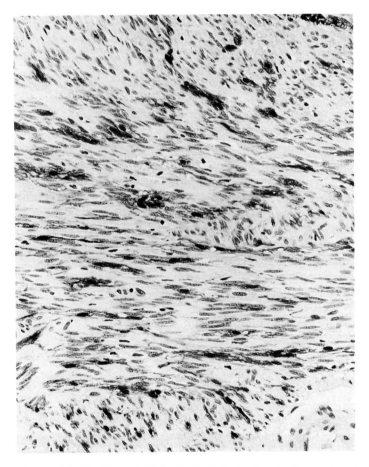

Fig. 10. S-100 in MPNST. Note the typically focal positivity one sees in MPNST: in many convincingly positive cases fewer than 20% of cells stain with this antibody. ABC; ×250

sarcoma. It has become apparent, in recent years, that no more than about 50% of MPNSTs are S-100 positive (DAIMARU et al. 1985; MATSUNOU et al. 1985; WICK et al. 1987). The basis for this has recently been demonstrated in several elegant studies of MPNST, comparing immunophenotype with ultrastructural features (JOHNSON et al. 1991; FISHER et al. 1992; HIROSE et al. 1992), from which it appears that S-100 positivity largely reflects the extent of true Schwannian differentiation: only those tumours in which the majority of cells are actual Schwann cells show reliable S-100 positivity (Fig. 10).

Cases in which there are substantial populations of perineurial cells or undifferentiated cells seem sometimes to be Leu-7 positive, although not on a reliable basis, and, to date, only one group has consistently claimed to demonstrate epithelial membrane antigen (EMA) positivity in largely perineurial MPNSTs (HIROSE et al. 1989, 1992), despite the fact that EMA reliably decorates perineurial cells in benign lesions (THEAKER et al. 1988; THEAKER and FLETCHER 1989). The hope that immunohistochemistry would facilitate the accurate recognition of a greater proportion of MPNSTs without resort to electron microscopy, particularly those with limited Schwannian differentiation, has not been realised to date.

There have been attempts to use other markers in the diagnosis of MPNST, most notably Leu-7 (SWANSON et al. 1987) and myelin basic protein (MOGOLLON et al. 1984; WICK et al. 1987), but, in truth, neither of these has proved to be specific or sensitive enough to be of any appreciable value.

The immunohistochemistry of epithelioid MPNST presents certain specific problems, particularly since S-100 will not distinguish MPNST from malignant melanoma. However, although epithelioid MPNST stains with neuron-specific enolase as well as S-100, personal experience and that of others (LASKIN et al. 1991) suggests that HMB-45, a melanoma antigen, is negative in most cases. Like most antigens, HMB-45 is not at all specific, but it may be of help in this particular context. As would be anticipated, epithelioid MPNST is keratin negative, allowing ready distinction from an epithelial metastasis. Previous reports of keratin positivity in rare cases of conventional MPNST (GRAY et al. 1989; HIROSE et al. 1992) are of uncertain significance and do not correlate with epithelioid morphology.

6 Electron Microscopy

Given that electron microscopy is not routinely available in many hospitals and that the ultrastructure of nerve sheath neoplasms has been the subject of many previous publications, this is not the place for a detailed account. Basically MPNST consists of variable proportions of three principal cell types: Schwann cells, perineurial cells and undifferentiated cells (TAXY et al.

1981; JOHNSON et al. 1991; FISHER et al. 1992; HIROSE et al. 1992). In our experience and that of many other authors, it seems that most cases show a reasonably widespread degree of evident neural differentiation and hence sampling error is not usually a problem in the ultrastructural examination of this particular group of sarcomas.

The key features indicative of Schwannian differentiation are: (a) elongated, complex interdigitating cell processes of varying diameter; and (b) well-formed, often continuous external lamina, sometimes showing reduplication. Additional features in limited degree are sparse pinocytotic vesicles, primitive junctions and occasional bundles of randomly arranged filaments. Long-spaced collagen (so-called Luse bodies), often seen in benign schwannomas, is uncommon in MPNST and in any case is not entirely specific. The features of perineurial differentiation are somewhat similar and include cell processes (in smaller number and usually with little interdigitation), a less well-formed external lamina, prominent intercellular junctions and numerous pinocytotic vesicles. In other words, the differences between Schwann cells and perineurial cells are a matter of degree (rather like myofibroblasts and smooth muscle cells!), and many people believe these cells to be closely related, with the same precursor. These similarities mean that it is almost impossible to reliably assess the relative extents of Schwannian or perineurial differentiation in a given neoplasm, especially if the lesion is not well differentiated.

Epithelioid MPNST, when examined ultrastructurally, usually shows remarkably well-formed features of Schwann cell differentiation (LODDING et al. 1986; LASKIN et al. 1991), which is somewhat surprising given its light-microscopic cytomorphology. This, in some cases, may prove to be the only convincing means of distinction from melanoma.

7 Conclusion

Malignant peripheral nerve sheath tumour is not especially rare and does not merit the enigmatic reputation which it seems to have acquired. With care, the majority of cases can be accurately and reproducibly identified. The real challenge now is to try and improve the currently rather poor clinical outcome in these cases.

References

Brooks JSJ, Freeman M, Enterline HT (1985) Malignant "Triton" tumors. Natural history and immunohistochemistry of nine new cases with literature review. Cancer 55: 2543–2549
Carney JA (1990) Psammomatous melanotic schwannoma. A distinctive heritable tumor with special associations, including cardiac myxoma and the Cushing syndrome. Am J Surg Pathol 14: 206–222

Chaudhuri B, Ronan SG, Manaligod JR (1980) Angiosarcoma arising in a plexiform neuro-fibroma. A case report. Cancer 46: 605–610

Christensen WN, Strong EW, Bains MC, Woodruff JM (1988) Neuroendocrine differentiation in the glandular peripheral nerve sheath tumor. Pathologic distinction from the biphasic synovial sarcoma with glands. Am J Surg Pathol 12: 417–426

Cross PA, Clarke NW (1988) Malignant nerve sheath tumour with epithelial elements. Histopathology 12: 547–549

D'Agostino AN, Soule EH, Miller RH (1963a) Primary malignant neoplasms of nerves (malignant neurilemmomas) in patients without manifestations of multiple neurofibromatosis (von Recklinghausen's disease). Cancer 16: 1003–1014

D'Agostino AN, Soule EH, Miller RH (1963b) Sarcomas of the peripheral nerves and somatic soft tissues associated with multiple neurofibromatosis (von Recklinghausen's disease). Cancer 16: 1015–1027

Daimaru Y, Hashimoto H, Enjoji M (1984) Malignant "Triton" tumors: a clinicopathologic and immunohistochemical study of nine cases. Hum Pathol 15: 768–778

Daimaru Y, Hashimoto H, Enjoji M (1985) Malignant peripheral nerve sheath tumors (malignant schwannomas). An immunohistochemical study of 29 cases. Am J Surg Pathol 9: 434–444

DiCarlo EF, Woodruff JM, Bansal M, Erlandson RA (1986) The purely epithelioid malignant peripheral nerve sheath tumor. Am J Surg Pathol 10: 478–490

Ducatman BS, Scheithauer BW (1983) Postirradiation neurofibrosarcoma. Cancer 51: 1028–1033

Ducatman BS, Scheithauer BW (1984) Malignant peripheral nerve sheath tumors with divergent differentiation. Cancer 54: 1049–1057

Ducatman BS, Scheithauer BW, Piepgras DG, Reiman HM (1984) Malignant peripheral nerve sheath tumors in childhood. J Neurooncol 2: 241–248

Ducatman BS, Scheithauer BW, Piepgras DG, Reiman HM, Ilstrup DM (1986) Malignant peripheral nerve sheath tumors. A clinicopathologic study of 120 cases. Cancer 57: 215–226

Enjoji M, Hashimoto H (1984) Diagnosis of soft tissue sarcomas. Pathol Res Pract 178: 215–226

Enzinger FM, Weiss SW (1988) Soft tissue tumors, 2nd edn. Mosby, New York, pp 781–800

Fisher C, Schofield JB (1991) S-100 protein positive synovial sarcoma. Histopathology 19: 375–377

Fisher C, Carter RL, Ramachandra S, Thomas DM (1992) Peripheral nerve sheath differentiation in malignant soft tissue tumours: an ultrastructural and immunohistochemical study. Histopathology 20: 115–125

Fletcher CDM (1992) Pleomorphic malignant fibrous histiocytoma: fact or fiction? A critical reappraisal based upon 159 tumors diagnosed as pleomorphic sarcoma. Am J Surg Pathol 16: 213–228

Fletcher CDM, Fernando IN, Braimbridge MV, McKee PH, Lyall JRW (1988) Malignant nerve sheath tumour arising in a ganglioneuroma. Histopathology 12: 445–448

Foley KM, Woodruff JM, Ellis FT, Posner JB (1980) Radiation-induced malignant and atypical peripheral nerve sheath tumors. Ann Neurol 7: 311–318

Ghali VS, Gold JE, Vincent RA, Cosgrove JM (1992) Malignant peripheral nerve sheath tumor arising spontaneously from retroperitoneal ganglioneuroma: a case report, review of the literature and immunohistochemical study. Hum Pathol 23: 72–75

Ghosh BC, Ghosh L, Huvos AG, Forster JG (1973) Malignant schwannoma. A clinicopathologic study. Cancer 31: 184–190

Goodlad JR, Fletcher CDM (1991) Malignant peripheral nerve sheath tumour with annulate lamellae mimicking pleomorphic malignant fibrous histiocytoma. J Pathol 164: 23–29

Gray MH, Rosenberg AE, Dickersin GR, Bhan AK (1989) Glial fibrillary acidic protein and keratin expression by benign and malignant nerve sheath tumours. Hum Pathol 20: 1089–1096

Guccion JG, Enzinger FM (1979) Malignant schwannoma associated with von Recklinghausen's neurofibromatosis. Virchows Arch [A] 383: 43–57

Herrera GA, Reimann BEF, Salinas JA, Turbat EA (1982) Malignant schwannomas presenting as malignant fibrous histiocytomas. Ultrastruct Pathol 3: 253–261

Hirose T, Sumimoto M, Kudo E, Hasegawa T, Teramae T, Murase M, Higasa Y, Ikata T, Hizawa K (1989) Malignant peripheral nerve sheath tumor (MPNST) showing perineurial cell differentiation. Am J Surg Pathol 13: 613–620

Hirose T, Hasegawa T, Kudo E, Seki K, Sano T, Hizawa K (1992) Malignant peripheral nerve sheath tumors: an immunohistochemical study in relation to ultrastructural features. Hum Pathol 23: 865–870

Hruban RH, Shiu MH, Senie RT, Woodruff JM (1990) Malignant peripheral nerve sheath tumours of the buttock and lower extremity. Cancer 66: 1253–1265

Janzer RC, Makek M (1983) Intraoral malignant melanotic schwannoma. Ultrastructural evidence for melanogenesis by Schwanns cells. Arch Pathol Lab Med 107: 298–301

Johnson TL, Lee MW, Meis JM, Zarbo RJ, Crissman JD (1991) Immunohistochemical characterization of malignant peripheral nerve sheath tumours. Surg Pathol 4: 121–135

Kahn HJ, Marks A, Thom H, Baumal R (1983) Role of antibody to S-100 protein in diagnostic pathology. Am J Clin Pathol 79: 341–347

Killeen RM, Davy CL, Bauserman SC (1988) Melanocytic schwannoma. Cancer 62: 174–183

Krausz T, Azzopardi JG, Pearse E (1984) Malignant melanoma of the sympathetic chain with a consideration of pigmented nerve sheath tumours. Histopathology 8: 881–894

Laskin WB, Silverman TA, Enzinger FM (1988) Postradiation soft tissue sarcomas. An analysis of 53 cases. Cancer 62: 2330–2340

Laskin WB, Weiss SW, Bratthauer GL (1991) Epithelioid variant of malignant peripheral nerve sheath tumor (malignant epithelioid schwannoma). Am J Surg Pathol 15: 1136–1145

Lodding P, Kindblom L-G, Angervall L (1986) Epithelioid malignant schwannoma. A study of 14 cases. Virchows Arch [A] 409: 433–451

Matsunou H, Shimoda T, Kakimoto S, Yamashita H, Ishikawa E, Mukai M (1985) Histopathologic and immunohistochemical study of malignant tumors of peripheral nerve sheath (malignant schwannoma). Cancer 56: 2269–2279

Meis JM, Enzinger FM, Martz KL, Neal JA (1992) Malignant peripheral nerve sheath tumors (malignant schwannomas) in children. Am J Surg Pathol 16: 694–707

Mennemeyer RP, Hammar SP, Tytus JS, Hallman KO, Raisis JE, Bockus D (1979) Melanotic schwannoma. Clinical and ultrastructural studies of three cases with evidence of intracellular melanin synthesis. Am J Surg Pathol 3: 3–10

Mogollon R, Penneys N, Albores-Saavedra J, Nadji M (1984) Malignant schwannoma presenting as a skin mass. Confirmation by the demonstration of myelin basic protein within tumor cells. Cancer 53: 1190–1193

Newman PL, Fletcher CDM (1991) Malignant mesenchymoma: clinicopathologic analysis of a series with evidence of low grade behaviour. Am J Surg Pathol 15: 607–614

Ooi A, Nakanishi I, Kojima M (1992) Malignant schwannoma with rhabdomyoblastic and melanocytic differentiation. Pathol Res Pract 188: 770–774

Ordonez NG, Mahfouz SM, Mackay B (1990) Synovial sarcoma: an immunohistochemical and ultrastructural study. Human Pathol 21: 733–749

Rasbridge SA, Browse NL, Tighe JR, Fletcher CDM (1989) Malignant nerve sheath tumor arising in a benign ancient schwannoma. Histopathology 14: 525–528

Rowlands D, Edwards C, Collins F (1987) Malignant melanotic schwannoma of the bronchus. J Clin Pathol 40: 1449–1455

Sordillo PP, Helson L, Hajdu SI, Magill GB, Kosloff C, Golbey RB, Beattie EJ (1981) Malignant schwannoma – clinical characteristics, survival and response to therapy. Cancer 47: 2503–2509

Sorensen SA, Mulvihill JJ, Nielsen A (1986) Long-term follow-up of von Recklinghausen neurofibromatosis. Survival and malignant neoplasms. N Engl J Med 314: 1010–1015

Stefansson K, Wollmann R, Jerkovic M (1982) S-100 protein in soft tissue tumors derived from Schwann cells and melanocytes. Am J Pathol 106: 261–268

Storm FK, Eilber FR, Mirra J, Morton DL (1980) Neurofibrosarcoma. Cancer 45: 126–129

Swanson PE, Manivel JC, Wick MR (1987) Immunoreactivity for Leu-7 in neurofibrosarcoma and other spindle cell sarcomas of soft tissue. Am J Pathol 126: 546–560

Takahashi K, Isobe T, Ohtsuki Y, Akagi T, Sonobe H, Okuyama T (1984) Immunohistochemical study on the distribution of alpha and beta subunits of S-100 protein in human neoplasms and normal tissues. Virchows Arch [B] 45: 385–396

Taxy JB, Battifora H, Trujillo Y, Dorfman HD (1981) Electron microscopy in the diagnosis of malignant schwannoma. Cancer 48: 1381-1391

Theaker JM, Fletcher CDM (1989) Epithelial membrane antigen expression by the perineurial cell: further studies of peripheral nerve lesions. Histopathology 14: 581–592

Theaker JM, Gatter KC, Puddle J (1988) Epithelial membrane antigen expression by the perineurium of peripheral nerve and in peripheral nerve tumours. Histopathology 13: 171–179

Tsuneyoshi M, Enjoji M (1979) Primary malignant peripheral nerve tumors (malignant schwannomas). A clinicopathologic and electron microscopic study. Acta Pathol Jpn 29: 363–375

Warner TFCS, Louie R, Hafez RG, Chandler E (1983) Malignant nerve sheath tumor containing endocrine cells. Am J Surg Pathol 7: 583–590

Weiss SW, Langloss JM, Enzinger FM (1983) Value of S-100 protein in the diagnosis of soft tissue tumors with particular reference to benign and malignant Schwann cell tumors. Lab Invest 49: 299–308

Wick MR, Swanson PE, Scheithauer BW, Manivel JC (1987) Malignant peripheral nerve sheath tumor. An immunohistochemical study of 62 cases. Am J Clin Pathol 87: 425–433

Woodruff JM (1976) Peripheral nerve tumors showing glandular differentiation (glandular schwannomas). Cancer 37: 2399–2413

Woodruff JM (1991) Tumors and tumorlike conditions of the peripheral nerve. In: Ninfo V, Chung EB, Cavazzana AO (eds) Tumors and tumorlike lesions of soft tissue. Churchill Livingstone, New York, pp 205–228

Rare Soft Tissue Sarcomas

C.D.M. FLETCHER

1 Introduction

In many ways the title "rare soft tissue sarcomas" is tautologous since, in relative terms, soft tissue sarcomas as a whole are comparatively uncommon. It is an interesting anomaly that the lesions to be covered in this chapter, while collectively accounting for only around 3%–4% of sarcomas and less than 0.04% of all malignancies, are, at least in some cases, often readily recognised by the general surgical pathologist. The diastase/PAS-positive crystals of alveolar soft part sarcoma are extremely well known and, at one time, it was almost traditional for an example of epithelioid sarcoma to be included in the British final postgraduate pathology examinations. Viewed logically, this seems somewhat inappropriate but probably reflects the philatelic tendency shared by many of us who work in diagnostic histopathology.

Current Topics in Pathology
Volume 89, Eds. D. Harms/D. Schmidt
© Springer-Verlag Berlin Heidelberg 1995

However, many of the tumours discussed in this chapter, which have sometimes been described as "tumours of uncertain histogenesis", have posed very considerable problems and controversies both nosologically and scientifically. To some extent this has been due to the relative paucity of material available for study but it also has much to do with the considerable ignorance (from which we still suffer) concerning the mechanisms which determine patterns of differentiation in soft tissue neoplasia. As a consequence we often have difficulty in defining differences between subgroups with overlapping morphological features, for example between epithelioid sarcoma and extrarenal rhabdoid tumour. At the present time it is both safer and more logical to classify lesions on the basis of their definable phenotype rather than on "questionable assumptions about their origins" (GOULD 1986) since, in the main, histogenetic theories of soft tissue neoplasia are untenable (FLETCHER and MCKEE 1990).

2 Alveolar Soft Part Sarcoma

The term alveolar soft part sarcoma (ASPS) was first coined for this distinctive neoplasm by CHRISTOPHERSON et al. in 1952; prior to that time a series of cases had been described as a form of malignant paraganglioma (SMETANA and SCOTT 1951) and other preceding cases had most often been reported as the malignant counterpart of granular cell "myoblastoma". The "histogenesis" or line of differentiation shown by ASPS has been the source of considerable controversy for the succeeding 40 years but currently seems likely to be resolved with increasing support for its rhabdomyoblastic nature.

2.1 Clinical Features

Alveolar soft part sarcoma may present over a wide age range but is most frequent in young adults. It is most common in females and this sex difference is especially marked in childhood/adolescent cases (LIEBERMAN et al. 1966, 1989). The majority of cases arise in or adjacent to skeletal muscle, especially of the proximal lower limb, and, in total, more than 70% of cases arise in the limbs (LIEBERMAN et al. 1989). Uncommon sites are the head and neck region, including the orbit (FONT et al. 1982) and retroperitoneum. Rare cases have also been described at visceral locations (GRAY et al. 1986; ABELER and NESLAND 1989; GUILLOU et al. 1991; YAGIHASHI et al. 1991); in some other reported examples there has probably been overlap with true paragangliomas. There are no distinctive clinical presenting features but a significant proportion of patients have pulmonary metastases when first seen (LIEBERMAN et al. 1989). Overall, however, it is common experience that

ASPS tends to pursue an indolent clinical course: the majority of patients eventually develop metastases and succumb to tumour but, in up to 50% of cases, this may be delayed for 10 years or more (AUERBACH and BROOKS 1987; LIEBERMAN et al. 1989). In comparison to many cancers, this may not seem too bad but it poses undoubted problems when advising generally young patients on the need for long-term follow up and the likely outcome.

2.2 Pathological Features

In "classical" cases the appearances of ASPS are very distinctive and only rarely cause diagnostic problems. As has often been observed, these lesions in fact have a pseudoalveolar (rather than truly alveolar) architecture and

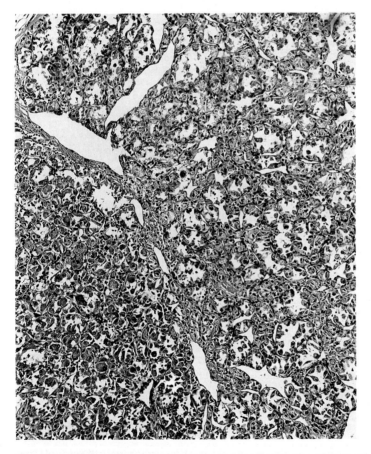

Fig. 1. Alveolar soft part sarcoma. A typical medium power view showing central loss of cohesion in tumour cell lobules. H&E; ×100

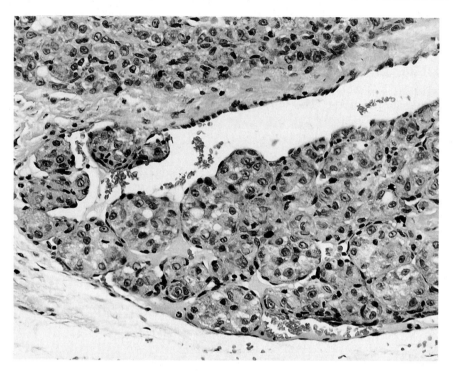

Fig. 2. Alveolar soft part sarcoma. This higher power view shows the typical cytomorphological features and also that tumour is filling an ectatic vein. H&E; ×250

are composed of round to ovoid cellular lobules, which show loss of cohesion or necrosis centrally (Fig. 1). The lobules are demarcated by delicate fibrovascular septa, the vascular element of which is often dilated and into which the tumour appears to bulge. The tumour, as a whole, has generally well-circumscribed margins.

Cytologically, tumour cells are rounded and typically have copious granular eosinophilic cytoplasm and a vesicular nucleus containing one or more prominent nucleoli. Mitoses tend to be remarkably scarce (Fig. 2). Adjacent to the degenerate centre of lobules ("alveoli"), the cells often appear to have clear cytoplasm but this is almost certainly degenerative. A small proportion of cases pose problems because the tumour cells are arranged only in small clusters or in diffuse sheets (LIEBERMAN et al. 1989) but, in this author's experience, true resemblance to a paraganglioma is very uncommon. In older patients confusion with a metastatic renal carcinoma is more likely. A characteristic feature, in most cases, is the presence of massive vascular (usually venous) invasion at the periphery of the tumour (Fig. 2).

As is well known, effectively all cases show granular intracytoplasmic PAS-positive/diastase-resistant material but in only around 20% of cases

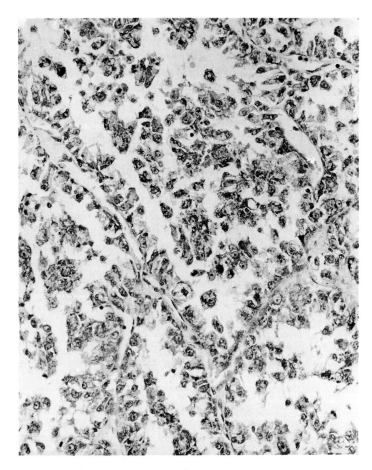

Fig. 3. Alveolar soft part sarcoma. Note the granular cytoplasmic positivity for sarcomeric actin. This often parallels the distribution of D/PAS-positive material. ABC method; ×250

does this have a crystalline appearance by light microscopy. Ultrastructurally, however, almost all cases contain rhomboidal or rectangular crystalline structures which appear to be formed from granular material derived from secretory granules adjacent to a prominent Golgi apparatus (PERSSON et al. 1988; LIEBERMAN et al. 1989; ORDONEZ et al. 1989). Some authors have shown these crystals to have a filamentous structure, most probably composed of actin (FISHER and REIDBORD 1971; MUKAI et al. 1984, 1990): importantly, similar crystalline structures have been found in a human muscle spindle (CARSTENS 1990).

With regard to differentiation in these lesions, much interest in recent years has centred on their immunophenotype, particularly with regard to myogenic antigens. An early study which showed renin positivity (DESCHRYVER-KECSKEMETI et al. 1982) has never been substantiated. Initial immunohistochemical studies could find no convincing evidence of either muscular or neuroectodermal differentiation (Mukai et al. 1983; Auerbach and Brooks 1987), but subsequently more sophisticated analyses using a wider range of antibodies, supported by immunoassay and immunoelectron microscopy, have repeatedly demonstrated convincing myogenic differentiation (Mukai et al. 1986; Foschini et al. 1988; Persson et al. 1988; Ordonez et al. 1989; Hirose et al. 1990; Miettinen and Ekfors 1990). It seems likely that much of the initial controversy related to differing antibodies and fixatives (Mukai et al. 1989) but it now appears, at least in our routine experience, that around 50% of cases are desmin positive and almost all cases show positive staining for sarcomeric actin in paraffin sections (Fig. 3). Further strong support for rhabdomyoblastic differentiation in ASPS has come more recently from the demonstration of MyoD1 expression (by immunohistochemistry and Western blotting) in these lesions (Rosai et al. 1991), since this protein (to date) is regarded as absolutely specific for cells showing genotypic evidence of skeletal muscle differentiation. Perhaps predictably, but not very convincingly, some authors have already cast doubt on this finding (Cullinane et al. 1992), thus ensuring that this saga will persist a little longer.

3 Clear Cell Sarcoma (Malignant Melanoma of Soft Parts)

Clear cell sarcoma was first recognised and so named by Enzinger in 1965. Despite minor nosological skirmishes during the 1970s, when some authors grouped this entity with synovial sarcoma (Hajdu et al. 1977; Tsuneyoshi et al. 1978), it is now generally accepted that this is a distinctive neuroectodermal neoplasm which shows melanogenesis in most cases and is better known as "malignant melanoma of soft parts" (Chung and Enzinger 1983).

3.1 Clinical Features

In a manner similar to ASPS, melanoma of soft parts shows a predilection for adolescents and young adults, although the absolute age range is wide (Chung and Enzinger 1983; Eckardt et al. 1983). The overwhelming majority of cases arise in the extremities, especially distally in the feet or hands. Isolated cases arising at more central locations often suggest the alternative diagnoses of either malignant melanotic schwannoma (Parker et al. 1980) or metastatic mucocutaneous melanoma. Melanoma of soft parts often grows quite slowly and the preoperative duration is commonly several years (Chung and Enzinger 1983; Kindblom et al. 1983; Sara et al. 1990). In our experience pain is a quite frequent presenting symptom. Because of their distal location, these tumours rarely reach a considerable size and most measure less than 5 cm in diameter. They are typically deep-seated and, as was accurately suggested in their original name (ENZINGER 1965), they are most often closely associated with tendoaponeurotic or fascial structures.

Apart from a tendency to repeated local recurrence (attributable to their surgically precarious location), the behaviour of malignant melanoma of soft parts is somewhat similar to melanomas elsewhere – in that the course is often hard to predict and metastases may be long delayed, albeit they usually develop in around 60% of cases and the overall mortality is at least 50%. A further melanomatous feature, which contrasts with most sarcomas, is that metastases commonly involve regional lymph nodes. Attempts to identify prognostic criteria in relatively small series have suggested small size (SARA et al. 1990) and DNA diploidy (EL-NAGGAR et al. 1991) as potentially useful parameters.

3.2 Pathological Features

In contrast to cutaneous melanoma, malignant melanoma of soft parts is morphologically quite homogeneous and tends to show reproducible features. It is characterised by nests, lobules or fascicles of usually spindle-shaped cells which most often have palely eosinophilic (rather than clear) cytoplasm (Fig. 4). In less than half the cases clear or vacuolated tumour cells are the dominant feature (Fig. 5). Tumour cell nests are separated by fibrous septa of varying thickness and the growth pattern is generally infiltrative. Perhaps most distinctive are the typically melanoma-like vesicular nuclei with a prominent eosinophilic nucleolus. In at least 50% of cases there are scattered distinctive multinucleate giant cells, the nuclei again being melanoma-like and often arranged in a wreath-like manner beneath the cell membrane. The number of giant cells is very variable and they may be hard to find. Similarly, mitoses tend to be suprisingly limited in number.

Although there is also often iron (haemosiderin) deposition in these lesions, around 50% of cases show intracytoplasmic melanin pigment but this may require a Masson Fontana or Warthin Starry stain for its convincing demonstration. Depending on fixation, most cases also show PAS-positive intracytoplasmic glycogen. Immunohistochemically S-100 protein and melanoma antigens (such as HMB-45) are positive in the majority of cases (KINDBLOM et al. 1983; SWANSON and WICK 1989). This technique is therefore of no use in making the distinction from metastatic mucocutaneous melanoma, nor indeed is ultrastructural examination by which many authors have repeatedly demonstrated typical melanosomes (BEARMAN et al. 1975; EKFORS and RANTAKOKKO 1979; BENSON et al. 1985). Therefore, in occasional cases, only careful clinicopathological correlation, aided by suggestive morphological features, will allow this distinction to be made. In-

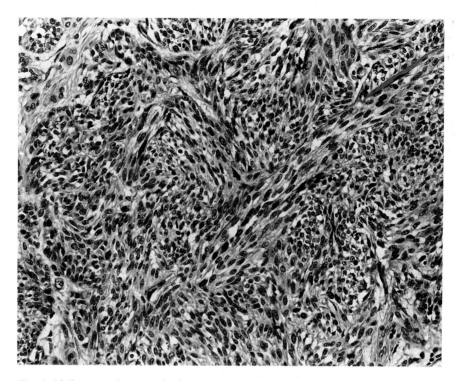

Fig. 4. Malignant melanoma of soft parts. In most cases the tumour has a fascicular pattern with palely eosinophilic cytoplasm. Note the vesicular nuclei. H&E; ×250

terestingly, there are also cytogenetic overlaps with conventional melanoma, especially involving structural abnormalities of chromosomes 7 and 8, but, in addition, malignant melanoma of soft parts appears to show a distinctive non-random (12;22) translocation (BRIDGE et al. 1990, 1991; REEVES et al. 1993) which is not seen in cutaneous lesions.

4 Epithelioid Sarcoma

Epithelioid sarcoma was first accurately delineated by ENZINGER in 1970. This, too, is a very distinctive and discrete entity but, despite the best efforts of many workers worldwide, the histogenesis or differentiation pattern of this lesion remains enigmatic.

4.1 Clinical Features

As with the first two tumour types described in this chapter, epithelioid sarcoma also shows a wide age range but a characteristic striking predilec-

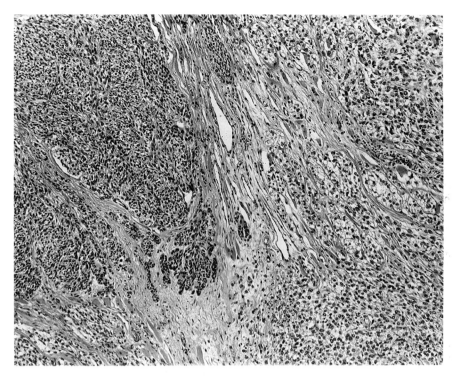

Fig. 5. Malignant melanoma of soft parts. In this field there is transition from spindle-celled (*left*) to clear-celled nests. H&E; ×100

tion for adolescents and young adults, with a male predominance (CHASE and ENZINGER 1985). Like malignant melanoma of soft parts, it is especially common in the distal extremities, particularly around the hand and wrist, although isolated cases have been reported at a wide variety of sites – but, interestingly, never within the abdominal cavity or retroperitoneum. The majority of cases are superficially located, often with cutaneous involvement, and less than a third involve deeper tissue such as skeletal muscle.

Classically, epithelioid sarcoma presents with one or more slowly growing nodules which are often painful and frequently ulcerate. This latter feature often stimulates initial confusion with a granulomatous or infective process. Thereafter the clinical course depends largely upon the extent of treatment undertaken. If, as is commonly the case, only local excision(s) is/are undertaken, this tumour shows a typical propensity for the most remarkable locally infiltrative spread (generally impalpable), which results in the development of satellite lesions ("recurrences") in the same region or, more often, proximally along the affected limb. Such spread is usually along tendo-fascial planes or is perineural and not infrequently occurs along the full length of a limb. It is this tendency which underscores the necessity for radical surgery at the time of first presentation, since adjuvant radiotherapy or chemotherapy are usually of little or no use.

The overall clinical course is often protracted and recurrences typically develop over a period of very many years. At least 50% of patients eventually develop metastases, most commonly in lymph nodes or the lungs (PRAT et al. 1978; CHASE and ENZINGER 1985). The eventual mortality is very hard to assess accurately since the very prolonged clinical course necessitates at least 20 years' follow up before a cure can be claimed (CHASE and ENZINGER 1983). While the very large AFIP study quoted above stated that only around a third of patients die from tumour, personal experience and that of others (DABSKA and KOSZAROWSKI 1982) would suggest that this rate is much higher.

4.2 Pathological Features

The majority of primary tumours are small (less than 3 cm) and only the uncommon deep-seated lesions tend to attain a large size. In most cases the histological features are remarkably homogeneous, as has been emphasised not only in larger series but in the very considerable number of published single case reports of epithelioid sarcoma. These lesions are characteristically ill defined and have a diffusely infiltrative, seemingly discohesive growth pattern. They are composed of relatively bland, monomorphic eosinophilic cells, the majority of which tend to be rounded or ovoid while a smaller proportion are spindled. The recently proposed existence of a very bland purely spindled variant (MIRRA et al. 1992) has yet to be substantiated. The cell cytoplasm is often somewhat hyaline in appearance and in some cases may be vacuolated or contain inclusions reminiscent of rhabdoid tumour (see below). Nuclei tend to be rounded and somewhat vesicular. In most cases there is little or no pleomorphism, giant cells are very rare and mitoses are relatively infrequent, most often numbering fewer than five per 10 HPF.

Architecturally, it is characteristic of epithelioid sarcoma that, in at least 50% of cases, tumour cells are arranged around nodular foci of necrosis/ necrobiosis (Fig. 6), hence another reason for confusion with a granulomatous lesion in times past (ENZINGER 1970). In addition to irregular infiltration into adjacent hyaline fibrous tissue, these tumours also often show cleft-like or even cavernous slits and spaces within tumour cell islands, and, in combination with cytoplasmic vacuolation, this may closely simulate an epithelioid endothelial neoplasm (WICK and MANIVEL 1987; HOCHSTETTER et al. 1991). Another quite common feature is osseous metaplasia, especially at the tumour periphery, where there is frequently also a marked chronic inflammatory infiltrate.

Immunohistochemically epithelioid sarcoma lives up to its name since, in almost all cases, there is striking keratin positivity (Fig. 7) (CHASE et al.

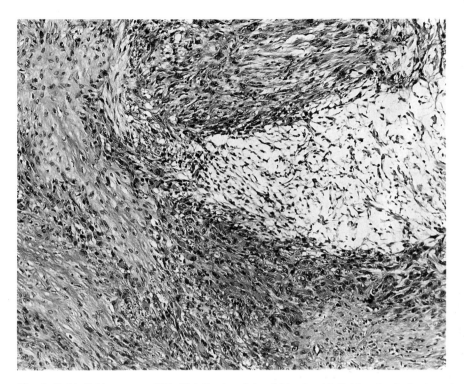

Fig. 6. Epithelioid sarcoma. This ill-defined nodule of bland epithelioid and spindle-shaped cells shows typical central degeneration. H&E; ×100

1984; MANIVEL et al. 1987; DAIMARU et al. 1987) and many cases also show epithelial membrane artigen (EMA) positivity. Interestingly, this contrasts with synovial sarcoma, in which EMA is generally the more sensitive marker. Ultrastructurally tumour cells are relatively undifferentiated (or at least non-specialised) leading to variable interpretation of the features (FISHER and HORVAT 1972; MUKAI et al. 1985; FISHER 1988; EYDEN et al. 1989) but relatively consistent findings are moderate amounts of rough endoplasmic reticulum, prominent intermediate filaments often in paranuclear whorls, short cell processes and subplasmalemmal densities.

Factors such as size, depth and mitotic activity appear to provide some guide to prognosis (CHASE and ENZINGER 1985), while ploidy and S-phase fraction have proved to be virtually useless (EL-NAGGAR and GARCIA 1992; PASTEL-LEVY et al. 1992). It has been proposed that those cases arising in the vulva have a more rapidly aggressive clinical course (ULBRIGHT et al. 1983) but it now appears that lesions at this and other proximal truncal locations may show greater morphological overlap with extrarenal rhabdoid tumour, along with immunophenotypic heterogeneity (PERRONE et al. 1989; MOLENAAR et al. 1989; GERHARZ et al. 1990). At present this remains a source of unresolved controversy.

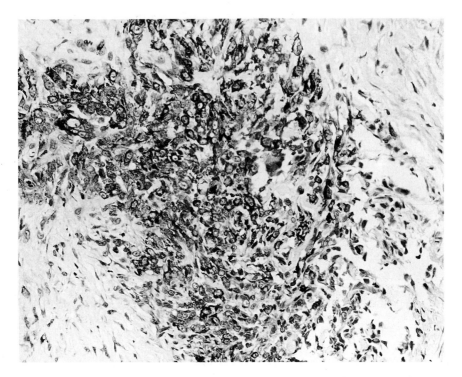

Fig. 7. Epithelioid sarcoma. Typically strong cytokeratin (CAM 5.2) positivity in both epithelioid and spindle-shaped cells. ABC method; ×250

5 Extrarenal Rhabdoid Tumour

The existence of extrarenal rhabdoid tumour was proposed on the basis of lesions presenting in soft tissue (LYNCH et al. 1983) (or at other non-renal sites) with morphological similarities to the distinctive malignant rhabdoid tumours of the kidney in children (HAAS et al. 1981; WEEKS et al. 1989a). While the concept of the paediatric renal neoplasms has remained discrete and definable, albeit with potential mimics (WEEKS et al. 1991), the extrarenal lesions have proved to be a source of confusion and controversy and most probably do *not* represent a specific entity, for reasons of heterogeneity described below.

5.1 Clinical Features

Extrarenal rhabdoid tumour, while most common in infancy and childhood, has been described over a wide age range and at almost every conceivable anatomical site. While deep soft tissue might be the most frequent location (TSUNEYOSHI et al. 1985; KODET et al. 1991a), other sites have included the liver (SOTELO-AVILA et al. 1986; PARHAM et al. 1988), bladder (CARTER et al. 1989), brain (BIGGS et al. 1987), orbit (WALFORD et al. 1992), vulva (PERRONE et al. 1989) and skin (DABBS and PARK 1988). By contrast with the renal lesions (WEEKS et al. 1989a), there is no convincing association with primitive neuroectodermal tumours of the central nervous system. Perhaps the only clinically distinctive features are the development of a rapidly enlarging mass and the almost equally rapid progression to metastases and death within 2 years in the vast majority of patients.

5.2 Pathological Features

At whatever primary site, extrarenal rhabdoid tumour tends to be a large mass showing extensive necrosis (Fig. 8). Histologically it has only three reproducible features and in some published cases these have not been reliably demonstrated. These features (Fig. 9) are (a) the presence of rounded

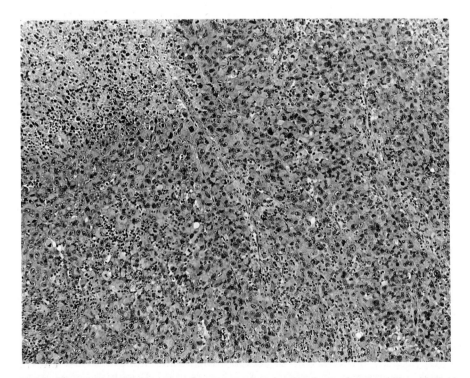

Fig. 8. Extrarenal rhabdoid tumour. Low power view showing sheets of eosinophilic epithelioid cells and adjacent necrosis (*top left*). H&E; ×100

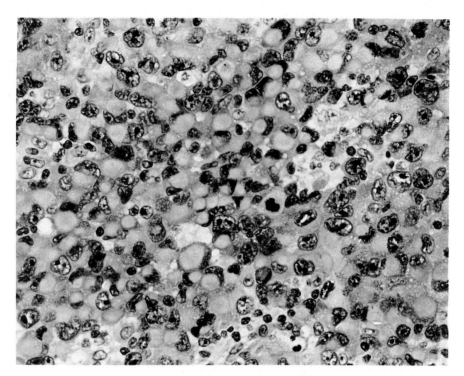

Fig. 9. Extrarenal rhabdoid tumour. Note the striking hyaline intracytoplasmic inclusions and characteristic nuclear morphology. H&E; ×400

intracytoplasmic hyaline inclusions (which correspond ultrastructurally to usually paranuclear filamentous whorls); (b) the presence of vesicular nuclei with a large, usually central, eosinophilic nucleolus; and (c) eosinophilic tumour cell cytoplasm. The main problems are that (a) these "typical" morphological features may only be focal and other areas of tumour may show a bewildering array of patterns (usually rather undifferentiated); and (b) that these same, supposedly distinctive, features may be seen focally in a wide range of other completely different definable tumour types. Common among the latter are synovial sarcoma, epithelioid sarcoma (as mentioned above), myxoid chondrosarcoma, mesothelioma (Tsuneyoshi et al. 1987), as well as melanoma (Bittesini et al. 1992) and even rhabdomyosarcoma (Kodet et al. 1991b). The notion of a "rhabdoid rhabdomyosarcoma" is, of course, laughable, given the original definition of rhabdoid tumour (Haas et al. 1981).

Some authors have suggested that the immunophenotype may be reproducible, in that many cases seem to show vimentin, cytokeratin and EMA positivity (Tsuneyoshi et al. 1985; Berry and Vujanic 1992), but, in reality, the patterns of antigen expression in tumours with these morphological features are almost unlimited in their heterogeneity (Schmidt et al.

1989; Tsokos et al. 1989; Fletcher and McKee 1990). In view of these many signs of anaplasia, it is remarkable that these tumours often seem to have a diploid DNA content (Schmidt et al. 1989) and a frequently normal karyotype (Douglass et al. 1990). On the basis of this clinical and immunophenotypic heterogeneity, it is believed increasingly that extrarenal rhabdoid tumour is *not* a distinct entity but rather that it represents the shared morphological pattern of a diverse range of poorly differentiated neoplasms (Weeks et al. 1989b; Fletcher and McKee 1990; Berry and Vujanic 1992).

6 Epithelioid Angiosarcoma

Since this chapter is devoted to the uncommon sarcomas and there is no separate chapter on vascular tumours, it was decided to include this recently characterised variant of angiosarcoma here, not least because it is a common source of diagnostic difficulty.

6.1 Clinical Features

While the well-known cutaneous angiosarcomas of the head and neck region in elderly patients quite frequently may show focally epithelioid features (Rosai et al. 1976; Cooper 1987), pure epithelioid angiosarcoma is actually very uncommon in the skin, both in our experience and that of others (Marrogi et al. 1990). It is more frequently encountered in deep soft tissue (Fletcher et al. 1991) or in the thyroid (Eusebi et al. 1990); the latter group of lesions, which are most common in areas of endemic goitre, are beyond the scope of this book. Deep-seated epithelioid angiosarcoma rises almost exclusively in adults, shows a male predominance and typically presents as a large circumscribed mass in limb musculature. In common with epithelioid haemangioendothelioma, some cases arise from large blood vessels. In most patients the clinical course is characterised by the rapid development of metastases and death within 2–3 years, but this is by no means an absolute rule. In up to a third of cases metastatic sites include lymph nodes.

6.2 Pathological Features

Epithelioid angiosarcoma is usually characterised by a diffuse, sheet-like growth pattern, and obvious vasoformative differentiation is typically minimal or absent. Tumour cells are large, rounded and have copious eosinophilic

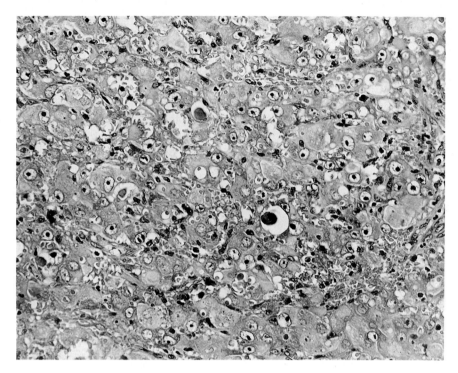

Fig. 10. Epithelioid angiosarcoma. Note the intracytoplasmic lumina and very distinctive nuclear morphology. H&E; ×250. (From FLETCHER et al. 1991)

(or amphophilic) cytoplasm, in which vacuoles (or "lumina") are evident in around 5% of cells (Fig. 10) The nuclei are especially distinctive in this context by being large and vesicular with a prominent, somewhat basophilic, nucleolus – almost a caricature of malignant melanoma. Mitoses tend to be frequent. Despite the misleadingly diffuse architecture, reticulin staining typically demonstrates vasoformative tubular structures, which exceed in size and complexity the packeting seen in any metastatic carcinoma (Fig. 11).

Perhaps thankfully for diagnostic pathologists, this variant of angiosarcoma is consistently Factor V111 RAg positive (Fig. 12), as well as usually also being positive for other endothelial antigens such as CD31, CD34 and UEA-I. The latter two, of course, are not specific and, in particular, the Ulex lectin is commonly positive in carcinomas which highlights the misleading aspect of epithelioid angiosarcoma – it is frequently (but not invariably) cytokeratin, and sometimes EMA, positive (GRAY et al. 1990; EUSEBI et al. 1990; FLETCHER et al. 1991). Whether or not this is related to the high content of intermediate filaments in these cells or is related to endothelial ontogenesis (JAHN et al. 1987) is unknown, but clearly this increases the risk of confusion with epithelioid sarcoma or an epithelial neoplasm. Ultrastruc-

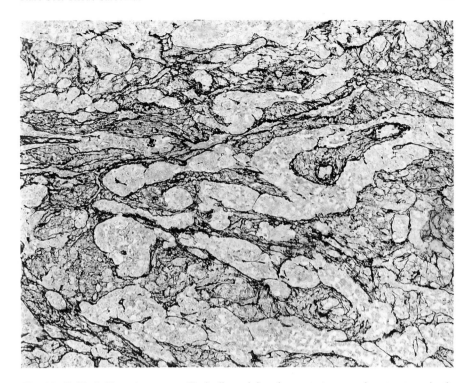

Fig. 11. Epithelioid angiosarcoma. Reticulin staining demonstrates vascular structures in the solid, sheet-like areas. Retic; ×100. (From FLETCHER et al. 1991)

turally, however, convincing features of vascular endothelial differentiation can usually be found. In purely morphological terms, although initially we felt that there was little overlap with epithelioid haemangioendothelioma (FLETCHER et al. 1991), this was probably mistaken as we have since seen rare cases showing an undoubted spectrum between these two entities.

7 Malignant Mesenchymoma

This enigmatic neoplasm has received little attention, other than in often rather dubious case reports, since STOUT's original series in 1948 and his subsequent paper on comparable lesions in childhood 13 years later (NASH and STOUT 1961). This probably reflects inadequate or inconsistently applied diagnostic criteria and the genuine rarity of these lesions. This author defines malignant mesenchymoma as a sarcoma which shows at least two distinct types of malignant mesenchymal differentiation, in addition to (or other than) undifferentiated, fibrosarcomatous, MFH-like or haemangiopericytoma-like

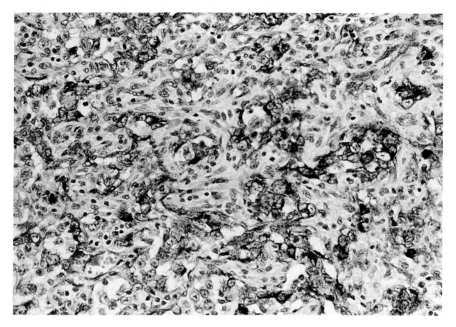

Fig. 12. Epithelioid angiosarcoma. The consistency with which these lesions are FV111 RAg-positive contrasts with the much more variable findings in conventional head and neck angiosarcoma. ABC method; ×250. (From FLETCHER et al. 1991)

areas (NEWMAN and FLETCHER 1991). By long tradition, malignant peripheral nerve sheath tumours showing heterologous differentiation (see the preceding chapter) are excluded from this category.

7.1 Clinical Features

Adopting the above strict criteria, malignant mesenchymoma is virtually confined to adults (of either sex) and shows a predilection for the retroperitoneum (NEWMAN and FLETCHER 1991), where, like many sarcomas, it often reaches a large size. A further third of cases arise in the lower limb. There are no clinically distinctive features at the time of presentation but what appears to be remarkable about this sarcoma type is its clinical behaviour. Given that, in almost all cases, one (or more) of the histological components is high grade (see below), malignant mesenchymoma appears to show a very low metastatic rate (NEWMAN and FLETCHER 1991), although the number of accurately reported cases is low. However, further personal experience and longer follow up since the series above was described has done nothing to change this view.

7.2 Pathological Features

Given the potentially wide range of elements that might theoretically be identified, the types of specific differention seen in malignant mesenchymoma are surprisingly limited. With very rare exceptions, the only definable constituents found are rhabdomyosarcoma, liposarcoma and osteo/chondrosarcoma (NEWMAN and FLETCHER 1991). We have now also encountered isolated cases with a leiomyosarcomatous component. The single most common combination is liposarcoma plus rhabdomyosarcoma (Fig. 13): most often the former component is well differentiated while the latter is typically pleomorphic and MFH-like (not to be mistaken for dedifferentiated liposarcoma), or fascicular. Osteoblastic differentiation is more common than chondroblastic. Most often the transition between differentiation types

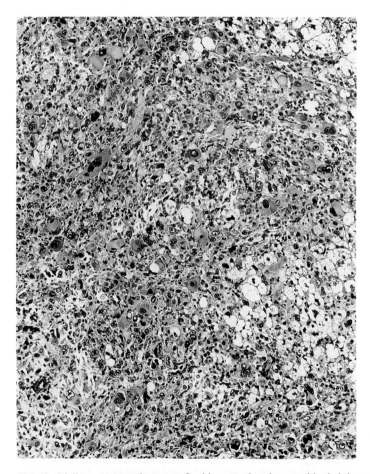

Fig. 13. Malignant mesenchymoma. In this example, pleomorphic rhabdomyoblasts are closely admixed with multivacuolated lipoblasts. Normally the transition is more abrupt. H&E; ×100

is abrupt. Although malignant mesenchymoma, when carefully defined, is rare, its limited phenotypic capacity may yet provide valuable clues to the molecular genetic basis of at least some types of mesenchymal differentiation.

8 Intraabdominal Desmoplastic Small Cell Tumour

This distinctive neoplasm was first recognised in 1989 (GERALD and ROSAI 1989) and it was delineated fully and definitively in a series of 19 cases published in mid-1991 by GERALD et al. Despite warning comments by Dr. Juan Rosai, at the International IAP Congress in October 1992, that extraabdominal, non-desmoplastic and larger cell varieties of this entity exist, the majority of cases show very reproducible features, as described herein. It seems probable that some of the polyphenotypic small round cell tumours described in recent years (SWANSON et al. 1988; PARHAM et al. 1992) may fall within this spectrum.

8.1 Clinical Features

Intraabdominal desmoplastic small cell tumour (IDSCT) arises almost exclusively in children, adolescents or young adults, with a striking male predominance, and presents with multiple large intraabdominal masses located on peritoneal surfaces. Less frequent female patients may show massive ovarian involvement (YOUNG et al. 1992). No single primary site can be identified. The majority of patients succumb within 3–4 years to the effects of extensive intraabdominal spread. Relatively few patients develop systemic metastases but this probably reflects their short survival time. Only isolated cases have shown any significant response to chemotherapy (GONZALEZ-CRUSSI et al. 1990; VARIEND et al. 1991).

8.2 Pathological Features

Intraabdominal desmoplastic small cell tumour consists of an admixture of clusters or sheets of small basophilic cells and a bland spindled desmoplastic stroma in variable proportions (Fig. 14). Most often the small round cell component is arranged in discrete clusters or nests, showing focal central necrosis. The cells are uniform in appearance, often have a very small amount of pale or clear cytoplasm and have small densely hyperchromatic nuclei (Fig. 15) which show a high mitotic rate. Rosettes have only very rarely been described (VARIEND et al. 1991) but in some cases there may be

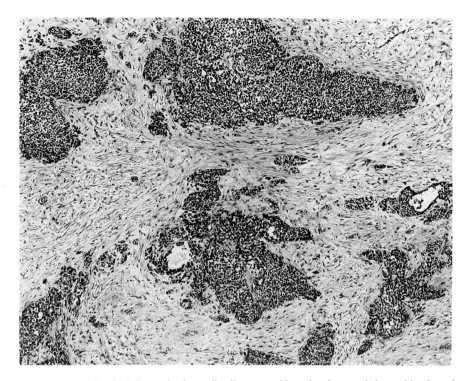

Fig. 14. Intraabdominal desmoplastic small cell tumour. Note the characteristic combination of small cell islands in an ãbdundant desmoplastic stroma. H&E; ×63

a hint of tubule formation (GONZALEZ-CRUSSI et al. 1990; YOUNG et al. 1992). The desmoplastic component resembles that of any desmoplastic carcinoma and is characterised by plump but bland myofibroblasts in a variably collagenous stroma.

The immunophenotype of the small cell component is the most characteristic feature of this tumour: in almost all cases these cells are keratin, EMA, desmin, neuron-specific enolase and vimentin positive. Depending upon one's initial morphological diagnosis, it is clear that this pattern of antigen expression may easily cause confusion with small cell carcinoma, rhabdomyosarcoma or a primitive neuroectodermal tumour – in other words, with all the likely differential diagnoses! Awareness of the entity of IDSCT is therefore essential. Ultrastructurally these tumours are largely undifferentiated and their only common feature seems to be the presence of paranuclear filamentous aggregates. The true nature of these neoplasms has been discussed in detail (GERALD et al. 1991; NIKOLAOU et al. 1992) but remains controversial. The peritoneal location, diffuse manner of growth and immunophenotype would all tend to favour a form of "mesothelioblastoma" (GERALD et al. 1991). However, reported cytogenetic findings in two cases (addendum to GERALD et al. 1991; SAWYER et al. 1992) have revealed an

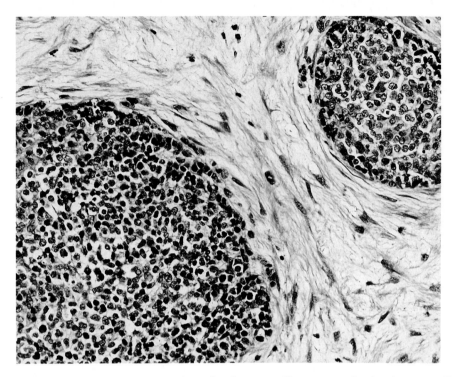

Fig. 15. Intraabdominal desmoplastic small cell tumour. The tumour cells often have a small amount of clear cytoplasm, giving a somewhat epithelial appearance. H&E; ×250

(11;22) translocation similar, but not identical, to that seen in primitive neuroectodermal tumours. This matter therefore awaits further resolution.

References

Abeler V, Nesland JM (1989) Alveolar soft part sarcoma in the uterine cervix. Arch Pathol Lab Med 113: 1179–1183

Auerbach HE, Brooks JJ (1987) Alveolar soft part sarcoma. A clinicopathologic and immunohistochemical study. Cancer 60: 66–73

Bearman RM, Noe J, Kempson RL (1975) Clear cell sarcoma with melanin pigment. Cancer 36: 977–984

Benson JD, Kraemer B, Mackay B (1985) Malignant melanoma of soft parts: an ultrastructural study of four cases. Ultrastruct Pathol 8: 57–70

Berry PJ, Vujanic GM (1992) Commentary: malignant rhabdoid tumour. Histopathology 20: 189–193

Biggs PJ, Garen PD, Powers JM, Garvin AJ (1987) Malignant rhabdoid tumor of the central nervous system. Hum Pathol 18: 332–337

Bittesini L, dei Tos AP, Fletcher CDM (1992) Metastatic malignant melanoma showing a rhabdoid phenotype: further evidence of a non-specific histological pattern. Histopathology 20: 167–170

Bridge JA, Brook DA, Neff JR, Huntrakoon M (1990) Chromosomal abnormalities in clear cell sarcoma. Implications for histogenesis. Am J Clin Pathol 93: 25–31

Bridge JA, Sreekantaiah C, Neff JR, Sandberg AA (1991) Cytogenetic findings in clear cell sarcoma of tendons and aponeuroses. Malignant melanoma of soft parts. Cancer Genet Cytogenet 52: 101–106

Carstens PHB (1990) Membrane-bound cytoplasmic crystals, similar to those in alveolar soft part sarcoma, in a human muscle spindle. Ultrastruct Pathol 14: 423–428

Carter RL, McCarthy KP, Al-Sam SZ, Monaghan P, Agrawal M, McElwain TJ (1989) Malignant rhabdoid tumour of the bladder with immunohistochemical and ultrastructural evidence suggesting histiocytic origin. Histopathology 14: 179–190

Chase DR, Enzinger FM (1985) Epithelioid sarcoma. Diagnosis, prognostic indicators and treatment. Am J Surg Pathol 9: 241–263

Chase DR, Enzinger FM, Weiss SW, Langloss JM (1984) Keratin in epithelioid sarcoma. An immunohistochemical study. Am J Surg Pathol 8: 435–441

Christopherson WM, Foote FW, Stewart FW (1952) Alveolar soft part sarcomas: structurally characteristic tumors of uncertain histogenesis. Cancer 5: 100–111

Chung EB, Enzinger FM (1983) Malignant melanoma of soft parts. A reassessment of clear cell sarcoma. Am J Surg Pathol 7: 405–413

Cooper PH (1987) Angiosarcomas of the skin. Semin Diagn Pathol 4: 2–17

Cullinane C, Thorner PS, Greenberg ML, Ng YK, Kumar M, Squire J (1992) Molecular genetic, cytogenetic and immunohistochemical characterization of alveolar soft part sarcoma. Implications for cell of origin. Cancer 70: 2444–2450

Dabbs DJ, Park HK (1988) Malignant rhabdoid skin tumor: an uncommon primary skin neoplasm. Ultrastructural and immunohistochemical analysis. J Cutan Pathol 15: 109–115

Dabska M, Koszarowski T (1982) Clinical and pathologic study of aponeurotic (epithelioid) sarcoma. Pathol Annu 17(1): 129–153

Daimaru Y, Hashimoto H, Tsuneyoshi M, Enjoji M (1987) Epithelial profile of epithelioid sarcoma. An immunohistochemical study of eight cases. Cancer 59: 134–141

DeSchryver-Kecskemeti K, Kraus FT, Engleman BA (1982) Alveolar soft part sarcoma – a malignant angioreninoma. Histochemical, immunocytochemical and electron microscopic study of four cases. Am J Surg Pathol 6: 5–18

Douglass EC, Valentine M, Rowe ST, Parham DM, Wilimas JA, Sanders JM, Houghton PJ (1990) Malignant rhabdoid tumor: a highly malignant childhood tumor with minimal karyotypic changes. Genes Chrom Cancer 2: 210–216

Eckardt JJ, Pritchard DJ, Soule EH (1983) Clear cell sarcoma. A clinicopathologic study of 27 cases. Cancer 52: 1482–1488

Ekfors TO, Rantakokko V (1979) Clear cell sarcoma of tendons and aponeuroses: malignant melanoma of soft tissues? Report of four cases. Pathol Res Pract 165: 422–428

El-Naggar AK, Garcia GM (1992) Epithelioid sarcoma. Flow cytometric study of DNA content and regional DNA heterogeneity. Cancer 69: 1721–1728

El-Naggar AK, Ordonez NG, Sara A, McLemore D, Batsakis JG (1991) Clear cell sarcomas and metastatic soft tissue melanomas. A flow cytometric comparison and prognostic implications. Cancer 67: 2173–2179

Enzinger FM (1965) Clear cell sarcoma of tendons and aponeuroses. An analysis of 21 cases. Cancer 18: 1163–1174

Enzinger FM (1970) Epithelioid sarcoma. A sarcoma simulating a granuloma or a carcinoma. Cancer 26: 1029–1041

Eusebi V, Carcangiu ML, Dina R, Rosai J (1990) Keratin-positive epithelioid angiosarcoma of thyroid. A report of four cases. Am J Surg Pathol 14: 737–747

Eyden BP, Harris M, Banerjee SS, McClure J (1989) The ultrastructure of epithelioid sarcoma. J Submicrosc Cytol Pathol 21: 281–293

Fisher C (1988) Epithelioid sarcoma: the spectrum of ultrastructural differentiation in seven immunohistochemically defined cases. Hum Pathol 19: 265–275

Fisher ER, Horvat B (1972) The fibrocytic derivation of the so-called epithelioid sarcoma. Cancer 30: 1074–1081

Fisher ER, Reidbord H (1971) Electron microscopic evidence suggesting the myogenous derivation of the so-called alveolar soft part sarcoma. Cancer 27: 150–159

Fletcher CDM, McKee PH (1990) Pathobiology of soft tissue tumours. Churchill Livingstone, Edinburgh

Fletcher CDM, Beham A, Bekir S, Clark EA, Marley NJE (1991) Epithelioid angiosarcoma of deep soft tissue: a distinctive tumor readily mistaken for an epithelial neoplasm. Am J Surg Pathol 15: 915–924

Font RL, Jurco S, Zimmerman LE (1982) Alveolar soft part sarcoma of the orbit: a clinico-pathologic analysis of seventeen cases and a review of the literature. Hum Pathol 13: 569–579

Foschini MP, Ceccarelli C, Eusebi V, Skalli O, Gabbiani G (1988) Alveolar soft part sarcoma: immunological evidence of rhabdomyoblastic differentiation. Histopathology 13: 101–108

Gerald WL, Rosai J (1989) Desmoplastic small cell tumor with divergent differentiation. Pediatr Pathol 9: 177–183

Gerald WL, Miller HK, Battifora H, Miettinen M, Silva EG, Rosai J (1991) Intra-abdominal desmoplastic smalll round cell tumor. Report of 19 cases of a distinctive type of high grade polyphenotypic malignancy affecting young individuals. Am J Surg Pathol 15: 499–513

Gerharz CD, Moll R, Meister P, Knuth A, Gabbert H (1990) Cytoskeletal heterogeneity of an epithelioid sarcoma with expression of vimentin, cytokeratins and neurofilaments. Am J Surg Pathol 14: 274–283

Gonzalez-Crussi F, Crawford SE, Sun CCJ (1990) Intraabdominal desmoplastic small cell tumors with divergent differentiation. Observations on three cases of childhood. Am J Surg Pathol 14: 633–642

Gould VE (1986) Histogenesis and differentiation: a re-evaluation of these concepts as criteria for the classification of tumours. Hum Pathol 17: 212–215

Gray GF, Glick AD, Kurtin PJ, Jones HW (1986) Alveolar soft part sarcoma of the uterus. Hum Pathol 17: 297–300

Gray MH, Rosenberg AE, Dickersin GR, Bhan AK (1990) Cytokeratin expression in epithelioid vascular neoplasms. Hum Pathol 21: 212–217

Guillou L, Lamoureaux E, Masse S, Costa J (1991) Alveolar soft part sarcoma of the uterine corpus: histological, immunocytochemical and ultrastructural study of a case. Virchows Arch [A] 418: 467–471

Haas JE, Palmer NF, Weinberg AG, Beckwith JB (1981) Ultrastructure of the malignant rhabdoid tumor of the kidney. A distinctive renal tumor of children. Hum Pathol 12: 646–657

Hajdu SI, Shiu MH, Fortner JG (1977) Tendosynovial sarcoma. A clinicopathologic study of 136 cases. Cancer 39: 1201–1217

Hirose T, Kudo E, Hasegawa T, Abe J-I, Hizawa K (1990) Cytoskeletal properties of alveolar soft part sarcoma. Hum Pathol 21: 204–211

Hochstetter ARV, Meyer VE, Grant JW, Honegger HP, Schreiber A (1991) Epithelioid sarcoma mimicking angiosarcoma: the value of immunohistochemistry in the differential diagnosis. Virchows Arch [A] 418: 271–278

Jahn L, Fouquet B, Rohe K, Franke WW (1987) Cytokeratins in certain endothelial and smooth muscle cells of two taxonomically distant vertebrate species, Xenopus laevis and man. Differentiation 36: 234–254

Kindblom L-G, Lodding P, Angervall L (1983) Clear cell sarcoma of tendons and aponeuroses. An immunohistochemical and electron microscopic analysis indicating neural crest origin. Virchows Arch [A] 401: 109–128

Kodet R, Newton WA, Sachs N, Hamoudi AB, Raney RB, Asmar L, Gehen EA (1991a) Rhabdoid tumors of soft tissue: a clinicopathologic study of 26 cases enrolled on the Intergroup Rhabdomyosarcoma Study. Hum Pathol 22: 674–681

Kodet R, Newton WA, Hamoudi AB, Asmar L (1991b) Rhabdomyosarcomas with intermediate filament inclusions and features of rhabdoid tumors. Light microscopic and immuno-histochemical study. Am J Sug Pathol 15: 257–267

Lieberman PH, Foote FW, Stewart FW, Berg JW (1966) Alveolar soft part sarcoma. J Am Med Assoc 198: 1047–1057

Lieberman PH, Brennan MF, Kimmel M, Erlandson RA, Garin – Chesa P, Flehinger BY (1989) Alveolar soft-part sarcoma. A clinicopathologic study of half a century. Cancer 63: 1–13

Lynch HT, Shurin SB, Dahms BB, Izant RJ, Lynch J, Danes BS (1983) Paravertebral malignant rhabdoid tumor in infancy. In vitro studies of a familial tumor. Cancer 52: 290–296.

Manivel JC, Wick MR, Dehner LP, Sibley RK (1987) Epithelioid sarcoma. An immuno-histochemical study. Am J Clin Pathol 87: 319–326

Marrogi AJ, Hunt SJ, Santa Cruz DJ (1990) Cutaneous epithelioid angiosarcoma. Am J Dermatopathol 12: 350–356

Miettinen M, Ekfors T (1990) Alveolar soft part sarcoma. Immunohistochemical evidence for muscle cell differentiation. Am J Clin Pathol 93: 32–38

Mirra JM, Kessler S, Bhuta S, Eckardt J (1992) The fibroma-like variant of epithelioid sarcoma. A fibrohistiocytic/myoid cell lesion often confused with benign and malignant spindle cell tumors. Cancer 69: 1382–1395

Molenaar WM, De Jong B, Dam-Meiring A, Postma A, Devries J, Hoekstra HJ (1989) Epithelioid sarcoma or malignant rhabdoid tumor of soft tissue? Epithelioid phenotype and rhabdoid karyotype. Hum Pathol 20: 347–351

Mukai M, Iri H, Nakajima T, Hirose S, Torikata C, Kageyama K, Ueno N, Murakimi K (1983) Alveolar soft part sarcoma. A review on its histogenesis and further studies based on electron microscopy, immunohistochemistry and biochemistry. Am J Surg Pathol 7: 679–689

Mukai M, Torikata C, Iri H, Mikata A, Sakamoto T, Hanaoka H, Shinohara C, Baba N, kanaya K, Kagayama K (1984) Alveolar soft part sarcoma. An elaboration of a three-dimensional configuration of the crystalloids by digital image processing. Am J Pathol 116: 398–406

Mukai M, Torikata C, Iri H, Hanaoka H, Kawai T, Yakumaru K, Shimoda T, Mikata A, Kageyama K (1985) Cellular differentiation of epithelioid sarcoma. An electron microscopic, enzyme histochemical and immunohistochemical study. Am J Pathol 119: 44–56

Mukai M, Torikata C, Iri H, Mikata A, Hanaoka H, Kato K, Kagayama K (1986) Histogenesis of alveolar soft-part sarcoma. An immunohistochemical and biochemical study. Am J Surg Pathol 10: 212–218

Mukai M, Torikata C, Shimoda T, Iri H (1989) Alveolar soft part sarcoma. Assessment of immunohistochemical demonstration of desmin using paraffin sections and frozen sections. Virchows Arch [A] 414: 503–509

Mukai M, Torikata C, Iri H (1990) Alveolar soft part sarcoma: an electron microscopic study especially of uncrystallised granules using a tannic acid-containing fixative. Ultrastruct Pathol 14: 41–50

Nash A, Stout AP (1961) Malignant mesenchymomas in children. Cancer 14: 524–533

Newman PL, Fletcher CDM (1991) Malignant mesenchymoma: clinicopathologic analysis of a series with evidence of low grade behaviour. Am J Surg Pathol 15: 607–614

Nikolaou I, Barbatis C, Laopodis V, Bekir S, Fletcher CDM (1992) Intra-abdominal desmoplastic small cell tumour with divergent differentiation. Report of two cases and review of the literature. Pathol Res Pract 188: 981–988

Ordonez NG, Ro JY, Mackay B (1989) Alveolar soft part sarcoma. An ultrastructural and immunocytochemical investigation of its histogenesis. Cancer 63: 1721–1736

Parham DM, Peiper SC, Robicheaux G, Riberio RC, Douglass EC (1988) Malignant rhabdoid tumor of the liver. Evidence for epithelial differentiation. Arch Pathol Lab Med 112: 61–64

Parker JB, Marcus PB, Martin JH (1980) Spinal melanotic clear cell sarcoma: a light and electronic microscopic study. Cancer 46: 718–724

Pastel-Levy C, Bell DA, Rosenberg AE, Preffer F, Colvin RB, Flotte TJ (1992) DNA flow cytometry of epithelioid sarcoma. Cancer 70: 2823–2826

Perrone T, Swanson PE, Twiggs L, Ulbright TM, Dehner LP (1989) Malignant rhabdoid tumor of the vulva: is distinction from epithelioid sarcoma possible? A pathological and immuno-histochemical study. Am J Surg Pathol 13: 848–858

Persson S, Willems J-S, Kindblom L-G, Angervall L (1988) Alveolar soft part sarcoma. An immunohistochemical, cytologic and electron-microscopic study and a quantivative DNA analysis. Virchows Arch [A] 412: 499–513

Prat J, Woodruff JM, Marcove RC (1978) Epithelioid sarcoma. An analysis of 22 cases indicating the prognostic significance of vascular invasion and regional lymph node metastases. Cancer 41: 1472–1487

Reeves BR, Fletcher CDM, Gusterson BA (1992) The translocation t(12;22)(q13;q13) is a non-random rearrangement in clear cell sarcoma. Cancer Genet Cytogenet 64: 101–103

Rosai J, Sumner HW, Kostianovsky M, Perez-Mesa C (1976) Angiosarcoma of the skin. A clinicopathologic and fine structural study. Hum Pathol 7: 83–109

Rosai J, Dias P, Parham DM, Shapiro DN, Houghton P (1991) MyoD1 protein expression in alveolar soft part sarcoma as confirmatory evidence of its skeletal muscle nature. Am J Surg Pathol 15: 974–981

Sara AS, Evans HL, Benjamin RS (1990) Malignant melanoma of soft parts (clear cell sarcoma). A study of 17 cases, with emphasis on prognostic factors. Cancer 65: 367–374

Sawyer JR, Tryka AF, Lewis JM (1992) A novel reciprocal chromosome translocation t(11;22)(p13;q12) in an intra-abdominal desmoplastic small round cell tumor. Am J Surg Pathol 16: 411–416

Schmidt D, Leuschner I, Harms D, Sprenger E, Schafer HJ (1989) Malignant rhabdoid tumor. A morphological and flow cytometric study. Pathol Res Pract 184: 202–210

Smetana HG, Scott WF (1951) Malignant tumors of nonchromaffin paraganglia. Milit Surg 109: 330–349

Sotelo-Avila C, Gonzalez-Crussi F, deMello D, Vogler C, Gooch WM, Gale G, Pena R (1986) Renal and extrarenal rhabdoid tumors in children: a clinicopathologic study of 14 patients. Semin Diagn Pathol 3: 151–163

Stout AP (1948) Mesenchymoma, the mixed tumor of mesenchymal derivatives. Ann Surg 127: 278–290

Swanson PE, Wick MR (1989) Clear cell sarcoma. An immunohistochemical analysis of six cases and comparison with other epithelioid neoplasms of soft tissue. Arch Pathol Lab Med 113: 55–60

Swanson PE, Dehner LP, Wick MR (1988) Polyphenotypic small cell tumors of childhood. Lab Invest 58: 9P (abstract)

Tsokos M, Kouraklis G, Chandra RS, Bhagavan BS, Triche TJ (1989) Malignant rhabdoid tumor of the kidney and soft tissues. Evidence for a diverse morphologic and immuno-cytochemical phenotype. Arch Pathol Lab Med 113: 115–120

Tsuneyoshi M, Enjoji M, Kubo T (1978) Clear cell sarcoma of tendons and aponeuroses. A comparative study of 13 cases with a provisional subgrouping into the melanotic and synovial types. Cancer 42: 243–252

Tsuneyoshi M, Daimaru Y, Hashimoto H, Enjoji M (1985) Malignant soft tissue neoplasms with the histologic features of renal rhabdoid tumors: an ultrastructural and immuno-histochemical study. Hum Pathol 16: 1235–1252

Tsuneyoshi M, Daimaru Y, Hashimoto H, Enjoji M (1987) The existence of rhabdoid cells in specified soft tissue sarcomas. Histopathological, ultrastructural and immunohistochemical evidence. Virchows Arch [A] 411: 509–514

Ulbright TM, Brookaw SA, Stehman FB, Roth LM (1983) Epithelioid sarcoma of the vulva. Evidence suggesting a more aggressive behaviour than extragenital epithelioid sarcoma. Cancer 52: 1462–1469

Variend S, Gerrard M, Norris PD, Goepel JR (1991) Intra-abdominal neuroectodermal tumour of childhood with divergent differentiation. Histopathology 18: 45–51

Walford N, Deferrai R, Slater RM, Delemarre JFM, Dingemans KP, Weerman MAV, Voute PA (1992) Intraorbital rhabdoid tumour following bilateral retinoblastoma. Histopathology 20: 170–173

Weeks DA, Beckwith JB, Mierau GW, Luckey DW (1989a) Rhabdoid tumor of kidney. A report of 111 cases from the National Wilm's Tumor Study Pathology Center. Am J Surg Pathol 13: 439–458

Weeks DA, Beckwith JB, Mierau GW (1989b) Rhabdoid tumor. An entity or a phenotype? Arch Pathol Lab Med 113: 113–114

Weeks DA, Beckwith JB, Mierau GW, Zuppan CW (1991) Renal neoplasms mimicking rhabdoid tumor of kidney. A report from the National Wilms Tumor Study Pathology Center. Am J Surg Pathol 15: 1042–1054

Wick MR, Manivel JC (1986) Epithelioid sarcoma and epitheliod hemangioendothelioma: an immunocytochemical and lectin histochemical comparison. Virchows Archiv [A] 410: 309–316

Yagihashi S, Yagihashi N, Hase Y, Nagai K, Alguacil-Garcia A (1991) Primary alveolar soft part sarcoma of stomach. Am J Surg Pathol 15: 399–406

Young RH, Eichhorn JH, Dickersin GR, Scully RE (1992) Ovarian involvement by the intra-abdominal desmoplastic small round cell tumor with divergent differentiation. A report of three cases. Hum Pathol 23: 454–464

Subject Index

tumor heterogeneity (*Contd.*)
–, ultrastructural level   127
tumor-suppressor genes   48

unclassified sarcoma   4, 13

von Recklinghausen's disease   334

Wilms' tumor, rhabdomyosarcomatous
component   253

Printing: Druckerei Zechner, Speyer
Binding: Buchbinderei Schäffer, Grünstadt